# Acute Neuro Care

Prasanna Udupi Bidkar
Ponniah Vanamoorthy
Editors

# Acute Neuro Care

## Focused Approach to Neuroemergencies

Springer

BYWORD BOOKS™

*Editors*
Prasanna Udupi Bidkar
MBBS, MD, DNB, DM
(Neuroanaesthesiology), MNAMS, MBA
Division of Neuroanaesthesiology
Department of Anaesthesiology
and critical care
Jawaharlal Institute of Postgraduate Medical
Education and Research
Puducherry
India

Ponniah Vanamoorthy
MBBS, MD, DNB
Senior consultant and Head
Neuroanaesthesiology & Neurocritical care
MGM Healthcare Pvt Ltd
Chennai, Tamil Nadu
India

ISBN 978-981-15-4073-8 ISBN 978-981-15-4071-4 (eBook)
https://doi.org/10.1007/978-981-15-4071-4



Co-publishing partnership between Byword Books Private Limited and Springer Nature India Private Limited.
This Springer imprint is published by the registered company Springer Nature Singapore Pte Ltd.
The registered company address is: 152 Beach Road, #21-01/04 Gateway East, Singapore 189721, Singapore

# Foreword

Neurocritical Care (NCC) is a subspecialty of Critical Care. NCC encompasses the care of patients with neurological and neurosurgical emergencies such as traumatic brain injury, subarachnoid hemorrhage, severe acute ischemic stroke, status epilepticus, and infectious conditions among others. The field of NCC has evolved tremendously in the past few decades. The advent of novel therapies and dedicated neurocritical care units have contributed to improved outcomes of neurocritically-ill patients. NCC is delivered in a more organized fashion around the globe and is now possible for neurointensivists to collaborate to further both clinical and research knowledge in this field. The creation of the Neurocritical Care Society (NCS) in the early 2000s has made such partnerships possible. NCS advocates for the highest quality of care for patients with critical neurological illnesses. NCS has collaborated with various organizations from all corners of the world to enhance education of neurological emergencies.

An important aspect of excellent NCC is the education of neurointensivists and critical care practitioners on the intricacies of these complex disorders. Drs. Prasanna Udupi Bidkar and Ponniah Vanamoorthy have edited an excellent textbook titled "Acute Neuro Care: A Focused Approach to Neuroemergencies." They have brought together a group of distinguished group of neuroanesthesiologists and neurointensivists from established academic centers in India. The chapters cover practical but important material including airway management, ultrasound techniques, neuropharmacology, and more in-depth look at the most common disorders. This endeavor will contribute a great deal to the enhancement of knowledge in NCC. I recommend this book for practitioners caring for patients with acute neurological emergencies, particularly those working in countries with emerging economies.

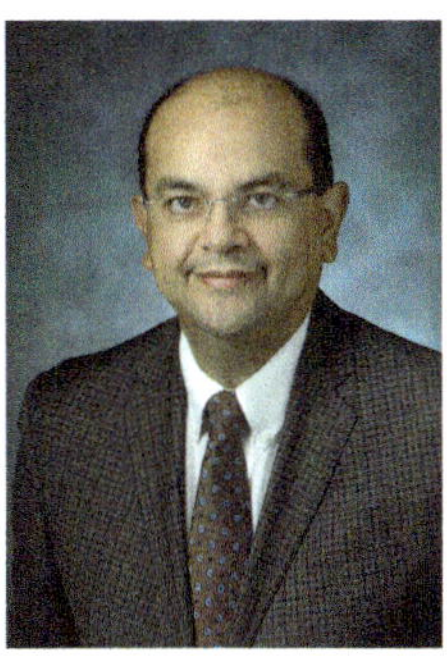

Jose I. Suarez, MD, FNCS, FANA, FAAN
Neurosciences Critical Care,
Departments of Anesthesiology
and Critical Care Medicine,
Neurology, and Neurosurgery
The Johns Hopkins University School of Medicine
Baltimore, MD, USA

Neurocritical Care Society
Chicago, IL, USA

# Preface

Neuro-Emergencies are time-sensitive situations in which effective therapies given during critical hours greatly improve the outcomes. A collaborative interdisciplinary approach with practical set of protocols, decision points, and communication is the key to good patient management.

Time is Brain and time lost is brain lost. Early recognition and neuroimaging are the essentials to institute time-sensitive effective treatment strategies in Neuro-Emergencies. With advances in medical sciences and upgradation of concepts, there is a pressing need to unwind a new outcome-centric approach in place of the traditional approach. Acute Neuro Care (ANC) explores the possibility of this approach and tries to simplify neuro-emergency care in a practical set of protocols. The learners will have the opportunity to absorb and implement these protocols in their day-to-day practice for improving patient outcomes.

Establishing systems of care, collaborating with primary centers, creating public awareness, enhancing clinical pathways, and implementing patient education form the crux of a strong survival chain in Neuro-Emergencies. The main objective of this endeavor is to inculcate and disseminate outcome-centric focused approach of history taking, clinical examination, and rapid imaging in everyday clinical practice among physicians and nursing personnel involved in the acute care of neurological patients.

A wide spectrum of topics are covered in this book such as neurotrauma, stroke, status epilepticus, coma, neuromuscular weakness, neuroinfections, and neuropharmacology and importantly include algorithmic approaches for easy understanding. With contributions from authors across various institutions in India, this book will provide a diverse yet focused set of learning material for easy adoption into daily clinical practice. In short, Acute Neuro Care is the one-stop destination to gain practical knowledge in management of Neuro-Emergencies.

Puducherry, India — Prasanna Udupi Bidkar
Chennai, India — Ponniah Vanamoorthy

# Contents

# About the Editors

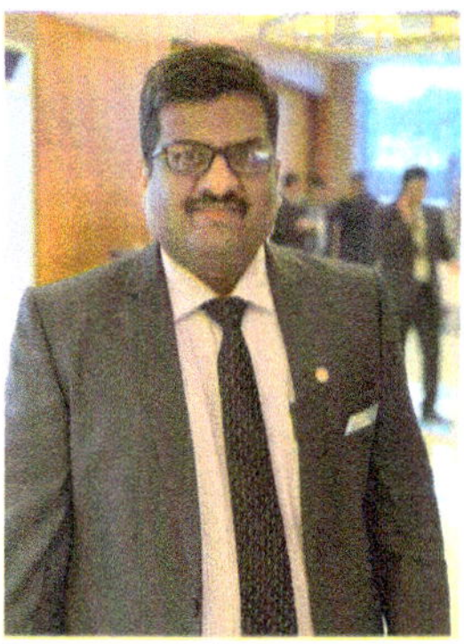

**Prasanna Udupi Bidkar** is incharge of the Division of Neuroanesthesiology at Jawaharlal Institute of Postgraduate Medical Education and Research (JIPMER), Pondicherry, and was instrumental in setting up the DM Neuroanesthesiology course at the institute. He has been working in neuroanesthesiology and neurocritical care for 15 years. He completed his DM in Neuroanesthesiology at the All India Institute of Medical Sciences (AIIMS), New Delhi. He has published more than 50 papers in reputed national and international journal and has written 12 chapters in various textbooks in the field of Neuroanaesthesiology and Neurocritical care. He is an active member and current treasurer of the Indian Society of Neuroanesthesiology and Critical Care (ISNACC). He is founding member and current treasurer of Neurocritical care society of India (NCSI).

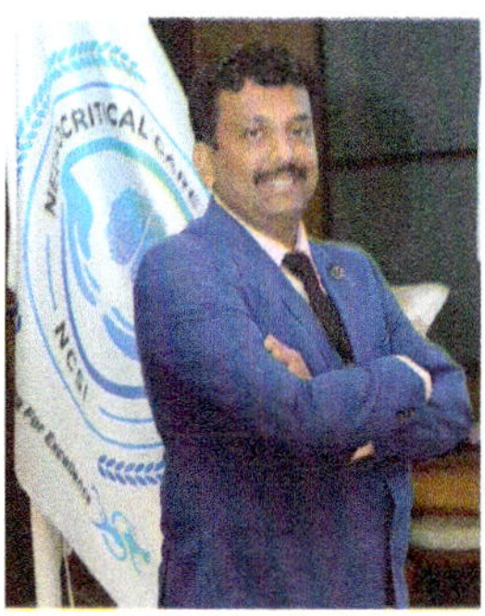


**Ponniah Vanamoorthy** is Chief of Neuroanesthesiology and Neurocritical Care Services at MGM Healthcare, Chennai. He was instrumental in setting up the Department of Neurosciences at Global Hospital, Chennai. He received advanced training in neuroanesthesiology and neurocritical care at the All India Institute of Medical Sciences (AIIMS), New Delhi. He is an authority on acute stroke management in India. He is an active member and current secretary of the Indian Society of Neuroanesthesiology and Critical Care (ISNACC). He is founding member and current secretary of Neurocritical care society of India (NCSI).

# Abbreviations

| | |
|---|---|
| ABC | Airway, breathing, and circulation |
| ACA | Anterior cerebral artery |
| AED | Antiepileptic drug |
| AFP | Acute flaccid paralysis |
| AIS | Acute ischemic stroke |
| BA | Bioavailability |
| BP | Blood pressure |
| CBC | Complete blood count |
| CBF | Cerebral blood flow |
| $CMRO_2$ | Cerebral metabolic rate of oxygen |
| CN | Cranial nerve |
| CNS | Central nervous system |
| CPP | Cerebral perfusion pressure |
| CSF | Cerebrospinal fluid |
| CT | Computed tomography |
| CVS | Cardiovascular system |
| DTR | Deep tendon reflex |
| ECG | Electrocardiography |
| ED | Emergency Department |
| EDH | Extradural hematoma |
| EEG | Electroencephalogram |
| EMS | Emergency medical services |
| ETT | Endotracheal tube |
| EVD | External ventricular drain |
| FFP | Fresh frozen plasma |
| GCS | Glasgow coma scale |
| HR | Heart rate |
| HTS | Hypertonic saline |
| ICA | Internal carotid artery |
| ICH | Intracranial hemorrhage |
| ICP | Intracranial hemorrhage |
| ICU | Intensive care unit |
| IVC | Inferior vena cava |
| LL | Lower limb |

| | |
|---|---|
| LMA | Laryngeal mask airway |
| LMN | Lower motor neuron |
| MAP | Mean arterial pressure |
| MCA | Middle cerebral artery |
| MILS | Manual in line stabilization |
| MRI | Magnetic resonance imaging |
| NCCT | Noncontrast CT |
| NCSE | Nonconvulsive status epilepticus |
| NOAC | Novel oral anticoagulants |
| ONSD | Optic nerve sheath diameter |
| P/A | Per abdomen |
| $PaCO_2$ | Partial pressure of carbon dioxide |
| PCA | Posterior cerebral artery |
| PEEP | Positive end expiratory pressure |
| $PO_2$ | Partial pressure of oxygen |
| POCUS | Point of care ultrasound |
| RS | Respiratory system |
| RSI | Rapid sequence induction |
| SAH | Subarachnoid hemorrhage |
| SCI | Spinal cord injury |
| SDH | Subdural hematoma |
| SE | Serum electrolytes |
| SPO2 | Oxygen saturation |
| TBI | Traumatic brain injury |
| TCCD | Transcranial colour duplex |
| TCD | Transcranial Doppler |
| TIA | Transient ischemic attack |
| UL | Upper limb |
| UMN | Upper motor neuron |
| USG | Ultrasonography |

# Airway and Breathing

# 1

Gyaninder Pal Singh, Surya Kumar Dube,
and Devika Bharadwaj

**Key Points**

- Airway management is one of the keystones of resuscitation
- Inability to maintain a patent airway for more than a few minutes may lead to an irreversible hypoxic insult to the brain
- Rapid assessment of the airway is important to identify patients with unprotected airways at risk of aspiration
- Neck movements should be restricted in patients in whom cervical spine injury has not been ruled out. Manual inline stabilisation should be used in these patients.
- Factors that may lead to an increase in intracranial pressure such as hypoxia, hypercarbia and hypotension should be avoided
- Adequate planning for the management of the difficult airway cannot be over emphasized

**Case**

A 48-year-old male patient, weighing 105 kg, presented to the emergency department with sudden onset severe headache and decreased sensorium. On admission, his heart rate was 114/min, blood pressure 196/112 mmHg, oxygen saturation 92%, respiratory rate 34/min with laboured breathing and gurgling sound and the ECG showed sinus tachycardia. His admission GCS was E2, V3, M4 with left sided hemiparesis and unequal pupils. Right pupil was mid-dilated sluggishly reacting to light and left pupil was constricted. He had a short neck with large jaw, beard and submandibular fat.

G. P. Singh (✉) · S. K. Dube · D. Bharadwaj
All India Institute of Medical Sciences, New Delhi, India


P. U. Bidkar, P. Vanamoorthy (eds.), *Acute Neuro Care*,
https://doi.org/10.1007/978-981-15-4071-4_1

## 1.1 Introduction

The ability to manage the airway appropriately is fundamental to resuscitation. Failure to maintain a patent airway for more than a few minutes can lead to brain injury or death. The goal of airway management is to maintain adequate oxygenation and ventilation and prevent aspiration. Even a single episode of hypoxia is shown to increase mortality in patients with neurological injury such as traumatic brain injury [1, 2]. Patients presenting with a neurological emergency have several unique airway and ventilation concerns. These include:

- Hypoxia and/or hypercarbia can increase the damage to already ischemic brain tissue (secondary brain injury).
- An unconscious patient is at risk of aspiration pneumonitis due to unprotected airway.
- Intracranial pressure (ICP) can be raised at the time of presentation.
- Intracranial injury can cause abnormal breathing patterns.
- Cervical spine (C-spine) injury can lead to intercostal muscle paralysis, diaphragmatic breathing, and interfere with the ability to meet oxygen demand.
- Head injured patients may have associated unstable cervical spine, facial/airway trauma, hypovolemia due to blood loss because of other injuries (e.g., fracture femur).

While prompt diagnosis and management of a neurological/neurosurgical emergency is essential, providing a protected, unobstructed airway and adequate ventilation takes priority over the management of neurological emergencies.

1. Airway and ventilation are the priorities
2. The aim is rapid stabilization of a patient with the neurological emergency
3. Do a rapid assessment of the airway
4. Plan for airway management and increase chances of first-pass intubation
5. Backup plan for managing a difficult airway

## 1.2 Rapid Airway Assessment

### 1.2.1 Need for Tracheal Intubation

An obtunded patient with unknown pathophysiology awaiting imaging must be assessed for need for airway protection and ventilation. Emergency care physician must assess for the following to decide whether the patient requires intubation.

(a) **Oxygenation**: Pulse oximetry, arterial blood gases or visual appearance (cyanosis) can be used to assess a patient for the adequacy of oxygenation.
(b) **Ventilation**: An unconscious patient with a head injury, may be obtunded due to use of alcohol or other drugs and those with neuromuscular weakness can have compromised ventilatory effort as well. Waveform capnography or arterial $PaCO_2$ can help assess whether the patient has normal ventilation/hypoventilation or respiratory failure. In the absence of these parameters, clinical assessment for signs of respiratory distress can be used to guide the need for intubation.
(c) **Patency of airway and risk of aspiration**: A quick neurological assessment should be done to assess if the airway is patent or compromised. A positive and appropriate verbal response indicates that the airway is patent with intact ventilation and brain perfusion. The Protection of the airway is the most important indication for intubation in an unconscious patient. In general, patient with Glasgow Coma Scale (GCS) score of 8 or less should be intubated. It is important to anticipate vomiting in such patients if the patient has raised ICP at the time of presentation to the emergency. The patient may have already aspirated before arrival and needs intubation to protect the airway. Blood or vomitus if present in the mouth should be suctioned immediately to prevent aspiration. Listening to sounds carefully can help to know the cause of airway obstruction; gurgling sound (fluid in the pharynx), snoring sound (soft tissue obstruction), crowing sound (obstruction at the level of larynx). Palpate the larynx for any surgical emphysema or anatomical disruption (may suggest laryngeal fracture).

In a patient with neurological compromise the purpose of securing the airway is to

- Deliver supplemental oxygen
- Support ventilation and
- Prevent aspiration

(d) **Circulation**: Assess the patient for hemodynamic instability or cardiac arrest.

If the patient is conscious or a relative is available one must also elicit a history of previous airway management and difficulty encountered. A quick history of previous medical illnesses and drug allergies helps to choose appropriate drugs for facilitating intubation. While assessing a patient for the need for intubation it is important to ask about the time of taking the last meal. The mnemonic SAMPLE can help you remember what to ask a patient's relative during your initial assessment.

**S** Signs and symptoms
**A** Allergies
**M** Medications (including the last dose taken)
**P** Past medical history
**L** Last meal taken
**E** Events

### 1.2.2 Assessment of Airway for Difficult Ventilation and/or Intubation

Assessing the airway for difficulty (i.e., predicted difficult mask ventilation and/or intubation) and formulating the plan accordingly increases the chance of successful airway management. Failure to intubate a patient is one of the most feared situations especially in an emergency when a patient needs urgent airway management [3, 4]. The inability to ventilate or intubate can be catastrophic without good planning. With little time to plan during an emergency, using quick assessment tools help to plan for appropriate backup in terms of skilled individuals (anesthetist, surgeon) and devices (fibreoptic, laryngeal mask airway, cricothyrotomy) [3–6]. Successful identification of features that are suggestive of the difficult airway allows planning towards safe airway management. In a review of 184 cases involving major airway complications by the Fourth National Audit Project of the Royal College of Anaesthetists and the Difficult Airway Society, patient-related factors were the most causal and contributory factor (77%) for airway complications [7]. Identifying such patients and preparing for the anticipated difficulty is key to successful airway management [7, 8].

There have been several attempts to device bedside tests and mnemonics to predict difficult airway. However, at times these bedside tests may fail due to unconscious or uncooperative patients in an emergency. Therefore there is a need to always plan for an alternative airway management technique before attempting intubation. Moreover, management of the airway in an emergency is always challenging due to tissue trauma, cardiovascular and respiratory instability and aspiration of pharyngeal and gastric contents [3, 5].

The "3-3-2 rule" can help in the quick assessment of a patient for potential airway difficulty [8] (three fingers into the mouth, three fingers under the chin and two fingers at the top of the neck.) Here, the first figure "3" refers to the ability to place three fingers (patient's fingers) in the patient's mouth. Adequate mouth opening should permit placement of the patient's three fingers between the upper and lower teeth. The next figure "3" refers to space from mentum to hyoid bone. Placement of three fingers side by side in the mandibular space indicates adequate mandibular dimension to permit access to the airway. The figure "2" in the rule requires placement of two fingers between the hyoid bone and the thyroid notch. Space less than 2 fingers indicate that the larynx is too high in the neck and direct laryngoscopy will be difficult/ impossible (as the angle between the base of the tongue to the larynx is too acute to be negotiated for direct visualization of the larynx).

The mnemonic **"MOANS"** (to predict difficult bag-mask ventilation)

**M** **M**ask seal
**O** **O**besity
**A** **A**dvanced age (>55 years)
**N** **N**o teeth
**S** **S**norer

Mnemonic **"LEMON"** (to predict difficult airway)

**L** **L**ook
**E** **E**valuate mouth opening and airway position
**M** **M**allampati score
**O** **O**bstruction
**N** **N**eck mobility

In a patient presenting with a neurological emergency Mallampati scoring, thyromental distance and neck mobility may be difficult to assess and often inaccurate if the patient is unconscious or drowsy [3]. Similarly patients with trauma in whom C-spine injury has not been ruled out, neck mobility should not be evaluated [5]. Patients anticipated to have difficult mask ventilation/intubation or both should prompt the emergency care physician to plan for appropriate backup skills and equipment before airway management.

## 1.3 Intubation in an Unconscious Patient

A patient can be unconscious due to a metabolic or structural lesion requiring urgent management. The diagnosis may be unclear at the time of initial resuscitation. With several differential diagnoses in mind (head injury, drug intoxication, stroke, aneurysm rupture, cerebral edema) the aim of airway management should be to protect the airway, prevent rise in ICP, prevent secondary injury to the brain [1] (hypoxemia, hypercarbia), maintain cerebral perfusion and avoid sudden rise or fall in blood pressure (may have disturbed autoregulation).

Currently, rapid sequence intubation (RSI) is considered the standard of care for intubation in emergencies [9]. The primary objective of RSI is to minimize the time interval between the loss of protective airway reflex and tracheal intubation with a cuffed endotracheal tube (ETT) in patients with a high risk of aspiration. The basic principle of RSI involves preoxygenation, administration of intravenous induction agent and neuromuscular blocking agent followed by rapid intubation and confirmation of ETT placement.

**Table 1.1** List of items for emergency airway cart

| | |
|---|---|
| 1. | Intravenous catheter (all sizes) |
| 2. | Syringes different sizes |
| 3. | Oropharyngeal and nasopharyngeal airway (all sizes) |
| 4. | Face masks (all sizes) |
| 5. | Laryngeal mask airway (all sizes) |
| 6. | Self-inflating resuscitating (AMBU) bag (adult and pediatric) |
| 7. | Laryngoscope with different size blades (Macintosh and Miller) |
| 8. | Endotracheal tubes (all sizes) |
| 9. | Stylet |
| 10. | Gum elastic bougie (adult and pediatric) |
| 11. | Airway exchange catheter (adult and pediatric) |
| 12. | Stethoscope |
| 13. | Magill forceps |
| 14. | Suction catheter (all sizes) |
| 15. | Nasogastric tube (different sizes) |
| 16. | Nasal cannula to supplement Oxygen |
| 17. | Emergency devices for failed intubation |
| (a) | Video laryngoscope with different blades |
| (b) | McCoy laryngoscope with blades |
| (c) | Intubating supraglottic airway devices (intubating-LMA, I-gel, air-Q) |
| (d) | Combitube/Laryngeal tubes of different sizes |
| (e) | Cricothyroidotomy set |
| (f) | Transtracheal jet ventilation device |
| (g) | Flexible fibreoptic laryngoscope |

*AMBU* Artificial Manual Breathing Unit or Air Mask Bag Unit, *LMA* Laryngeal Mask Airway

Steps for successful airway management in an unconscious patient:

### 1.3.1 Step 1: Assess and Prepare

Assess the patient for need of the intubation and any anticipated difficulty. Prepare your equipment and drugs before airway management. Check the availability of a working suction, oxygen source, and working intravenous access. Ensure monitoring for ECG, blood pressure, and $SpO_2$ monitoring before airway management. Call for help if the difficulty is anticipated. Suggested contents of the emergency airway cart are given in Table 1.1.

### 1.3.2 Step 2: Open and Maintain Patency of the Airway

Head tilt and chin lift/jaw thrust maneuver can be used to relieve the airway obstruction caused by tongue fall in an unconscious patient (due to loss of muscle tone in tongue and upper airway musculature). However, it causes movement at the atlantoaxial joint. If a C-spine injury has not been ruled out in trauma victims, jaw thrust maneuver should be used to open the airway [5]. Jaw thrust does not lead to the movement of the cervical spine.

The oropharyngeal or nasopharyngeal airway can be placed in an unconscious patient with absent cough or gag reflex to maintain the patency of airway. Do not use an oropharyngeal airway in a conscious or semiconscious patient as it can provoke vomiting; however, the nasopharyngeal airway can be used in these patients. Avoid a nasopharyngeal airway in a patient with suspected cribriform plate fracture (CSF leak from the nose) as this may cause intracranial injury and introduce infection into the cranium.

### 1.3.3 Step 3: Preoxygenate for 3–5 min

Administer 100% oxygen with a tight-fitting mask and bag for 3–5 min. It helps to build the oxygen reserve in the patient and allows more time to intubate, thus reducing the risk of desaturation. Desaturation is common during emergency intubation due to several reasons [10]. Decreased functional residual capacity may be present due to lung pathology such as pulmonary edema, pneumonia, pulmonary contusion, etc. Pulmonary aspiration and esophageal intubation can also lead to severe desaturation during intubation. Desaturation during RSI increases the risk of dysrhythmia, hemodynamic compromise, hypoxic brain injury, and death.

Preoxygenation is essential before RSI, anticipated difficult ventilation/ intubation, obese or pregnant patients with anticipated difficulty and in children [10]. Preoxygenation before RSI provides an oxygen reservoir in the lungs and helps to tide over the apnoeic spell during intubation. Preoxygenation for 3–5 min replaces the nitrogen content of the functional residual capacity of lungs with 100% oxygen [10].

**Cricoid Pressure Controversy** Cricoid pressure has been an essential part of RSI until recently. The original technique of cricoid pressure described by Sellick required the head and neck in extreme extension for the esophagus to be tethered against cervical vertebrae. The sniffing position used for laryngoscopy and intubation may not achieve the same success in occluding the esophagus. An unconscious patient requires maintaining the neck immobilized until C-spine injury has been ruled out. The efficacy of cricoid pressure in this position is unknown. ACLS 2015 guidelines suggest that cricoid pressure may offer some protection from aspiration and gastric insufflation. However, it may also impede ventilation and ETT insertion. A recent randomized trial reported increased difficulty in tracheal intubation (poor Cormack and Lehane (CL) grade on laryngoscopy and longer intubation time) with no benefit in preventing pulmonary aspiration with the application of cricoid pressure during RSI [11].

### 1.3.4 Step 4: Administer Induction Agent and Neuromuscular Blocking Agents

An ideal drug for RSI should achieve a rapid loss of consciousness, improve intubation conditions, induce minimum hemodynamic disturbances and blunt sympathetic responses to laryngoscopy and intubation. However, none of the anesthetic qualify the ideal drug description.

*Properties of an ideal RSI inducing agent*

- Rapid and smooth induction (smoothly and quickly render the patient unconscious, unresponsive and amnestic)
- Provide analgesia
- Maintain stable cerebral perfusion pressure
- Maintain stable cardiovascular hemodynamics
- Easily and immediately reversible
- Do not have any side effects

**Choice of Induction Agents** Several anesthetic drugs can be used for rapid sequence intubation. In the majority of patients, clinical condition of the patient dictates the choice of induction drug. Commonly used induction agents for RSI include etomidate, ketamine, propofol, and thiopentone. The doses, merits, and demerits of various induction agents are mentioned in Table 1.2. Similar intubating conditions have been noted regardless of the induction drug used during RSI.

**Choice of Muscle Relaxant** Succinylcholine (SCh) and rocuronium are the most suitable muscle relaxants that can be used for RSI. Both SCh and rocuronium have a rapid onset of action (Table 1.3). SCh causes a transient but clinically insignificant rise in ICP [12]. It may be used for RSI in a neurological emergency [12]. It is important to avoid coughing, bucking on ETT, hypoxia, and hypercarbia as it will cause a clinically significant rise in ICP (if not blunted with appropriate drug therapy).

**Table 1.2** Common induction agents used for rapid sequence intubation (RSI)

| Induction agents | Dose and Route | | Onset | Comments |
|---|---|---|---|---|
| Etomidate | 0.2–0.4 mg/kg | IV | <1 min | Maintain hemodynamic myoclonic activity, inhibit cortisol synthesis |
| Propofol | 1.5–2.5 mg/kg | IV | <1 min | Decrease CBF, $CMRO_2$ and ICP, hypotension, myocardial depression, pain on injection |
| Thiopentone | 3–5 mg/kg | IV | <1 min | Decrease CBF, $CMRO_2$, and ICP, hypotension, myocardial depression |
| Ketamine | 1–2 mg/kg | IV | <1 min | Tachycardia, hypertension, transient rise in ICP and IOP, hallucinations, increased secretions |
| Midazolam | 0.1–0.3 mg/kg | IV | 2–5 min | Slow onset, hypotension, respiratory depression, apnoea |

*ICP* intracranial pressure, *IOP* intraocular pressure, *CBF* cerebral blood flow, $CMRO_2$ cerebral metabolic rate of oxygen, *IV* intravenous route

**Table 1.3** Paralytic agents used for rapid sequence intubation

| Paralytic agents | Dose and Route | | Onset and Duration | Comments |
|---|---|---|---|---|
| Succinylcholine | 1.5–2.0 mg/kg | IV | 45–60 s; 5–10 min | Hyperkalaemia, bradycardia, transient rise in ICP and IOP |
| Rocuronium | 0.6–1.2 mg/kg | IV | 60–90 s; 45–90 min | Pain on injection, anaphylaxis, Reversed by Sugammadex |

*ICP* intracranial pressure, *IOP* intraocular pressure, *IV* intravenous route

**Table 1.4** Drugs to prevent response to laryngoscopy and intubation

| Drugs | Dose and Route | Onset | Duration of action |
|---|---|---|---|
| Esmolol | 1 mg/kg IV | 2 min | 10 min |
| Lidocaine | 1.5 mg/kg IV | 45–90 s | 10–20 min |
| Fentanyl | 3 μg/kg IV | 2–3 min | 30–50 min |

SCh has a faster recovery time as compared to rocuronium if allowed to spontaneously recover from neuromuscular blockade. However Sugammadex 16 mg/kg can be used for faster reversal of rocuronium 1.2 mg/kg, as compared to spontaneous recovery from Sch (6.2 ± 1.8 min vs 10.9 ± 2.4 min, respectively) [13]. Therefore rocuronium increases the margin of safety for the resumption of spontaneous ventilation after RSI if sugammadex is available for reversal.

### 1.3.5 Step 5: Blunting Laryngoscopic Response Before Intubation

Laryngoscopy can lead to intense sympathetic and parasympathetic stimulation and a rise in ICP [14]. Drugs and their doses used for blunting the laryngoscopic response are given in Table 1.4. These drugs should be administered before intubation [14] depending on their time of onset of action to adequately blunt the response.

### 1.3.6 Step 6: Tracheal Intubation

The patient is placed in sniffing position (neck flexed with head extended) and the mandible is lifted forward with the help of a laryngoscope (this aligns the oral, pharyngeal, and laryngeal axes so that the pathway from lips to glottis is in a straight line). After the patient is relaxed intubate the trachea with proper size ETT, inflate the cuff and check for successful intubation (Table 1.5). Secure the ETT with adhesive tapes.

However, if the C-spine injury is suspected or has not been ruled out, then manual inline stabilization (MILS) should be applied during laryngoscopy and intubation to stabilize the neck movements.

**Table 1.5** Evidence of successful endotracheal intubation

| | |
|---|---|
| **Clinical signs** | |
| 1. | Direct visualization of ETT passing through vocal cords |
| 2. | Chest rise during ventilation |
| 3. | Moisture on the wall of ETT (tube condensation) during expiration |
| 4. | Breath sounds heard over the chest and no sound heard over epigastrium on auscultation |
| **Monitoring parameters** | |
| 1. | Persistent Capnogram reading and/or waveform |
| 2. | Maintenance of oxygen saturation |
| **Other evidence** | |
| 1. | Fibreoptic confirmation |
| 2. | Radiological confirmation of ETT on X-ray chest |
| 3. | Ultrasonographic confirmation of ETT in the trachea |

#### 1.3.6.1 Nasotracheal or Orotracheal Intubation?

Use of both the techniques are safe and effective if performed properly, although the orotracheal route is more commonly used. Fractures of facial bone and frontal sinus, basilar skull fractures, and cribriform plate fractures are contraindications to nasotracheal intubation. Nasal fracture, raccoon eyes (ecchymosis in the periorbital region), Battle sign (postauricular ecchymosis), cerebrospinal fluid rhinorrhea or otorrhea are signs of such injuries. C-spine immobilization should be maintained during nasotracheal intubation as with orotracheal intubation.

### 1.3.7 Step 7: Post-tracheal Intubation Care

Properly secure the ETT with adhesive tapes/ ETT holders. Start mechanical ventilation and reassess the vitals (heart rate, rhythm, blood pressure, and $SpO_2$). Suction the ETT using suction catheter if blood/ secretions/ vomitus noted in the ETT.

## 1.4 Management of Difficult Airway

### 1.4.1 Basic Preparation for Difficult Airway Management

American Society of Anesthesiologists (ASA) [15] recommends the following preparation if a difficult airway is suspected:

1. Inform the patient (or responsible person) about the procedures and of the special risks about the management of the difficult airway.
2. At least one additional individual who is immediately available to serve as an assistant in difficult airway management should be available.
3. Always preoxygenate the patient before initiating management of the difficult airway (uncooperative or pediatric patients may impede opportunities for preoxygenation).

4. Actively consider giving supplemental oxygen throughout the process of difficult airway management. Opportunities for supplemental oxygen administration include (but are not limited to) oxygen delivery by nasal cannulae, facemask or laryngeal mask airway (LMA), insufflation; and oxygen delivery by facemask, blow-by or nasal cannulae after extubation of the trachea.

Mnemonic **"SOAPME"** may be used to help guide preparation before securing difficult airway:

**S: Suction** (working suction and different size suction catheter)
**O: Oxygen** (uninterrupted supply of oxygen)
**A: Airway equipment** (working laryngoscope with all size blades, nasal prongs, different size masks, ETTs & LMAs, Oro- and nasopharyngeal airway, stylet/bougie, stethoscope, self-inflating resuscitation bag, difficult airway cart with all emergency airway devices)
**P: Patient position** (sniffing position, head neutral with MILS in C-spine injury)
**M: Monitors and Medications** (cardiac monitor/ pulse-oximeter, drugs and syringes)
**E: Esophageal detection device** (capnograph, end-tidal $CO_2$ detectors)

### 1.4.2 Ensure Adequate Facemask Ventilation

Patient may be positioned in sniffing position (head tilt - chin lift) to open the airway, if a C-spine injury is not suspected or has been ruled out. If still not able to ventilate adequately, LMA, combitube or laryngeal tube airway can be inserted in such a situation. Appropriate size LMA (sizes are according to patient's weight) should be inserted. LMA may be used as a rescue device in cannot ventilate, cannot intubate (CVCI) situation but it may not be suitable as a definitive airway and proper placement requires appropriate training [16]. Intubating-LMA (I-LMA) and other supraglottic airway devices (SADs) like I-gel and air-Q may also be used for rescue ventilation and may later also act as a conduit for tracheal intubation [16]. However, a major disadvantage with SADs is the pressure exerted on the cervical spine during insertion which can increase the secondary injury in patients with C-spine injury [17]. Laryngeal tube airway and combitube have the advantage of blind insertion, however, they cannot be used as definitive airway (a definitive airway requires a tube placed in the trachea with the cuff inflated below the vocal cords and connected to some form of oxygen-enriched assisted ventilation).

### 1.4.3 Improve the Chances of Successful Intubation

The patient should be placed in "sniffing position", if C-spine injury has been ruled out. If required, BURP (Backward Upward Rightward Pressure) may be applied on thyroid cartilage to help visualize the vocal cords [18]. In case the larynx is anteriorly placed, a stylet or gum elastic bougie may be used to aid the ETT pass through vocal cords [19]. If unable to intubate the trachea, ask for experienced help (e.g., Anaesthesiologist or experienced person) and advanced equipment (e.g., McCoy laryngoscope blades/Video laryngoscope/ fibreoptic).

Continue ventilation with cricoid pressure (to prevent gastric content aspiration) till the help arrive. Avoidance of positive pressure ventilation before intubation has been the cornerstone of Rapid sequence intubation (RSI). Advocates of this approach claim that positive pressure ventilation increases the risk of gastric insufflation and aspiration. Currently, it is recommended to use positive pressure ventilation during RSI in some special patient groups such as obese, pregnant, pediatric, and critically ill patients before securing the airway. These patients are likely to develop hypoxemia very rapidly in a difficult airway situation due to low functional residual capacity. Avoiding the risk of hypoxemia outweighs the potential risk of gastric insufflation.

**Practical tips for airway management in all neurological emergencies**

- Consider all patients full stomach and plan for rapid sequence intubation (RSI).
- The priority is always bag-mask ventilation. Do not rush to intubate.
- Do not hesitate to call for help.
- Always use manual inline stabilization (MILS) in head injury patients during intubation if C-spine injury is not ruled out.
- Use the most familiar device for intubation first.
- If ventilation or intubation fails, try something different next time. Always have an alternative plan ready in mind if unable to ventilate/ intubate.
- Avoid nasotracheal intubation in head injury patients.
- Keep track of time.

**Practical tips to avoid rise in ICP [20] during airway management**

- Avoid hypoventilation during mask ventilation. Carbon dioxide is a potent cerebral vasodilator and leads to rise in ICP [21].
- Never attempt laryngoscopy and intubation without medications even if the patient is unresponsive.
- Blunt the laryngoscopic response with lignocaine/esmolol/fentanyl.
- Avoid using tube-tie around the neck to secure the ETT as this can compress the internal jugular vein and decrease the cerebral venous drainage leading to rise in ICP.
- Avoid coughing and bucking on ETT. Maintain adequate analgesia and sedation after intubation.
- Elevate head end of the bed by 30° after intubation.

## 1.5 Airway Management in Specific Neurological Emergencies

### 1.5.1 Airway Management in Traumatic Head Injury

The primary injury due to mechanical impact may result in skull fracture, brain contusion, intracranial vascular, and parenchymal injuries. The intracranial bleed, cerebral edema, and inflammation following the intracranial injury can lead to raised intracranial pressure (ICP) and reduced cerebral perfusion pressure [22]. The goal of management in patients with traumatic brain injury (TBI) is to prevent secondary injury to the brain [1]. Hypoxia is an important cause of secondary brain injury in these patients and $SaO_2$ <60 mmHg is independently associated with increased morbidity and mortality from severe traumatic brain injury. Hence early resuscitation is an important aspect of management of TBI [23].

Airway management in TBI can be complicated by:

- Urgency of the situation due to pre-existing or worsening hypoxia
- Possibility of C-spine injury
- Airway compromise (blood/vomitus/debris in oral cavity, associated laryngotracheal injury)
- Full stomach
- Intracranial hypertension
- Skull base fracture (fracture of the cribriform plate, CSF rhinorrhoea/otorrhoea)
- Possibility of hypovolemia

The C-spine injury should be ruled out in all patients with traumatic brain injury. Until the C-spine injury has been ruled out, immobilization of cervical spine should be maintained during transport and airway management [24]. The technique of airway management of TBI patients described in the literature is a combination of rapid sequence intubation with cricoid pressure and MILS using a intubating device in according to individual expertise.

The AHA ACLS guidelines 2015 recommends the use of jaw thrust without head extension to open airway in patients with suspected C-spine injury. While spinal immobilization devices are useful during transport, manual spinal immobilization is required during airway management. Removing the anterior portion of the collar and performing MILS during intubation allows greater mouth opening and facilitates laryngoscopy. Nasal intubation should be avoided in patients with skull base fracture, severe facial fractures, and bleeding diathesis.

ICP is often raised in TBI patients due to intracranial space-occupying lesions such as hematoma or cerebral edema. Raised ICP leading to brain herniation present as altered mental status, unilaterally dilated pupil, decerebrates, or extensor posturing. Airway manipulation in such patients causes sympathetic response leading to a rise in heart rate, blood pressure, and ICP. Hence, blunting the laryngoscopic response in these patients is essential before attempting laryngoscopy and intubation.

The choice of appropriate anesthetic agents is essential while intubating such patients. The advantages and disadvantages of using various anesthetic drugs while intubating TBI patients are given in Table 1.2.

The muscle relaxants suitable for rapid sequence intubation are SCh and rocuronium. SCh can cause a transient rise in ICP. However, the clinical relevance of this transient rise in ICP is questionable. Moreover, hypoxia and hypercarbia can lead to a clinically significant increase in ICP [21]. Hence it has been suggested that Sch may be used in TBI patients if the difficult airway is anticipated.

### 1.5.2 Airway Management in Cervical Spine Injury

The unstable cervical spine can be an associated injury in trauma victims [24, 25]. 2–5% of blunt trauma patients have a cervical spine injury [25]. The odds of having a C-spine injury in a patient with trauma is 8.5 fold higher with GCS score of ≤8, 14 folds with persistent unconsciousness, obvious facial or head trauma, hypotension, and 58 folds with focal neurological deficit [25, 26]. Injuries to the upper cervical spine account for up to 80% mortality related to cervical spine trauma [25]. The National Emergency X-radiography Utilization Study [27] (NEXUS) identified the clinical criteria that put patients at low risk for C-spine instability. NEXUS criteria is a valuable clinical decision-making tool to rule out C-spine injuries in the general population without radiographic imaging. It includes five criteria (Table 1.6) and all must be present to rule out C-spine injuries.

Canadian CT Head and C-spine Study Group evaluated for low risk of C-spine injury using three questions. It evaluates the need for a CT spine based on the Yes or No question algorithm in patients with suspected cervical spine injury (Fig. 1.1) [28].

If there is no urgent need for intubation, the radiological clearance of C-spine may be obtained [29]. A missed C-spine injury can have serious consequences and hence until the cervical spine has been cleared, spine should be immobilized to maintain normal physiological alignment and to protect the spinal cord from secondary injury [24]. Besides the instability of C-spine, airway management in these patients may be complicated by full stomach, blood in the airway, and early phase of spinal shock with vasodilatation and bradycardia [30]. Profound bradycardia during laryngoscopy can be prevented by pretreatment with anticholinergic agents in these patients [30].

**Table 1.6** NEXUS low-risk criteria (to rule out C-spine injury without imaging)

| | |
|---|---|
| 1. | No posterior midline cervical spine tenderness |
| 2. | No focal neurological deficit |
| 3. | Normal level of alertness |
| 4. | No evidence of intoxication |
| 5. | No painful distracting injury |

*NEXUS* National Emergency X-radiography utilization study

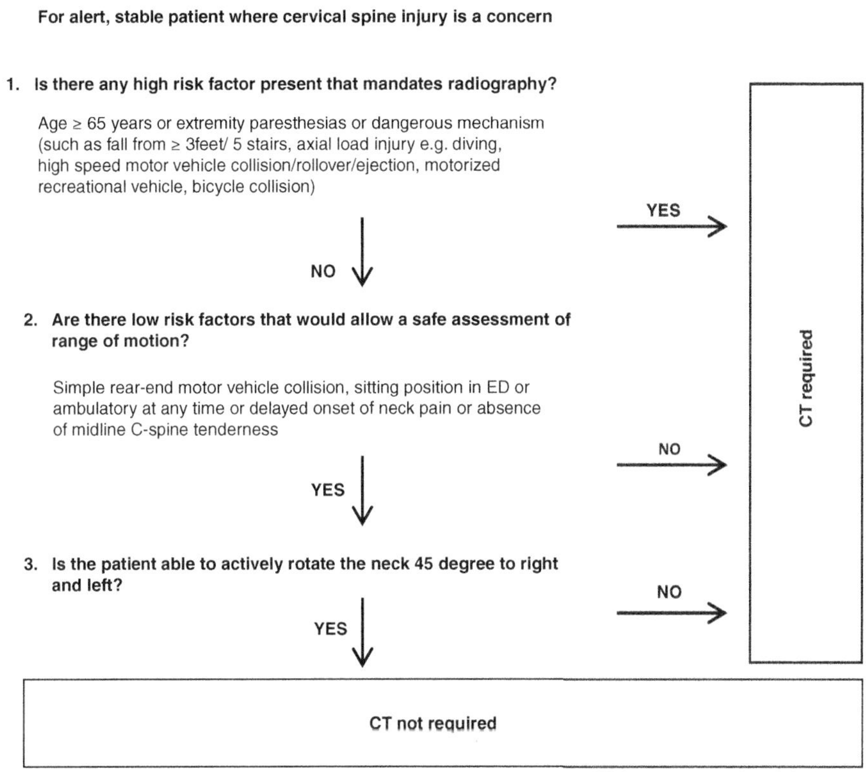


**Fig. 1.1** The Canadian C-spine rule

All airway maneuvers and airway management devices result in varying degrees of cervical spine motion even when the cervical spine is immobilized [31]. In a study on cadavers, chin lift and jaw thrust resulted in disc space expansion greater than 5 mm at the site of cervical injury [32]. Mask ventilation alone can cause up to 3 mm of cervical spine displacement. Cricoid pressure should not be used in patients with C-spine injury since it causes posterior displacement of cervical spine. In an emergency, advanced airway devices may not be readily available. Moreover, each airway management technique has its risks and benefits. A clinician must choose the one likely to be successful on the first attempt while applying MILS with each intubation when cervical spine instability is suspected.

The anterior portion of the cervical collar can be removed during airway management [33]. MILS must be applied by a second provider with two hands maintaining the cervical spine and head in a neutral position after the collar has been removed. MILS is easy to perform and is a widely accepted standard of care for airway management in cervical injury patients. It has been shown to limit head extension and decrease vertebral subluxation and angulation in C-spine injury models [34, 35]. However, it may decrease the mouth opening, provide a poor laryngoscopic view, and increase the time to intubation. While applying MILS,

**Table 1.7** Neurological disorders leading to respiratory dysfunction

| Site of lesion | Disease |
|---|---|
| Anterior horn cell | Spinal muscular atrophy<br>Post-polio syndrome<br>Amyotrophic lateral sclerosis |
| Peripheral nerve | Guillain-Barre syndrome<br>Porphyria<br>Critical illness polyneuropathy |
| Neuromuscular junction | Myasthenia gravis<br>Botulism |
| Myopathies | Congenital muscular dystrophy<br>Limb-girdle muscular dystrophy<br>Myotonic dystrophies<br>Duchenne muscular dystrophy<br>Polymyositis<br>Critical illness myopathy<br>Hypokalaemia Rhabdomyolysis |

Cormack-Lehane grade worsens by >1 grade in 35.6% patients and >2 grade in approximately 10% patients. Despite this disadvantages, MILS must be used for airway management of unstable C-spine to prevent secondary neurological injury.

### 1.5.3 Airway Management in Neuromuscular Weakness

Patients with neuromuscular weakness can present with respiratory failure due to the weakness of respiratory muscles [36, 37]. Neurological disorders that can lead to respiratory muscle weakness are summarised in Table 1.7.

Due to respiratory muscle weakness, these patients tend to hypoventilate and retain carbon dioxide leading to type 2 respiratory failure. Respiratory failure is not seen until the respiratory muscle strength has fallen to 25–30% of normal [38]. Some patients such as those with spina bifida, poliomyelitis, and some muscular dystrophies can have kyphoscoliosis that worsens the respiratory impairment.

Signs of respiratory failure

- Marked tachypnoea
- Bradypnea, apnoea (late)
- Increased, decreased or no respiratory efforts
- Poor to absent distal air movement
- Tachycardia (early)
- Bradycardia (late)
- Cyanosis
- Stupor, coma (late)

Patients with muscle weakness may have little or no respiratory efforts despite being in respiratory failure. Such patients may require confirmation by objective measurements such as pulse oximetry or blood gas analysis [37]. Respiratory failure can present with rise in arterial carbon dioxide levels (hypercarbia) or a drop in blood oxygenation (hypoxemia) or both. Such patients benefit from non-invasive ventilation combined with airway clearance by the frequent use of chest physiotherapy and cough assist devices [36–40]. Patients with rapidly progressive course not showing improvement in gas exchange and work of breathing with non-invasive ventilation will require intubation [36, 39].

Neurological illnesses are also associated with an increased risk of pneumonia. The weakness of facial, oropharyngeal, and laryngeal muscles lead to compromised swallowing and clearance of secretions. Weak cough reflex due to the weakness of abdominal muscles is another factor for increased risk of aspiration [37, 38]. Airway protection by ETT is required in patients with bulbar involvement and the risk of pulmonary aspiration. Bulbar involvement can be assessed by poor swallowing, dysarthria, weak mastication, facial weakness, nasal speech, and difficulty in protruding tongue [37, 38]. A single breath test is a useful method to assess the patient for the extent of respiratory impairment in patients with neuromuscular weakness. This test is performed by asking the patient to take a maximal inspiratory breath and begin counting. Normal patients can count up to 50 but a patient with severe impairment in vital capacity is indicated by a single breath count of <15 [39].

There are several concerns unique to patients with the neuromuscular weakness that should be kept in mind during airway management of these patients:

- These patients may have chronic silent aspiration leading to respiratory compromise.
- Succinylcholine is contraindicated in several neuromuscular diseases (amyotrophic lateral sclerosis, spinal muscular atrophy, 48 h after spinal injury up to 6 months, multiple sclerosis, Guillain-Barre syndrome (GBS)) due to the risk of severe hyperkalemia leading to cardiac arrest.
- Autonomic dysfunction may be an associated feature with weakness (spinal cord injury, multiple sclerosis, GBS, Eaton-lambert syndrome). Autonomic dysfunction leads to hemodynamic instability especially with the use of anesthetic drugs during intubation.

### 1.5.4 Airway Management in Stroke

Airway and ventilation is an essential part of supportive care in the management of stroke patients. As ACLS 2015 guidelines emphasise that "time is brain", assessment and stabilization of ABC (Airway, Breathing and Circulation) should be done in initial 10 min of receiving the patient in the emergency department. Maintaining tissue oxygenation is essential during cerebral ischemia due to stroke to prevent worsening of neurological injury [41]. Partial airway obstruction, hypoventilation, aspiration pneumonia and atelectasis are potential respiratory complications that can occur in patients presenting with stroke. Unconscious or brainstem stroke patients may also have impairment of oropharyngeal motility and loss of protective reflexes. Stroke leading to cerebral edema can cause a rise in ICP. These patients benefit from elective intubation and ventilation. Supplemental oxygen should be administered if hypoxia is evident on arterial blood gas or desaturation noted with pulse oximetry.

## 1.6 Summary

Airway management is the priority while managing a patient with a neurological emergency. A neurological emergency requires a rapid diagnosis and management with the aim of achieving a good outcome. "Time is brain" but only after the patient has been stabilized with a secure airway, ventilation, and circulation. Proper planning for the management of difficult airway and associated problems unique to patients with neurological/neurosurgical illness helps to prevent complications and mortality during airway management.

## Multiple Choice Question

1. Which of the following is NOT true. The goal of airway management is to
   (a) Maintain adequate oxygenation
   (b) Maintain adequate ventilation
   (c) Prevent regurgitation
   (d) Prevent aspiration
2. Which of the following about rapid sequence intubation (RSI) is correct
   (a) RSI should not be done in emergency situations.
   (b) The primary objective of RSI is to minimise the time of induction.
   (c) RSI should be preferred in patients with high risk of aspiration.
   (d) Preoxygenation is avoided during rapid sequence induction.
3. Identify the wrong statement
   (a) In emergency situation, consider all patients to be full stomach.
   (b) Avoid nasotracheal intubation in head injury patients with skull base fracture.
   (c) Always have an alternative plan ready in mind if unable to ventilate/intubate.
   (d) Always use manual inline stabilisation (MILS) in head injury patients during intubation if C-spine injury is ruled out.
4. In the "3-3-2 rule" for quick assessment of a patient for potential airway difficulty, the figure "2" refers to
   (a) placement of 2 fingers into the mouth of the patient between the upper and lower teeth
   (b) Placement of 2 fingers in the mandibular space (from mentum to hyoid bone)

(c) placement of 2 fingers between the hyoid bone and thyroid notch
(d) placement of 2 fingers between the thyroid and cricoid cartilage

5. Which of the following is incorrect.
   In a patient with neurological compromise the purpose of securing airway is to
   (a) Deliver supplemental oxygen
   (b) Perform neurological assessment
   (c) Support ventilation
   (d) Prevent aspiration
6. A patient of respiratory failure may present with
   (a) Hypercarbia and hyperoxemia
   (b) Hypocarbia and hypoxemia
   (c) Hypocarbia and hyperoxemia
   (d) Hypercarbia and hypoxemia
7. The induction agent of choice in a patient of head trauma with hypotension is
   (a) Propofol
   (b) Thiopentone
   (c) Etomidate
   (d) Midazolam
8. Which of the following statements is NOT correct.
   In a patient with suspected C-spine injury
   (a) To open the airway, use of jaw thrust without head extension is recommended.
   (b) Manual inline stabilisation (MILS) should always be used during airway management.
   (c) Cricoid pressure should not be used during tracheal intubation.
   (d) Radiological clearance of C-spine must be obtained in all cases prior to tracheal intubation.
9. Which of the following muscle relaxant is used for rapid sequence induction
   (a) Rocuronium
   (b) Vecuronium
   (c) Pancuronium
   (d) Atracurium
10. All of the following may be used to improve the chances of successful intubation except
    (a) Cricoid pressure may be applied to stabilize the trachea.
    (b) Place the patient in "sniffing position", if C-spine injury is ruled out.
    (c) BURP may be applied on thyroid cartilage to help visualise the vocal cords.
    (d) In case of anteriorly placed larynx, a stylet or gum elastic bougie may be used to pass the ETT through the vocal cords.

Answers : 1. (c), 2. (c), 3. (d), 4. (c), 5. (b), 6. (d), 7. (c), 8. (d), 9. (a), 10. (a)

## References


1. Chesnut RM, Marshall LF, Klauber MR, et al. The role of secondary brain injury in determining outcome from severe head injury. J Trauma. 1993;34:216–22.
2. Warner KJ, Cuschieri J, Copass MK, et al. The impact of prehospital ventilation on outcome after severe traumatic brain injury. J Trauma. 2007;62:1330–6.
3. Roppolo LP, Walters K. Airway management in neurological emergencies. Neurocrit Care. 2004;1:405–14.
4. Pierre EJ, McNeer RR, Shamir MY. Early management of the traumatized airway. Anesthesiol Clin. 2007;25:1–11.
5. Langeron O, Birenbaum A, Amour J. Airway management in trauma. Minerva Anestesiol. 2009;75:307–11.
6. Aziz M. Airway management in neuroanaesthesiology. Anesthesiol Clin. 2012;30:229–40.
7. Davies L, Benger JR. Audit of advanced airway management in UK emergency departments following the Fourth National Audit Project of the Royal College of Anaesthetists and Difficult Airway Society. Emerg Med J. 2013;30:427.
8. Murphy MF, Walls RM. Identification of the difficult and failed airway. In: Manual of emergency airway management. 3rd ed. Philadelphia: Lippincott Williams & Wilkins; 2008.
9. El-Orbany M, Connolly LA. Rapid sequence induction and intubation: current controversy. Anesth Analg. 2010;110:1318–25.
10. Pourmand A, Robinson C, Dorwart K, et al. Pre-oxygenation: implications in emergency airway management. Am J Emerg Med. 2017;35:1177–83.
11. Birenbaum A, Hajage D, Roche S, et al. Effect of cricoid pressure compared with a sham procedure in the rapid sequence induction of anesthesia: the IRIS randomized clinical trial. JAMA Surg. 2019;154:9–17.
12. Kovarik WD, Mayberg TS, Lam AM, et al. Succinylcholine does not change intracranial pressure, cerebral blood flow velocity, or the electroencephalogram in patients with neurologic injury. Anesth Analg. 1994;78:469–73.
13. Lee C, Jahr JS, Candiotti KA, et al. Reversal of profound neuromuscular block by sugammadex administered three minutes after rocuronium: a comparison with spontaneous recovery from succinylcholine. Anesthesiology. 2009;110:1020–5.
14. Lev R, Rosen P. Prophylactic lidocaine use preintubation: a review. J Emerg Med. 1994;12:499–506.
15. Apfelbau JL, Hagberg CA, Caplan RA, et al. Practice guidelines for management of the difficult airway: an updated report by the American Society of Anesthesiologists Task Force on management of the difficult airway. Anesthesiology. 2013;118:251–70.
16. Khan RM. Supraglottic airway devices. In: Khan RM, Maroof M, editors. Airway management: manual for clinical practitioners and examinees. 4th ed. Hyderabad: Paras Medical Publisher; 2011. p. 172–205.
17. Keller C, Brimacombe J, Keller K. Pressures exerted against the cervical vertebrae by the standard and intubating laryngeal mask airways: a randomized, controlled, cross-over study in fresh cadavers. Anesth Analg. 1999;89:1296–300.
18. Takahata O, Kubota M, Mamiya K, et al. The efficacy of the "BURP" maneuver during a difficult laryngoscopy. Anesth Analg. 1997;84:419–21.
19. Nolan JP, Wilson ME. Orotracheal intubation in patients with potential cervical spine injuries. An indication for the gum elastic bougie. Anaesthesia. 1993;48:630–3.
20. Rangel-Castillo L, Gopinath S, Robertson CS. Management of intracranial hypertension. Neurol Clin. 2008;26:521–41.

21. Marx P, Weinert G, Pfiester P, Kuhn H. The influence of hypercapnia and hypoxia on intracranial pressure and on CSF electrolyte concentrations. In: Schürmann K, Brock M, Reulen HJ, Voth D, editors. Brain edema/cerebello pontine angle tumors. Advances in neurosurgery, vol. 1. Berlin: Springer; 1973.
22. Werner C, Engelhard K. Pathophysiology of traumatic brain injury. Br J Anaesth. 2007;99:4–9.
23. Sharma D, Vavilala MS. Perioperative management of adult traumatic brain injury. Anaesthesiol Clin. 2012;30:333–46.
24. Crosby ET. Airway management in adults after cervical spine trauma. Anesthesiology. 2006;104:1293–318.
25. Holly LT, Kelly DF, Counelis GJ, et al. Cervical spine trauma associated with moderate and severe head injury: incidence, risk factors, and injury characteristics. J Neurosurg. 2002;96(3 Suppl):285–91.
26. Hackl W, Hausberger K, Sailer R, et al. Prevalence of cervical spine injuries in patients with facial trauma. Oral Surg Oral Med Oral Pathol Oral Radiol Endodontol. 2001;92:370–6.
27. Hoffman JR, Mower WR, Wolfson AB, et al. Validity of a set of clinical criteria to rule out injury to the cervical spine in patients with blunt trauma. National Emergency X-Radiography Utilization Study Group. N Engl J Med. 2000;343:94–9.
28. Stiell IG, Wells GA, Vandemheen KL, et al. The Canadian C-spine rule for radiography in alert and stable trauma patients. JAMA. 2001;286:1841–8.
29. Blackmore CC, Emerson SS, Mann FA, et al. Cervical spine imaging in patients with trauma: determination of fracture risk to optimize use. Radiology. 1999;211:759–65.
30. Bao FP, Zhang HG, Zhu SM. Anesthetic considerations for patients with acute cervical spinal cord injury. Neural Regen Res. 2017;12:499–504.
31. Donaldson WF III, Heil BV, Donaldson VP, Silvagglo VJ. The effect of airway maneuvers on the unstable C1-C2 segment: a cadaver study. Spine. 1997;22:1215–8.
32. Hauswald M, Sklar DP, Tandberg D, et al. Cervical spine movement during airway management: cinefluoroscopic appraisal in human cadavers. Am J Emerg Med. 1991;9:535–8.
33. Goutcher CM, Lochhead V. Reduction in mouth opening with semi-rigid cervical collars. Br J Anaesth. 2005;95:344–8.
34. Podolsky S, Baraff LJ, Simon RR, et al. Efficacy of cervical spine immobilization methods. J Trauma. 1983;23:461–5.
35. Aprahamian C, Thompson BM, Finger WA, et al. Experimental cervical spine injury model; evaluation of airway management and splinting techniques. Ann Emerg Med. 1984;13:584–7.
36. Overbeck MC. Airway management of respiratory failure. Emerg Med Clin North Am. 2016;34:97–127.
37. Mangera Z, Panesar G, Makker H. Practical approach to management of respiratory complications in neurological disorders. Int J Gen Med. 2012;5:255–63.
38. Nayak R. Practical approach to the patient with acute neuromuscular weakness. World J Clin Cases. 2017;5:270–9.
39. Davidson AC, Banham S, Elliott M, et al. BTS/ICS guideline for the ventilatory management of acute hypercapnic respiratory failure in adults. Thorax. 2016;71:ii1–ii35.
40. Brambrink AM, Kirsch JR. Perioperative care of patients with neuromuscular disease and dysfunction. Anesthesiol Clin. 2007;25:483–509.
41. Jauch EC, Saver JL, Adams HP, et al. Guidelines for the early management of patients with acute Ischemic Stroke. Stroke. 2013;44:870–947.

# Approach to a Patient with Coma

# 2

S. Srinivasan and Prasanna Udupi Bidkar

**Key Points**

- Coma is defined as a state of unresponsiveness of an individual to external or internal stimuli in which a patient lies with eyes closed unaware of the environment
- Vegetative state is an outcome after coma, where arousal and sleep–wake cycles return, unaccompanied by cognitive function
- GCS and AVPU are useful scales for assessment of neurological status
- Respiratory pattern and examination of pupils is important in the assessment of comatose patients
- Aetiology of coma is multifactorial
- Management begins with stabilization of the airway and cervical spine and includes conducting relevant laboratory and radiological investigations to facilitate institution of treatment of the causative factors

**Case Scenario**

A 25-year male was found lying in the ground, and was brought by bystanders to emergency department. No other history was available. The patient was not responding to commands and on painful stimuli withdraws hand, no vocalization. He was hypothermic. On examination, multiple ecchymotic patches in the forearm, heart rate 60/min, respiratory rate 8/min, SPO2 84% on room air and pupils bilaterally constricted.

S. Srinivasan · P. U. Bidkar (✉)
Jawaharlal Institute of Postgraduate Medical Education and Research, Pondicherry, India


P. U. Bidkar, P. Vanamoorthy (eds.), *Acute Neuro Care*,
https://doi.org/10.1007/978-981-15-4071-4_2

## 2.1 Introduction

Coma occurs secondary to many systemic conditions leading to neurological insult. Rapid diagnosis and treatment is essential in preventing any secondary brain injury and, aid in improving the outcome. In this chapter, we would like to discuss the various conditions mimicking coma, neurological examination patients in coma, diagnosis of the predisposing condition, and stepwise approach to the management of a comatose patient.

## 2.2 Coma

Coma is defined as a state where an individual is not responsive to external or internal stimuli. The lies with eyes closed and without any awareness of the environment. It is a state in which patient cannot be aroused. A patient is said to be in a stupor if he awakens briefly in response to stimulation and then goes back to sleep-like state [1]. The increasing degree of unresponsiveness can be graded from lethargy to coma.

## 2.3 Vegetative State

A vegetative state is one of the outcomes of coma. In a vegetative state, arousal and sleep-wake cycles return but are not accompanied by cognitive function. The will not be able to interact with the environment. The patient does not exhibit sustained, reproducible, purposeful, or voluntary behavioral responses to visual, auditory, tactile or noxious stimuli. If the vegetative state persists for more than 1 month, then it is termed as persistent vegetative state (PVS). The state can be declared as permanent if it persists beyond 3 months after nontraumatic injury and 12 months after traumatic injury in adults and children [2].

## 2.4 Neurological Examination of the Comatose Patient

Glasgow Coma Scale is a good indicator of neurological disability in comatose patients. In case of emergency neurological assessment can be done using **AVPU** (A—Alert, V—verbal commands, P—to Painful stimuli, U—Unresponsive) scale. The detailed examination of the central nervous system in comatose patients includes

1. Rating of consciousness
2. Respiratory pattern
3. Pupillary size and reactivity
4. Eye position and movement
5. Corneal reflex
6. Motor function

**Table 2.1** Glasgow Coma Scale (GCS) = E + M + V

| *Eye Opening (E)* | | *Verbal Response (V)* | |
|---|---|---|---|
| Spontaneous | 4 | Oriented | 5 |
| To loud voice | 3 | Confused disoriented | 4 |
| To pain | 2 | Inappropriate words | 3 |
| None | 1 | Incomprehensible sounds | 2 |
| | | None | 1 |
| *Motor Response (M)* | | Max score 15, Min score 3, Coma < 8 | |
| Obeys commands | 6 | | |
| Localizes pain | 5 | | |
| Withdraws from pain | 4 | | |
| Abnormal flexion posturing | 3 | | |
| Extensor posturing | 2 | | |
| None | 1 | | |

**Table 2.2** Respiratory patterns in coma

| | Pattern | Lesion |
|---|---|---|
| Cheyne–Stokes pattern | 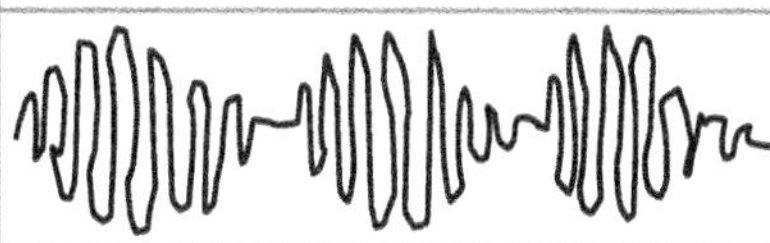 | Bilateral cortical and forebrain |
| Central neurogenic hyperventilation | 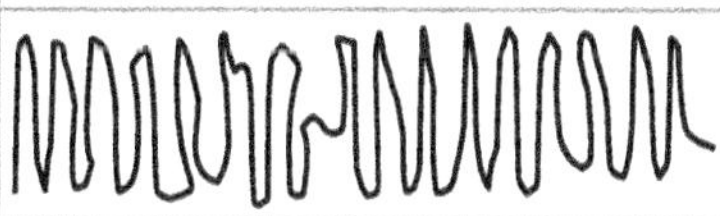 | Midbrain upper pons |
| Apneustic breathing | 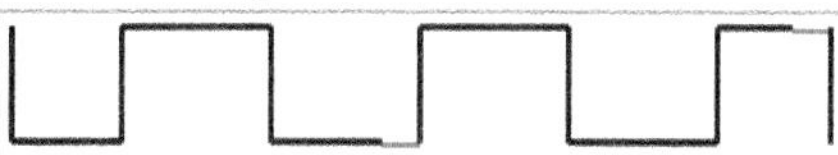 | Mid-lower pons |
| Ataxic breathing | 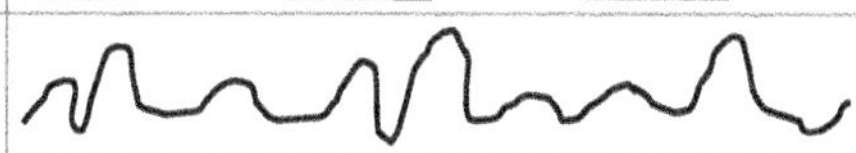 | Dorsomedial medulla |

**Rating of Consciousness** Glasgow Coma Scale (GCS) is commonly used to measure the level of unconsciousness [3–15]. A GCS of 15 means completely conscious and a GCS of 3 signifies deep coma. It is based on the assessment of three parameters: eye opening, motor response, and verbal response (Table 2.1).

### 2.4.1 Respiratory Pattern

The pattern of breathing is important in the assessment of comatose patients [14]. Assessment of breathing pattern may reveal the probable location of the lesion leading to coma (Table 2.2).

**Table 2.3** Pupillary examination and interpretation

| Pupil | Cause |
|---|---|
| Pinpoint | Opiate overdose, pontine haemorrhage |
| Small | N in bright room, Horner's syndrome, metabolic coma |
| Midposition-NR | Brain stem damage |
| Unilateral dilated | Abnormal, uncal herniation |
| Bilateral dilated and fixed | Brain death |

### 2.4.2 Pupillary Examination

Pupillary examination along with GCS forms an important part of the neurologic assessment of patients with coma (Table 2.3). Bilaterally dilated nonreactive pupils suggest extensive brain damage. Bilateral pinpoint pupils are seen in narcotic overdose or pontine hemorrhage. A unilateral dilated pupil is suggestive of intracranial space-occupying lesions like tumour or hematoma. Normal size reactive pupils generally indicate metabolic causes of coma.

### 2.4.3 Motor Examination

**Decorticate Posturing** It is a flexor response of upper limbs with the flexion at elbow joints and wrist joints with extension of both lower limbs. It denotes cortical damage.

**Decerebrate Posturing** It is an extensor response with the adduction of the upper limb with pronation. Extension of lower limbs is present. It denotes brainstem dysfunction.

Prognosis is poor in patients with decerebrate posturing.

## 2.5 Causes of Coma

Coma can be due to various intracranial pathologies or can be due to metabolic causes. Metabolic causes are the most common cause of coma in medical intensive care units. Hence during the evaluation of these patients, all the possibilities of coma should be carefully assessed and confirmatory tests should be done whenever necessary (Table 2.4).

### 2.5.1 Conditions Which Mimic Coma

Various neurological conditions mimic coma [15–20]. The physician needs to keep these differential diagnoses in mind during neurologic assessment of comatose patients (Table 2.5).

**Table 2.4** Causes of coma

| Structural brain injury | |
|---|---|
| Cerebral hemisphere | Brainstem |
| *Unilateral (with displacement)* | Pontine haemorrhage |
| Intraparenchymal haematoma | Basilar artery occlusion and brainstem infarct |
| Middle cerebral artery ischaemic stroke | Central pontine myelinolysis |
| Intracranial venous thrombosis | Brainstem haemorrhagic contusion |
| Haemorrhagic contusion | Cerebellum (with displacement of brainstem) |
| Cerebral abscess | Cerebellar infarct |
| Brain tumour | Cerebellar haematoma |
| Subdural or epidural haematoma | Cerebellar abscess |
| Bilateral | Cerebellar glioma |
| Subarachnoid haemorrhage | |
| Multiple traumatic brain contusions | |
| Penetrating traumatic brain injury | |
| Anoxic–ischaemic encephalopathy | |
| Multiple cerebral infarcts | |
| Bilateral thalamic infarcts | |
| Lymphoma | |
| Encephalitis | |
| Acute disseminated encephalomyelitis | |
| Cerebral edema | |
| Multiple brain metastases | |
| Acute hydrocephalus | |
| Acute leukoencephalopathy | |
| Air or fat embolism | |
| Diffuse physiological brain dysfunction | Acute metabolic–endocrine derangement |
| Generalized tonic–clonic seizures | Hypoglycaemia |
| Poisoning, illicit drug use | Hyperglycaemia (non-ketotic hyperosmolar) |
| Hypothermia | Hyponatraemia |
| Gas inhalation | Hypernatraemia |
| Acute (lethal) catatonia Malignant neuroleptic syndrome | Addison's disease |
| *Psychogenic unresponsiveness* | Hypercalcaemia |
| Hysterical coma | Acute hypothyroidism |
| Malingering | Acute panhypopituitarism |
| | Acute uraemia |
| | Hyperbilirubinaemia |
| | Hypercapnia |

### 2.5.2 Approach to a Comatose Patient

The initial management of the patients in coma begins by assessment of Airway (A), Breathing (B) and Circulation (C). If there is a possibility of cervical spine injury, the spine should be immobilized. The priority of an initial assessment is to maintain a patent airway, thus allowing optimal ventilation and oxygenation. All patients

**Table 2.5** Conditions mimicking coma

| Condition | Self-awareness | Sleep–wake cycles | Motor function | Experience suffering | EEG |
|---|---|---|---|---|---|
| PVS | No | Yes | No purposeful movement | No | δ or θ activity |
| Coma | No | No | No purposeful movement | No | δ or θ activity |
| Brain death | No | No | No purposeful movement | No | EEG silence |
| Locked- in syndrome | Present | Intact | Quadriplegia | Yes | Normal or minimally abnormal |
| Akinetic mutism | Present | Intact | Paucity of movement | yes | Non- specific slowing |

with head injury with <8 require endotracheal intubation for the protection of the airway. Hypotension and hypoxia aggravate secondary brain injury, hence it should be avoided. A rapid search for the involvement of other organ systems should be done following the stabilization of ABC. A detailed stepwise approach of these patients is presented in Table 2.6.

### 2.5.3 Investigations

Keeping in mind the preceding differential diagnosis for states of coma, the sequence of diagnostic studies becomes clear. Rapid identification of metabolic or toxic causes of coma are determined by laboratory testing of blood, urine, gastric aspirate, and cerebrospinal fluid (CSF).

### 2.5.4 Laboratory Investigations

1. Venous blood: hemoglobin (Hb) white blood count, platelets, glucose, electrolytes, calcium, blood urea nitrogen, creatinine, osmolality, coagulation studies, liver function tests, muscle enzymes, thyroid and adrenal functions, toxicology screen, blood cultures
2. Arterial blood: pH, $PCO_2$, $PO_2$, carboxyhemoglobin ammonia
3. Urine: toxicology, microscopic examination
4. Gastric aspirate: toxicology
5. Cerebrospinal fluid: cell count, protein, glucose, gram stain, culture, counterimmunoelectrophoresis, viral and fungal antigens, and antibody titers.

**Table 2.6** Approach to a patient with coma

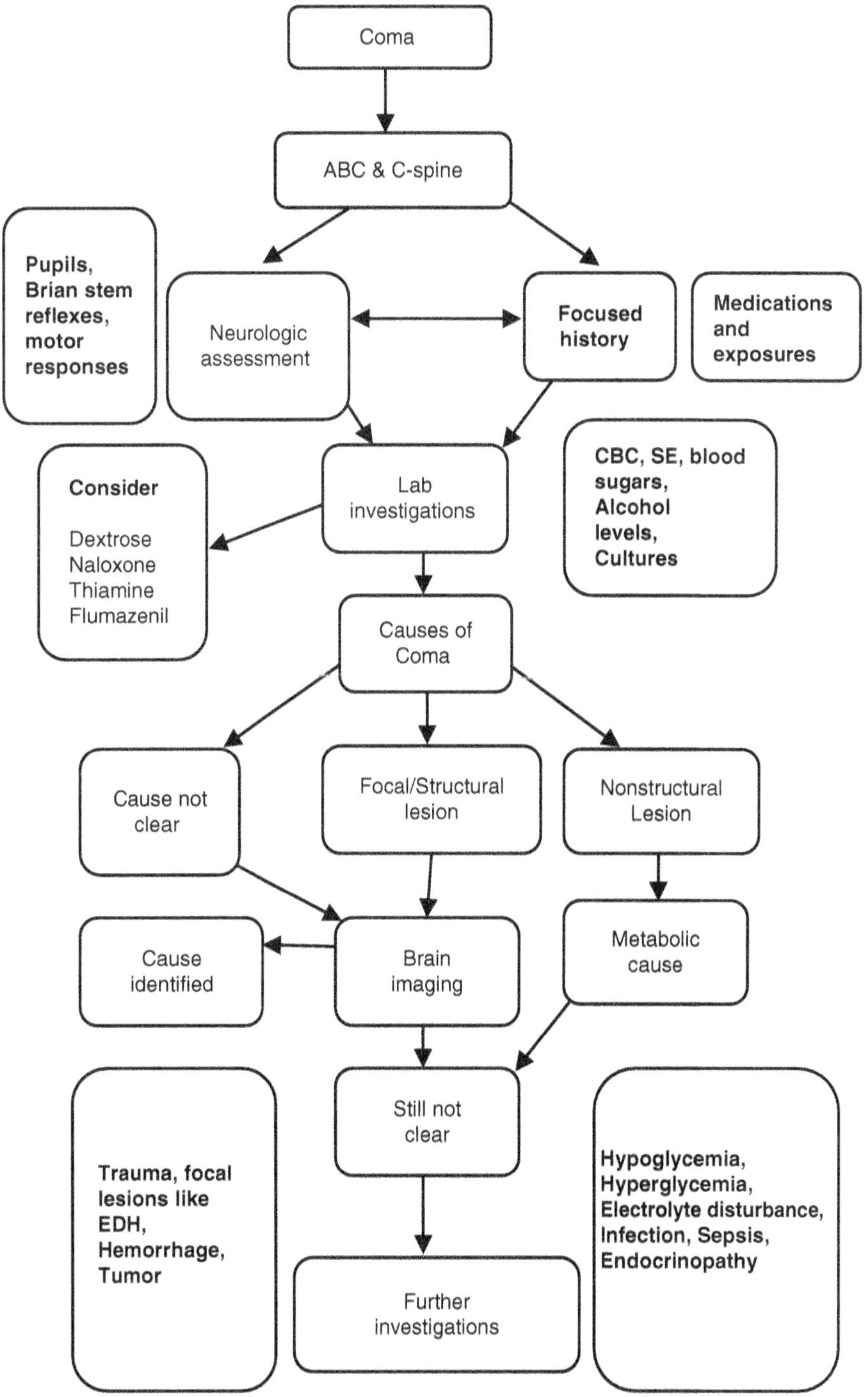

### 2.5.5 Radiological Examination

Noncontrast CT scan is the initial investigation of choice in patients with suspected/presumed structural lesion. An initial CT scan helps to rule out many structural causes like intracranial hematoma, subarachnoid hemorrhage cerebral infarction, cerebral edema, and brain neoplasm. However, in case of doubt additional investigations like MRI [21–24] and EEG [25–27] can be performed to rule out other causes of coma. Following are the some additional investigation needed to establish the cause of coma.

1. Computed tomography
2. Magnetic resonance imaging
3. Lumbar puncture
4. Electro-encephalography
5. Evoked potentials

## 2.6 Treatment of Coma

### 2.6.1 Initial Management

Treatment must be instituted immediately, even when the diagnosis is uncertain, to prevent further brain damage secondary to complications. Airway, breathing, and circulation should be assessed and every step should be taken to prevent hypoxemia. Airway should be secured with a cuffed endotracheal tube to prevent aspiration of gastric contents.

The cause of the coma should be investigated and treated accordingly. Supportive care with or without ventilator support should be instituted in vegetative patients. Comatose patients should be assessed frequently. By the end of the first hour of presentation, assessment, and management of ABC, toxicology screen, routing laboratory investigations and a CT scan should be done (Table 2.7).

### 2.6.2 Coma Cocktail

It involves administration of 50% dextrose (0.5–1 mg), oxygen, naloxone (0.4–2 mg), thiamine (100 mg) and flumazenil (0.2 mg) as an empiric treatment in comatose patients especially if the etiology is not known [28]. It helps in the correction of the reversible causes of coma including hypoglycemia, hypoxia, opioid, or benzodiazepine overdose or thiamine deficiency. Coma cocktail is not routinely recommended if early investigations point to a specific diagnosis [29].

**Table 2.7** Coma Checklist by the end of first hour

- ABC & Spine
- Blood sugar
- Narcotic overdose / Naloxone given
- SE, CBC, Toxicology screen & ABG
- Radiology (CT scan)

**Table 2.8** Outcome after coma

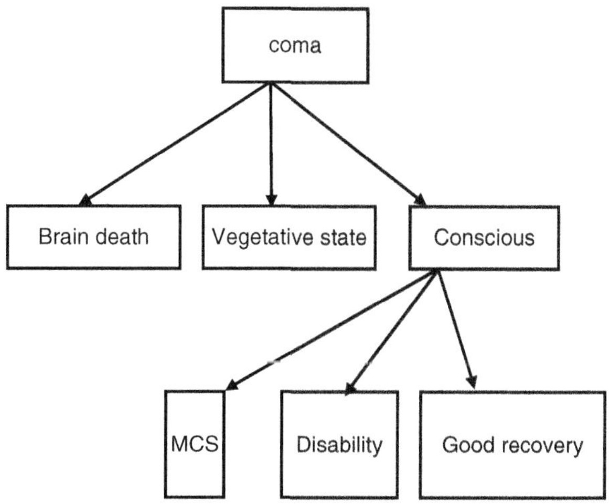


### 2.6.3 Outcome After Coma

Possible outcomes after coma include a good recovery with patient regaining full consciousness with good recovery, consciousness with some disability secondary to brain damage, or a minimally conscious state where a patient has limited awareness intermittently. Some patients may progress to a vegetative state remaining awake without any awareness of the environment. Brain death may be another possible outcome in severe cases (Table 2.8).

## Multiple Choice Questions

1. Pick out the correct statement about coma
   (a) Coma is a state of unresponsiveness to external and internal stimuli.
   (b) Patient does not have awareness of environment.
   (c) Sleep–wake cycle is absent
   (d) All of the above.
2. Pick out the wrong statement about vegetative state
   (a) Arousal and sleep–wake cycle return.
   (b) Cognitive function intact.
   (c) It is termed as persistent vegetative state if it persists for 1 month.
   (d) It can be declared permanent if it persists 3 months after non traumatic injury.
3. What are the disadvantages of Glasgow Coma Scale(GCS)
   (a) Pupillary examination not included.
   (b) Respiratory pattern not considered.
   (c) Not useful in intubated patients.
   (d) All of the above.
4. A patient with severe head injury got admitted in casualty. He was not having any eye opening even after painful stimuli, motor examination reveals abnormal flexion posturing of limbs and makes a verbal response with incomprehensible sounds. What will be the GCS score?
   (a) 6/15
   (b) 3/15
   (c) 12/15
   (d) 10/15
5. A comatose patient was observed with respiratory pattern of Cheyne–Stokes breathing. What could be the probable site of lesion in brain presenting with that pattern of breathing?
   (a) Bilateral cortical and forebrain
   (b) Midbrain
   (c) Dorsomedial medulla
   (d) Pons.
6. Normal, reactive pupils in a comatose patient is usually suggestive of:
   (a) Metabolic cause.
   (b) Pontine haemorrhage.
   (c) Narcotic overdose.
   (d) None of the above.
7. Characteristic features of locked-in syndrome include:
   (a) Self-awareness is present.
   (b) Sleep–wake cycle is intact.
   (c) Normal EEG.
   (d) All of the above.

8. Management of coma in the first hour includes:
   (a) Assessment of airway, breathing and circulation.
   (b) Blood sugar, serum electrolytes, toxicological screening.
   (c) CT brain
   (d) All the above.
9. Which of the following is not a part of coma cocktail :
   (a) 50% dextrose
   (b) Naloxone
   (c) Thiamine
   (d) IV magnesium.
10. Pick out the incorrect statement:
   (a) Decorticate posture involves flexion of upper limbs with flexion at elbow.
   (b) Decerebrate posturing is extensor response with adduction of upper limb with pronation.
   (c) Decerebrate posturing indicates brainstem damage.
   (d) Decorticate posturing carries a poorer prognosis than decerebrate posturing.

Answers: 1. (d), 2. (b), 3. (d), 4. (a), 5. (a), 6. (a), 7. (d), 8. (d), 9. (d), 10, (d)

## References

1. Weyhenmyeye JA, Gallman EA. Rapid review neuroscience. 1st ed. Maryland Heights: Mosby Elsevier; 2007. p. 177–9.
2. The Multi-Society Task Force on PVS. Medical aspects of the persistent vegetative state. N Engl J Med. 1994;330:1499–508.
3. Teasdale G, Jennett B. Assessment of coma and impaired consciousness. A practical scale. Lancet. 1974;2(7872):81–4.
4. The Brain Trauma Foundation: The American Association of Neurological Surgeons. The joint section on neurotrauma and critical care. Glasgow coma scale score. J Neurotrauma. 2000;17:563–71.
5. Booth CM, Boone RH, Tomlinson G, et al. Is this patient dead, vegetative, or severely neurologically impaired? Assessing outcome for comatose survivors of cardiac arrest. JAMA. 2004;291:870–9.
6. Winkler JV, Rosen P, Alfry EJ. Prehospital use of the Glasgow coma scale in severe head injury. J Emerg Med. 1984;2:1–6.
7. Baxt WG, Moody P. The impact of advanced prehospital emergency care on the mortality of severely brain-injured patients. J Trauma. 1987;27:365–9.
8. Massagli TL, Michaud LJ, Rivara FP. Association between injury indices and outcome after severe traumatic brain injury in children. Arch Phys Med Rehabil. 1996;77:125–32.
9. Servadei F, Nasi MT, Cremonini AM, et al. Importance of a reliable admission Glasgow Coma Scale score for determining the need for evacuation of posttraumatic subdural hematomas: A prospective study of 65 patients. J Trauma. 1998;44:868–73.
10. Howard RS, Hirsch NP, Miller DH, Raps E. Coma, vegetative state and locked in syndrome. In: Critical care neurology. Boston: Butterworth Heinemann; 1999. p. 91–120. (stupor).
11. Stevens RD, Bhardwaj A. Approach to the comatose patient. Crit Care Med. 2006;34(1):31–41.
12. Segatore M, Way C. The Glasgow coma scale: time for change. Heart Lung. 1992;21:548–57.
13. Sternbach GL. The Glasgow coma scale. J Emerg Med. 2000;19:67–71.

14. North JB, Jennett S. Abnormal breathing patterns associated with acute brain damage. Arch Neurol. 1974;31:338–44.
15. Cairns HWB, Whitteridge D. Akineticmutism with an epidermoid cyst of the 3rd ventricle. Brain. 1941;64:273–91.
16. Ackermann H, Ziegler W. Akineticmutism—a review of the literature. Fortschr Neurol Psychiatr. 1995;63:59–67.
17. Giacino JT, Zasler ND, Whyte J, Katz DI, Glen M, Andary M. Recommendations for use of uniform nomenclature pertinent to patients with severe alterations in consciousness: American Congress of rehabilitation medicine. Arch Phys Med Rehabil. 1995;76:205–9.
18. Cartlidge N. States related to or confused with coma. J Neurol Neurosurg Psychiatry. 2001;71:i18–9.
19. Smith E, Delargy M. Locked-in syndrome. BMJ. 2005;330:406–9.
20. Vargas F, Hilbert G, Gruson D, et al. Fulminant Guillain-Barre syndrome mimicking cerebral death: case report and literature review. Intensive Care Med. 2000;26:623–7.
21. Restrepo L, Wityk RJ, Grega MA, et al. Diffusion-and perfusion-weighted magnetic resonance imaging of the brain before and after coronary artery bypass grafting surgery. Stroke. 2002;33:2909–15.
22. Wityk RJ, Goldsborough MA, Hillis A, et al. Diffusion- and perfusion-weighted brain magnetic resonance imaging in patients with neurologic complications after cardiac surgery. Arch Neurol. 2001;58:571–6.
23. Finelli PF, Uphoff DF. Magnetic resonance imaging abnormalities with septic encephalopathy. J Neurol Neurosurg Psychiatry. 2004;75:1189–91.
24. Hollinger P, Zurcher R, Schroth G, et al. Diffusion magnetic resonance imaging findings in cerebritis and brain abscesses in a patient with septic encephalopathy. J Neurol. 2000;247:232–4.
25. Towne AR, Waterhouse EJ, Boggs JG, et al. Prevalence of nonconvulsive status epilepticus in comatose patients. Neurology. 2000;54:340–5.
26. Claassen J, Mayer SA, Kowalski RG, et al. Detection of electrographic seizures with continuous EEG monitoring in critically ill patients. Neurology. 2004;62:1743–8.
27. Varelas PN, Spanaki MV, Hacein-Bey L, et al. Emergent EEG: indications and diagnostic yield. Neurology. 2003;61:702–4.
28. Dana Bartlett RN. The coma cocktail: indications, contraindications, adverse effects, proper dose, and proper route. J Emerg Nurs. 2004;30:572–4.
29. Bledsoe BE. No more coma cocktails. Using science to dispel myths & improve patient care. J Emerg Med Serv. 2002;27(11):54–60.

# 3 Focused Neurological Evaluation

Ajay Prasad Hrishi and Manikandan Sethuraman

## Key Points

- Focused neurological examination starts with obtaining a detailed history including presenting complaints and relevant medical and surgical history
- Optimization of airway, breathing, and circulation is crucial before proceeding with neurological examination
- Various scoring systems are available for assessment of consciousness—GCS, AVPU, FOUR score
- Fundoscopic examination, evaluation of eye movements, and focal neurological deficits are essential components of neurological examination
- Testing for reflexes and tone helps in differentiating between upper and lower motor neuron lesions
- Examination of the sensory system, cerebellar signs complete a focused neurological examination

## Case Scenario

An 18-year-old boy is struck on the side of the head by a ball during a cricket match. He appears dazed for about 30 s, but is lucid for several minutes before he abruptly becomes stuporous. His limbs on the side opposite the site of the blow are more flaccid than those on the same side as the injury. On arrival in the emergency room 25 min after the accident, he is unresponsive to painful stimuli. His

A. P. Hrishi · M. Sethuraman (✉)
Sree Chitra Tirunal Institute of Medical Sciences and Technology, Trivandrum, India
e-mail: drajay@sctimst.ac.in


P. U. Bidkar, P. Vanamoorthy (eds.), *Acute Neuro Care*,
https://doi.org/10.1007/978-981-15-4071-4_3

pulse is 40 beats per minute, with an electrocardiography (ECG) revealing no arrhythmias. His blood pressure in both arms is 170/110 mmHg. You are called upon to assess the neurological status. How to proceed?

## 3.1 Introduction

A focused neurological examination is one of the essential parts of neurological examination in critically ill patients. It is akin to screening tests for the rapid diagnosis of any pathological disease of the patient and is very much a part of busy emergency department (ED). It is aimed to use highly sensitive tests for disease identification. It saves time and also helps in preventing unnecessary investigations for the patient who do not have the disease. Since "Time Is Brain," it is essential for every physician involved in the management of acute neurological disease to know how to conduct a focused neurological examination. This chapter is aimed to cover the diagnosis of acute neurological diseases presenting to ED as well as further management in intensive care units. An approach to a neurosurgical/neuro-medical emergency begins with an appropriate history of surrounding events followed by a general examination and a focused neurological examination.

## 3.2 Focused Clinical History

A detailed history of presenting events and a general medical history should be obtained from the patient (if possible), family members, or emergency service personnel. This should include the following facts:

Presenting events:

- Rapidity of symptom onset or neurological deterioration
- Seizures
- Nausea and vomiting
- Recent or previous trauma
- Recent febrile illness

Previous medical history:

- Hypertension
- Diabetes mellitus
- Epilepsy
- Known history of previous/underlying malignancy/pituitary tumor
- HIV and antiretroviral treatment
- History of anticoagulant use
- Compliance with treatment for co-morbidities mentioned above

Surgical history:

- Previous neurosurgery, e.g., ventriculoperitoneal shunt/endoscopic third ventriculostomy.

Patients may present with more than one neurological symptom. The timing of symptoms provide an essential clue to etiology; e.g., rapid onset of symptoms can occur in a stroke or subarachnoid hemorrhage, a relapsing/ remitting pattern could indicate multiple sclerosis and a more gradual decline could raise suspicion about an intracranial lesion or motor neuron disease. Ask specifically about the history of preceding and precipitating factors; if the headache started after a head injury in an elderly patient, the possibility of a subdural hematoma could be considered. If the patient is complaining of an intermittent problem, enquire about the frequency of attacks, duration of symptoms on each occasion and note if they have any pattern.

*The red flags in history (Warrants immediate admission and evaluation)*

- Headache of recent onset accompanied by features suggestive of raised intracranial pressure (ICP) (for example vomiting, drowsiness, posture-related headache).
- Focal or non-focal neurological symptoms (for example blackout or change in personality, cognitive function or memory)
- New, qualitatively different, unexplained headache that becomes progressively severe
- A new-onset seizure
- Progressive neurological deficit (sensory or motor)
- Cranial nerve palsy (for example: visual disturbances, diplopia, unilateral sensorineural deafness)

## 3.3 General Survey and Clinical Examination

The clinical examination focuses on the principles of standard ABCD (Airway, Breathing, Circulation, and Disability) approach and supportive management is instituted simultaneously as and when problems are identified.

1. **Inspection**

   Inspect for any evidence of trauma such as scalp bruising or laceration. Presence of periorbital (raccoon eyes) or retro-auricular bruising (Battle sign) or CSF leak from the nose or ear should raise the red flag to immediately screen for skull base fractures. Avoid nasal insertion of an airway, endotracheal tube or Ryle's tube, until skull base fracture, has been ruled out [1, 2].
2. **Airway and breathing**

   Ensure airway patency and that the patient is maintaining an oxygen saturation of above 95%. Consider intubation if the Glasgow coma scale (GCS) <8. Patients can have various abnormal patterns of breathing. Identifying the respiratory pattern helps in management as well as provides us with a clue as to the location of the lesion [1–3]. Cheyne Stokes respiration is the most common abnormal breathing pattern, characterized by periods of hyperventilation alternating with periods of apnea. It is seen in large bilateral supratentorial lesions. Central neurogenic hyperventilation characterized by rapid, regular, and sustained periods of hyperventilation is seen in large pontine lesions, hypoxia, and metabolic acidosis [3–5]. Apneustic breathing, where periods of inspiration ending with brief 2–3-s pauses and alternating irregularly with expiratory pauses is seen with large bilateral mid-pontine lesions. Ataxic breathing of irregular alternating deep and shallow breaths and irregular pauses may be seen in large bilateral posterior fossa lesions especially when associated with medullary compression.

3. **Circulation**

   Elevated blood pressure may be a reactive phenomenon or reflect the underlying cause. With increasing intracranial pressure, an acute rise in blood pressure maybe accompanied by bradycardia and decreased respiration (Cushing's reflex) and is a sign of impending tonsillar herniation.

4. **Temperature**

   Fever may indicate underlying CNS infection. However, hyperthermia can present in conditions like subarachnoid hemorrhage, intraventricular hemorrhage, and hypothalamic lesions.

## 3.4 Focused Neurological Examination

A focused neurological evaluation is an important diagnostic tool in the evaluation of any neurological problem.

### 3.4.1 Assessment of Level of Consciousness

(a) **AVPU—simple scoring system**

   The AVPU scale has four possible outcomes for recording with the best (A) to worst (U) score to avoid unnecessary tests on conscious patients. Alert (A): The patient is fully awake but not necessarily oriented. The patient will spontaneously open eyes, respond to voice, and will have a normal motor function. Verbal (V): The patient responds to verbal commands in any of the three component measures of eyes, voice, or motor—e.g., the patient's eyes open on verbal stimulus. Pain (P): The patient responds to a painful central stimulus like a sternal rub, supraorbital pressure, or a peripheral stimulus such as squeezing the fingers or nail bed. The patient may have some level of consciousness and may respond by using their voice, moving their eyes, or moving part of their body which includes abnormal posturing. Unresponsive (U): The patient does not have any eye, voice, or motor response to voice or pain.

(b) **Glasgow Coma Scale (GCS)**

   GCS can assess the depth of coma, and it consists of three components: eye-opening, best verbal, and best motor responses, with a total score ranging from 3 to 15 (Table 3.1). GCS should be assessed only after resuscitation and stabilization of hemodynamic and oxygenation status. One of the shortcomings of the GCS score is that the verbal component cannot be assessed in intubated patients. Also, patients with hypoxia, hypotension, facial swelling, alcohol, and drug intoxication may not be able to give responses in all components of GCS. The motor response has maximum weightage among the components, and the best motor response in any limb is acceptable.

**Table 3.1** Glasgow coma scale

| Score | 1 | 2 | 3 | 4 | 5 | 6 |
|---|---|---|---|---|---|---|
| Eye | No response | To pain | To speech | Opens eyes spontaneously | N/A | N/A |
| Best verbal response | No response | Incomprehensible sounds | Inappropriate words | Confused | Oriented to space time and person | N/A |
| Best motor response | No response | Abnormal extension (decerebrate) | Abnormal flexion (decorticate) | Flexion withdrawal to pain | Localizes pain | Obeys commands |

The severity of traumatic brain injury (TBI) is classified based on GCS as follows:

- GCS score < 8–9 - Severe TBI
- GCS score 8 or 9–12 - Moderate TBI
- GCS score ≥ 13 - Minor TBI

(c) **FOUR Score**

"FOUR" in the scoring system is an acronym for "Full Outline of UnResponsiveness." It assesses the main four domains of neurological function, i.e., eye responses, motor responses, brainstem reflexes, and the breathing pattern (Table 3.2). FOUR score has better sensitivity, specificity, accuracy, and positive predictive value in neurological and TBI settings and with better interobserver reliability as compared to the GCS. It is beneficial in testing intubated patients and detecting patients in "locked-in state."

### 3.4.2 Fundoscopy and Pupillary Response

Fundoscopic examination for papilledema is an essential clinical skill. Pupils are checked for both size and response to light. A unilateral dilated pupil suggests the presence of a structural lesion with uncal herniation. Uncal herniation happens as a result of the third nerve play due to compression of the nerve by the uncus and warrants immediate attention [3, 4]. The patient should preferably be immediately intubated, and control of ventilation is necessary to avoid further worsening. Pontine lesions result in pinpoint pupils, while midbrain lesions are associated with mid-position fixed pupils [3–5].

### 3.4.3 Eye Movements

Evaluation of spontaneous eye movements and ocular reflexes—oculocephalic (doll's eye) and oculovestibular reflex is done to evaluate the status of the brain stem. Hemispheric lesions involving the frontal eye fields result in deviation of the eyes away from the side of the associated hemiplegia. Brainstem lesions involving the reticular formation in the pons result in conjugate deviation of the eyes toward

**Table 3.2** FOUR score

| | Score | | Score |
|---|---|---|---|
| *Eye response* | | *Brainstem reflex* | |
| Eyes open, tracking or blinking to command | 4 | Pupil and corneal reflex present | 4 |
| Eyelids open but not tracking | 3 | One pupil wide and fixed | 3 |
| Eyelids closed, but opens to loud voice | 2 | Pupil or corneal reflex absent | 2 |
| Eyelids closed, but opens to pain | 1 | Pupil and corneal reflex absent | 1 |
| Eyelids remain closed for pain | 0 | Absent pupil, corneal or cough reflex | 0 |
| *Motor response* | | *Respiration* | |
| Thumbs up, fist or peace sign | 4 | Regular breathing pattern | 4 |
| Localizing pain | 3 | Cheyne stokes breathing | 3 |
| Flexion response to pain | 2 | Irregular breathing | 2 |
| Extension response | 1 | Triggers ventilator or breathes above the set ventilator rate | 1 |
| No response to pain or generalized myoclonus state | 0 | Apnea or breaths at the set ventilator rate | 0 |

**Table 3.3** Causes of neck stiffness

- Meningitis
- Subarachnoid hemorrhage
- Tonsillar herniation (raised intracranial pressure)
- Cervical spine trauma

the side of the associated hemiplegia. Nystagmus may indicate cerebellar lesions. The cervical spine should be cleared before attempting dolls eye reflex as sidewise head movements can worsen the insult to the spinal cord [3, 4].

### 3.4.4 Meningism

Remember that neck stiffness has several causes and does not always mean meningitis—performing a lumbar puncture in a patient with tonsillar herniation will have disastrous consequences [4] (Table 3.3).

### 3.4.5 Focal Neurological Deficits

Along with the assessment of the motor component of the Glasgow coma score, focal motor deficits including cranial, motor, or sensory system deficits should be documented.

(a) **Cranial nerve examination**

Third and sixth nerve palsies are common indicators of raised intracranial pressure. Other cranial nerve deficits may also be present depending on the location of the pathology. The detailed examination and the probable causes are given in the following Table 3.4.

**Table 3.4** Cranial nerve examination and suspected common etiologies for cranial nerve dysfunction

| Cranial nerve | Symptoms and signs | Suspected etiology |
|---|---|---|
| I Olfactory | Smell—test each nostril for the ability to differentiate different smells | Trauma, frontal lobe tumor, meningitis |
| II Optic | Acuity—Snellen chart<br>Visual fields—compare with your own visual fields by standing directly in front of the patient with your head at the same level<br>Pupils—size, shape, reaction to light, and accommodation<br>Ophthalmoscopy—darken room, dilate the pupil with one drop tropicamide 0.5% if needed, view optic disc (pale, swollen), follow each vessel outwards to view each quadrant, track outwards to check lens and cornea | Monocular blindness—lesion in one eye or optic nerve (e.g., multiple sclerosis, giant cell arteritis)<br>Bitemporal hemianopia—optic chiasm compression, e.g., pituitary apoplexy/adenoma, craniopharyngioma, internal carotid artery aneurysm<br>Homonymous hemianopia—affects half the visual field on the side opposite the lesion. Lesion beyond the optic chiasm, e.g., stroke, abscess, tumor |
| III Oculomotor | Ptosis, large pupil, eye down and out diplopia from a third nerve lesion may cause nystagmus (Fig. 3.1) | Posterior communicating artery aneurysm, idiopathic |
| IV Trochlear | Diplopia on looking down and in; may compensate by tilting head | Rare in isolation. May occur as a result of trauma to the orbit |
| V Trigeminal | Motor—open mouth—jaw deviates to the side of the lesion<br>Sensory—corneal reflex is lost first. Check all three divisions | Bulbar palsy, acoustic neuroma, trigeminal neuralgia, caroticocavernous fistula, skull base fracture |
| VI Abducens | Horizontal diplopia on looking outwards (Fig. 3.2) | Pontine stroke,<br>Raised intracranial pressure |
| VII Facial | Causes facial weakness and droop<br>Ask to raise eyebrows, show teeth, puff out cheeks:<br>Lower motor neuron (LMN) lesion: all one side of the face is affected<br>Upper motor neuron (UMN) lesion: lower two-thirds of the face affected only | LMN—Bell's palsy, polio, otitis media, skull fracture, cerebellopontine angle<br>Tumors, parotid tumors,<br>UMN—stroke, CP angle tumor |
| VIII Vestibulo-auditory | Auditory—ask to repeat a number whispered in one ear while you block the other<br>Vestibular—ask about balance, check for nystagmus—ask the patient to fix on finger 75 cm away—check gaze—upwards, downwards, lateral (both directions), keeping finger <30 from the midline | Acoustic neuroma,<br>Brainstem stroke |
| IX, X Glossopharyngeal, Vagus | Gag reflex, the soft-palate moves towards the normal side on saying "Aah" | Trauma, brainstem lesions, neck tumors |

(continued)

**Table 3.4** (continued)

| Cranial nerve | Symptoms and signs | Suspected etiology |
|---|---|---|
| XI Accessory | Trapezii—shrug shoulders against resistance<br>Sternomastoid—turn head to right/left against resistance | Skull base fracture near the jugular foramen, stroke, bulbar palsy |
| XII Hypoglossal | Tongue deviates to the side of the lesion | Trauma, brainstem lesions |

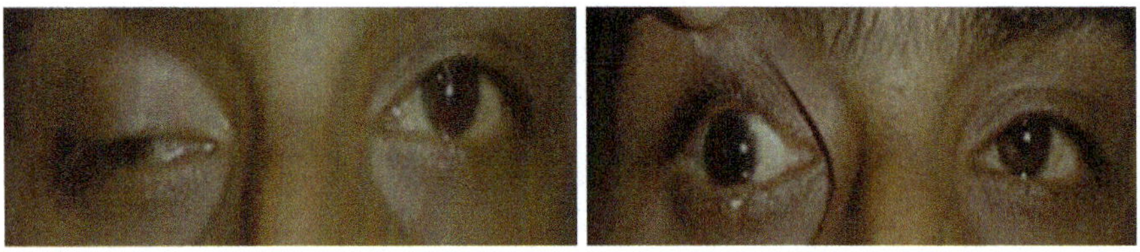

**Fig. 3.1** Third nerve palsy of the left eye resulting in ptosis, large pupil, eye down and out diplopia

**Fig. 3.2** Sixth cranial nerve palsy resulting in horizontal diplopia on looking outwards of the right eye

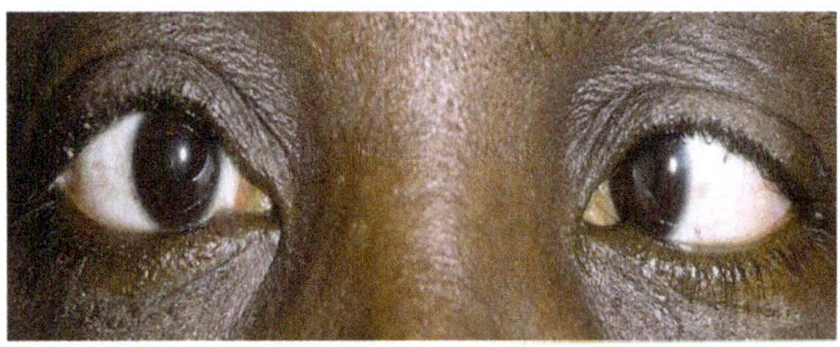

**(b) Motor system**

Check the tone of the limbs and record whether it is increased (suggesting a cerebral or pyramidal lesion), normal, or decreased (suggesting a lower motor neuron, neuromuscular junction, or muscle lesion) [4, 5]. Cogwheel and clasp-knife rigidity is typical of Parkinson's disease, while spasticity is associated with stroke and brain injury. The Medical Research Council (Medical Research Council, 1981) has developed a useful grading system for recording power on a scale from 0 to 5, where 0 indicates no movement; 1 indicates a flicker of movement; 2 indicates movement when gravity is eliminated; 3 indicates that movement can overcome gravity but not resistance; 4 indicates movement against resistance but with less strength than usual; and 5 indicates full, normal strength. The brief evaluation of motor power of upper and lower limbs is explained in Table 3.5.

**(c) Reflexes**

Reflexes are automatic responses [6]. The reflex arc goes from the stimulus via a sensory nerve to the spinal cord and then back along a motor nerve to cause muscle contraction, without brain involvement [7]. Record whether reflexes are absent, present with reinforcement, normal, or brisk (Table 3.6).

An absent or reduced reflex implies a breach in the reflex arc at any of the following locations:

- Sensory nerve or root, e.g., neuropathy, spondylosis
- Anterior horn cell, e.g., motor neurone disease, polio

**Table 3.5** Brief motor system examination

| Joint | Movement | Nerve roots | Joint | Movement | Nerve roots |
|---|---|---|---|---|---|
| Shoulder | Abduction | C5,6 | Hip | Flexion | L1-3 |
| | Adduction | C6-8 | | Extension | L4,5 and S1 |
| Elbow | Flexion | C5,6 | Knee | Flexion | L5 and S1 |
| | Extension | C7,8 | | Extension | L3,4 |
| Wrist | Flexion | C7,8 | Ankle | Dorsiflexion | L4,5 |
| | Extension | C6,7 | | Plantarflexion | S1,2 |
| Fingers | Flexion | C8 | Toes | Extensors | L5, S1 |
| | Extension | C7 | | Flexors | S2 |
| | Abduction | T1 | | | |

**Table 3.6** Reflexes—root values

| Reflex | Nerve root |
|---|---|
| Biceps | C5,6 |
| Triceps | C6,7 |
| Finger jerk/Hoffman | C8 |
| Abdominal (4 quadrants) | T7-12 |
| Knee | L3,4 |
| Ankle | S1,2 |
| Plantar | L5, S1,2 |

**Table 3.7** Upper motor neurone vs. lower motor neurone weakness

| Upper motor neuron (UMN) lesion | Lower motor neuron (LMN) lesion |
|---|---|
| Normal muscle bulk | Wasting and atrophy |
| Muscle tone—hypertonia | Muscle tone—hypotonia |
| Muscle power—reduced | Muscle power—reduced |
| Reflex— hyperreflexia | Reflex—reduced or absent |

- Motor nerve or root, e.g., neuropathy, spondylosis
- Nerve endings, e.g., myasthenia gravis
- Muscle, e.g., myopathy

An increased or brisk reflex implies lack of higher control indicating an upper motor neuron lesion, for example, after a stroke. Clonus is a rhythmic, involuntary muscle contraction due to abrupt tendon stretching (for example, by dorsiflexing the ankle). It is associated with upper motor neuron lesions (Table 3.7).

- *Sensory System*

  Any suspected sensory loss should be mapped. Test each sensory modality (light touch, pinprick, cold, vibration, and joint position sense) separately. Figure 3.3 demonstrates dermatomes and peripheral nerve distribution [5].

**(d) Coordination**

Coordination can be checked in several simple ways. Ask the patient to point to his or her nose and then to your finger held at arm's length away from the patient. Examine each arm separately and repeat several times. Rapid alternating movements, such as tapping the back of one hand with first the palm and

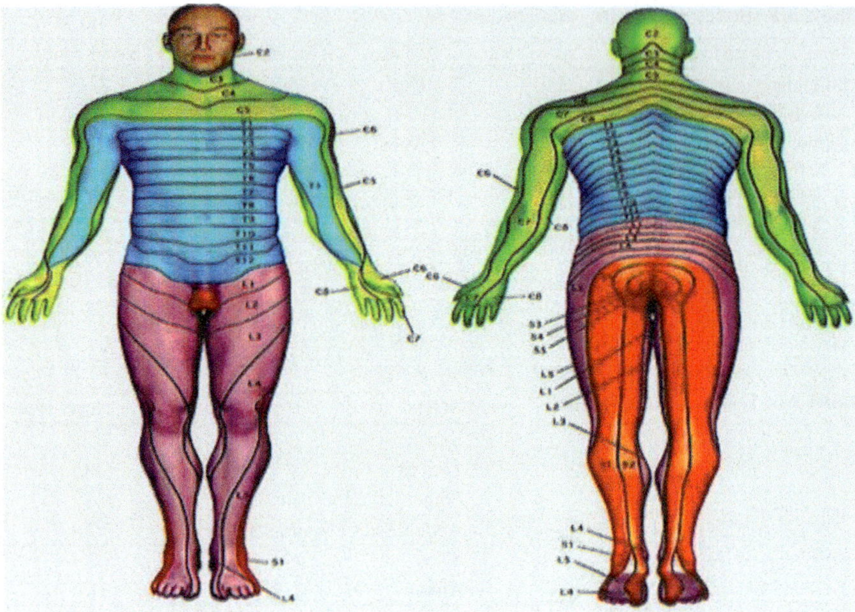

**Fig. 3.3** Dermatomal distribution of the human body and its innervation

then the back of the other hand, are also useful tests of upper limb coordination. Lower limb coordination can be checked when the patient is lying on the examination couch. Ask him or her to run the heel of one foot along the shin of the other leg. Again, examine each leg separately and repeat several times. Ataxia or lack of coordination can result from central lesions (mainly cerebellar lesions), peripheral sensory lesions or maybe a side effect of alcohol or certain drugs (for example, phenytoin or carbamazepine) [5, 6].

(e) **Cerebellar signs**
- Nystagmus—fast component towards the side of the lesion
- Intention tremor and dysmetria
- Speech—slow, slurred, explosive, scanning
- Hypotonia
- Pendular jerks—muscle contraction and relaxation is slow
- Past pointing
- Ataxia—present with eyes open or closed with a broad base gait

## 3.5 Common Neurological Emergencies and Its Clinical Presentations

1. **Acute loss of consciousness**

   Loss of consciousness is a presentation common to a variety of medical conditions and is best assessed using the GCS, as described above. Metabolic causes of acute loss of consciousness are more likely to produce symmetrical neurological deficits as compared with focal deficits seen in structural causes [5] (Table 3.8).

**Table 3.8** Causes of acute loss of consciousness

| Toxic/metabolic | Structural |
|---|---|
| 1. Electrolyte imbalance<br>Hypo/hypernatremia<br>2. Endocrine<br>Hypoglycemia<br>Diabetic ketoacidosis<br>Addison crisis<br>3. Toxins<br>Ethanol<br>Drug overdose<br>4. Organ failure<br>Uremia<br>Hypoxemia<br>Liver failure<br>5. Epilepsy | 1. Vascular<br>Bilateral cortical/subcortical infarcts<br>Bilateral carotid artery stenosis<br>Bilateral di-encephalic infarcts<br>2. Infectious<br>Abscess<br>Empyema<br>3. Trauma<br>4. Neoplastic<br>Primary<br>Secondary<br>5. Increased intracranial pressure<br>Herniation from mass effect |

**Table 3.9** Focal neurologic deficits without trauma

| Clinical condition | Specific history | Focused clinical examination |
|---|---|---|
| Acute presentation:<br>For example:<br>Intracerebral hematoma (ICH)/ischemic stroke | • Common in elderly patient<br>• H/o hypertension, ischemic heart disease, atrial fibrillation<br>• H/o use of oral anticoagulants<br>• Commonly present with headache, nausea, vomiting,<br>• Seizures<br>• Acute onset focal weakness | • Elevated blood pressure, atrial fibrillation, poor cardiac status.<br>• It may be attributed to the underlying chronic hypertension or as a result of raised intracranial pressure<br>• Excessive bruising or bleeding in the oral cavity or gastrointestinal system may indicate anticoagulant toxicity<br>• Focal neurological deficits vary in presentation depending on the location of the hematoma and include hemiparesis, gaze palsy or other cranial nerve palsies |
| Chronic presentation<br>For example: Intracranial space-occupying lesion (ICSOL) such as primary/metastatic tumors | • H/o previous or current underlying malignancies<br>• H/o unexplained weight loss, loss of appetite.<br>• Longstanding progressive headache<br>• Seizures<br>• Gradually progressive weakness | • Altered level of consciousness,<br>• Signs of raised ICP<br>• Focal neurological deficits depending on the location of the lesion.<br>• Systemic examination to screen for an occult primary tumor, e.g., breast, lung, liver, kidney |

2. Patients presenting with focal neurological deficits/ seizures without a history of trauma (Table 3.9)
3. Patients presenting with the focal neurological deficit with a history of trauma (Table 3.10)
4. Patients presenting with a history of sudden-onset severe headache (Table 3.11).
5. Meningism with fever (Table 3.12)
6. Neurological deficits with a history of previous neurosurgery (Table 3.13)

**Table 3.10** Focal neurologic deficits with trauma

| Clinical condition | Specific history | Focused clinical examination |
|---|---|---|
| Extradural hematoma (EDH) | • It is commonly caused by skull fractures with an associated blood vessel injury, following a direct blow to the head<br>• ±H/o of loss of consciousness<br>• Severe headache, vomiting<br>• Seizures<br>• Lucid interval in 20% of patients with EDH<br>• EDH can be missed if these patients present during the classic "lucid interval" between the initial trauma and neurological deterioration | • External evidence of trauma such as lacerations, bruising, palpable fractures<br>• ±CSF leak from the nose or ears suggestive of a base of skull fracture.<br>• Features of raised ICP<br>• Focal neurological deficits<br>• Signs of herniation (e.g.: Pupillary asymmetry, III and VICN palsy) |
| Subdural hematoma (SDH) | • Most common post-traumatic intracranial hematomas<br>• High-speed impact to the skull, which causes brain tissue to decelerate relative to the fixed dural structures, leading to tearing of blood vessels<br>• More severe presentation compared to EDH<br>• Commonly present with a decreased level of consciousness | |
| Chronic subdural hematoma | • Commonly seen in elderly population<br>• Typical history of minor head trauma few weeks before presentation<br>• Severe progressive headache, seizures and decreased level of consciousness | • Delayed onset of focal neurological deficits, features of raised ICP and CN palsy |

**Table 3.11** Conditions with sudden severe headache

| Clinical condition | Specific history | Focused clinical examination |
|---|---|---|
| Subarachnoid hemorrhage (SAH) | • Classical sudden-onset severe headache.<br>• "The worst headache of my life"<br>• Retro-orbital headache radiating to the neck<br>• H/o sentinel headache in the past weeks<br>• Associated with nausea, vomiting and dizziness, seizures, photophobia<br>• Can deteriorate within seconds or minutes following headache | • Decreased level of consciousness<br>• Neck stiffness<br>• Focal deficits may be due to mass effect from the aneurysm (e.g., third nerve palsy in posterior communicating artery aneurysms) or ICH |
| Pituitary apoplexy | • H/o pituitary tumor, pregnancy<br>• Acute onset headache, vomiting<br>• Acute deterioration of visual acuity or visual fields defects<br>• H/o suggestive of hypopituitarism (tiredness, weight gain, decreased libido, menstrual irregularities)<br>• Hyperpituitarism (e.g., Cushing's disease, acromegaly, or hyperthyroidism) | • Acute onset ophthalmoplegia<br>• Decreased visual acuity<br>• Visual field defects (bitemporal hemianopia)<br>• Hypotension<br>• Hypothermia |

**Table 3.12** Meningism with fever

| Clinical condition | Specific history | Focused clinical examination |
|---|---|---|
| Meningitis<br>Brain abscess<br>Subdural empyema | • H/o recent febrile illness, including dental infections, otitis media, mastoiditis or sinusitis 1–2 weeks before neurological deterioration<br>• Severe progressive headache (localized to the side of the abscess),<br>• Altered sensorium, high- or low-grade fever<br>• Seizures<br>• Nausea and vomiting | • Fever<br>• Neck stiffness<br>• Signs of raised ICP. Focal neurological deficits may be present (determined by the size and location of the infective foci)<br>• Infratentorial lesions present as cerebellar signs<br>• Supratentorial lesions can present as hemiparesis, mental status changes and speech difficulties<br>• Systemic examination—ENT, oral, cardiovascular and respiratory systems for primary foci |

**Table 3.13** Focal neurologic deficits after neurosurgery

| Clinical condition | Specific history | Focused clinical examination |
|---|---|---|
| 1. Ventriculoperitoneal shunt dysfunction<br>2. Failed endoscopic third ventriculostomy<br>3. Post-operative hydrocephalus | • History of neurosurgical intervention<br>• Progressive headache, vomiting, or drowsiness<br>• Rapid clinical deterioration | • Altered level of consciousness, papilledema<br>• Signs of raised ICP<br>• ± signs of inflammation or swelling around the scalp or abdominal incisions suggestive of shunt infection or obstruction<br>• Neck stiffness<br>• Palpate the shunt tract for possible disconnection or fractures |

## 3.6 Focused Neurological Examination of the Spinal Cord and Neuromuscular Disorders

Patients with spinal cord disorders and neuromuscular disease can present acutely to the emergency department with various neurological symptoms.

The following things need to be assessed when examining the patient with suspected spine pathology in ED:

- *Location of lesion*: It is important to differentiate whether the lesions are located in the sites like vertebral canal, spinal cord, nerve roots, neuromuscular junction, muscle. Within the spinal cord, it is crucial to locate the level of the spinal cord involvement. It helps in identifying patients who need airway management.
- Once the location of the lesion is identified along the pathway, it is essential to *confirm the diagnosis and find out the cause*. This is usually done using clinical examination, biochemical examination with supplementary radiological investigations like computed tomography (CT) scans, magnetic resonance imaging (MRI) [5, 8].

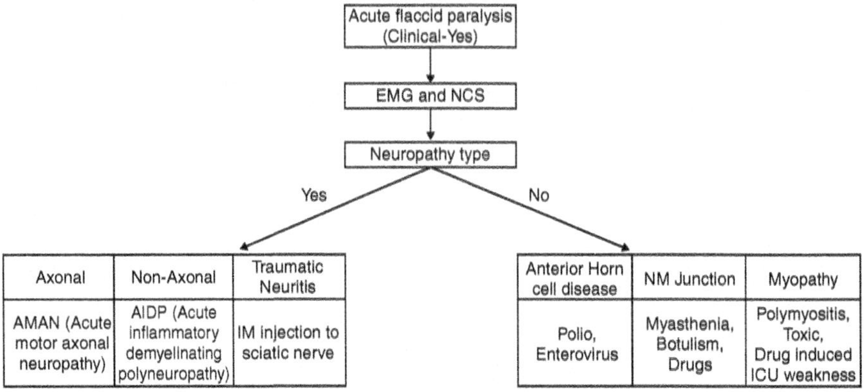


EMG - Electromyography, NCS - Nerve conduction studies, NM - Neuromuscular, ICU - Intensive care unit

**Fig. 3.4** Showing the flow chart for evaluation of Acute Flaccid Paralysis (AFP) patients

- Once the focused neurological examination is complete, the ED physician needs to identify the unstable patients, *stabilize* them, and refer the patients to appropriate centers or units for further management. The diseases involving the spinal cord can be broadly classified to examine as:
  (a) Acute flaccid paralysis,
  (b) Acute spastic paralysis,
  (c) Spinal cord trauma.

### 3.6.1 Acute Flaccid Paralysis (AFP)

AFP is a clinical syndrome characterized by the acute onset of muscle weakness starting with limb muscles with progression within days to weeks to respiratory muscles, bulbar muscles. Rapid assessment in the ED is required for prevention and diagnosis of respiratory paralysis, otherwise death can ensure [8]. The following stepwise approach can help in the rapid assessment of AFP patients (Fig. 3.4). Once the diagnosis of AFP is achieved the etiology of AFP needs to be established as described in Table 3.14.

1. Rapidly progressive limb weakness (History of: gait unsteadiness, difficulty in using limb muscles, bladder, bowel disturbances)—If Yes—neurological clinical exam.
2. Rapid neurological examination:
   (a) *History of (H/O) Breathing difficulties* If yes (Bedside evaluation of respiratory function—tachypnea, shallow breathing, Use of accessory respiratory muscles, abnormal breathing pattern, difficulty in sustained head lift).

**Table 3.14** Features of different conditions causing Acute Flaccid Paralysis. (AMAN—acute motor axonal neuropathy, AIDP—acute inflammatory demyelinating polyneuropathy, CSF—cerebrospinal fluid, NCS—nerve conduction studies, EMG—electromyography)

| Subtype | Motor | Sensory loss | CSF | Bowel and bladder | NCS | EMG |
|---|---|---|---|---|---|---|
| AMAN | Widespread weakness Bilateral facial and tongue | No Pain + | Normal | Nil | Reduced CMAP, axonal degeneration | Denervation potentials |
| AIDP | Ascending symmetric weakness, facial, bulbar | Present, pain+ | Albumino cytologic dissociation | Nil | Reduced CMAP, Demyelination | |
| Anterior horn cell disease (polio, enterovirus) | Rapid onset full paralysis, fever at onset | Nil, Pain+ | Aseptic meningitis | Nil | Reduced CMAP | Denervation |
| Traumatic neuritis | Acute asymmetric | Yes Pain + | Normal | Nil | Axonal degeneration | Denervation |
| Acute transverse myelitis | Preceding infection, lower limb symmetrical weakness | Yes Pain+ | Pleocytosis | Yes | Normal | Normal |
| Neuro-pathies (toxins, infection) | Bilateral symmetric rapidly progressive Descending (botulism), ascending type (tick infection) | ± | Normal | No | Facilitation with repetitive stimuli | Normal or denervation |
| Myasthenia gravis | Ocular, bulbar, Multifocal weakness | No | Normal | No | Decrement on repetitive stimuli | Normal |
| Myositis (viral, polio) | Asymmetric proximal > distal, fever at onset | No | Normal | No | Normal | Myopathic |

*If yes*—pulse oximetry, arterial blood gas analysis, bedside tests for vital capacity like single breath count, maximum voluntary ventilation (MVV), cough test. If positive for respiratory muscle involvement proceed for oxygenation/ ventilation management, stabilize the patient.
*If no*—no further evaluation.

(b) *H/O swallowing difficulties (alone or with respiratory difficulties),*
*If Yes*—evaluation of protective airway reflexes, rule out pulmonary aspiration—care for airway protection. Watch for respiratory involvement.
*If no*—no further neurological testing.

(c) *Spasticity present (hypertonia, hyperreflexia, clonus) AFP ruled out: Proceed for further evaluation.*

(d) Presence of weakness, atonia, hyporeflexia, absent clonus, fasciculations, atonic bladder, neurogenic bladder, bowel involvement, autonomic dysfunction, sensory involvement (loss of sensation, paresthesia, pain).
*If yes*—flaccid paralysis, *If no*—AFP ruled out.

(e) If Yes—identify the site of lesion, cause of AFP (Table 3.4).

### 3.6.2 Acute Spastic Paralysis (Related to Spinal Cord)

In contrast to AFP, patients can present with spastic paralysis which can be due to intracranial (cerebral hemisphere or brainstem lesions), cervicomedullary, or at spinal (extramedullary or intramedullary) regions. The patients usually will have muscle weakness of upper motor neuron type, increased DTR, clonus [8, 9]. Associated sensory, bladder, and autonomic dysfunction can coexist depending on the type and location of the lesion. History may help to identify the level of the lesion as well as to proceed for further investigations to confirm the diagnosis, identify the etiology and for treatment plans, as illustrated in Table 3.15 [10, 12, 13].

### 3.6.3 Spinal Cord Injury (SCI)

Spinal cord injury is one of the common conditions encountered by the ED physician. SCI can occur in automobile accidents, falls, hanging, vascular events. ED physicians can encounter patients with SCI alone or a part of polytrauma. The caregivers need to recognize the injury based on clinical and radiological features, stabilize, and prevent further secondary damage [10, 11]. It is also important to distinguish between hemodynamic and respiratory stability and neurological stability. Knowledge of a rapid and focused approach for examination of suspected spinal cord injured is highly desirable for the caregivers to help in the management of these patients especially in victims of mass casualties. This topic will be discussed in detail in the chapter on SCI.

**Table 3.15** The salient clinical features of patients presenting with acute spastic paralysis

| Level | History | Motor | Pain | Sensory | Bowel and bladder |
|---|---|---|---|---|---|
| Intracranial (vascular, tumor, trauma, degenerative, demyelinating) | Acute to subacute onset, H/O loss of consciousness, headache, seizures, features of raised ICP, papilledema | Mostly unilateral, upper motor type, associated cranial nerve involvement | Absent | ± (depends on somatosensory area involvement) usually unilateral | Rarely involved |
| Cervicomedullary | More common in children<br>Can be intramedullary (gliomas, AVMs, vascular) or extramedullary (AAD, basilar invagination, Arachnoid cysts, Chiari malformation, trauma) | Usually UMN type quadriparesis/quadriplegia, (Elsberg phenomenon) (symmetrical or asymmetrical UL weakness > LL) lower cranial nerve involvement, altered breathing, diaphragm weakness, cerebellar signs<br>Horizontal nystagmus | Radiation to occiput ± back of neck | Paraesthesia, loss of sensations (UL > LL), loss of pain and temperature with preserved sensations (IM lesions) or loss of sensation in EM lesions<br>C1 lesion-hypoaesthesia at occiput | Incontinence of bowel and bladder |
| Spinal cord (extramedullary) | Acute to subacute to chronic | Similar to above without cerebellar/cranial nerve involvement. Above C4- weakness and wasting of sub occipital region, diaphragm weakness | Present can be radicular or vertebral | Dermatomal loss at the level of lesion. Loss of proprioception, touch. Pain and temperature may be preserved. Sacral involved early | Usually late involvement |
| Spinal cord (intramedullary) | | LMN type weakness | Nonspecific diffuse pain, absent radicular pain | Dissociative sensory loss, sacral sparing | Early involvement |

## 3.7 Summary

The focused neurological examination helps in rapid assessment, triage of patients with polytrauma as well as acute neurological conditions since time is crucial for both brain and spinal cord. However, the limitation is adequate training of personnel involved in the care of such patients. A high index of suspicion, detailed history, and focused neurological assessment of these patients will ensure rapid diagnosis and prompt referral to a neurosurgeon/physician.

## Multiple Choice Questions

1. A 60-year-old right-handed man has presented with gradually progressive hearing loss of the right ear. No h/o worsening balance or ringing in his ears and not associated with pain. A vibrating tuning fork is applied to the center of his forehead. The sound is louder in his left ear. This finding suggests which of the following?
   (a) Bilateral sensorineural hearing loss
   (b) Bilateral conductive hearing loss
   (c) Right ear conductive hearing loss
   (d) Left ear sensorineural hearing loss
   (e) Right ear sensorineural hearing loss
2. A 51-year-old woman is being evaluated for gait difficulties. On examination, it is found that her ability to walk along a straight line touching the heel of one foot to the toe of the other is impaired. This finding is most common with which of the following?
   (a) Cerebellar dysfunction
   (b) Parietal lobe damage
   (c) Temporal lobe damage
   (d) Ocular motor disturbances
   (e) Dysesthesias in the feet
3. A 32-year-old biker lower back pain radiating down the posterior aspect of his left leg and paresthesias in the lateral aspect of his left foot for the past 6 months. Motor power, bowel and bladder function is normal. Examination would be most likely to show which of the following?
   (a) Left Babinski sign
   (b) Loss of pinprick sensation over the web space between the first and second digits of the left foot
   (c) Hyperreflexia at the left knee jerk
   (d) Hyporeflexia in the left Achilles tendon reflex
   (e) Decreased rectal tone

4. A 22-year-old man sustained multiple injuries in an automobile accident. After orthopedic surgery, he is not awakening. If his brainstem function is intact, when he is lying supine with his head slightly elevated (30°) and one external auditory meatus is irrigated with warm water, which of the following would be expected?
   (a) Tonic deviation of the eyes toward the ear that is stimulated
   (b) Nystagmus in both eyes toward the ear that is stimulated
   (c) Tonic deviation of the ipsilateral eye toward the ear that is stimulated
   (d) Nystagmus in both eyes away from the ear that is stimulated
   (e) Tonic deviation of both eyes away from the ear that is stimulated
5. Following cardiac catheterization, a 60-year-old right-handed man acutely develops a loss of sensation involving the entire left side of his body (face, arm, and leg). Which of the following structures has most likely been damaged?
   (a) Internal capsule
   (b) Thalamus
   (c) Hippocampus
   (d) Globus pallidus
   (e) Pons
6. A 65-year-old diabetic man with h/o cerebellar stroke 5 years back says that he has now fully recovered. His medical records state that he presented with left-sided dysdiadochokinesia. Which of the following was most likely impaired?
   (a) Successive finger movements
   (b) Heel-to-toe walking
   (c) Rapid alternating movements
   (d) Tremor suppression
   (e) Conjugate eye movements
7. A 33-year-old woman has an acute onset of headache with blurring of vision. On examination, she has a right ptosis and anisocoria. This could be due to the insult to which of the following structures?
   (a) Optic tract
   (b) Optic chiasm
   (c) CN III
   (d) T1 nerve root
   (e) Superior cervical ganglion
8. A 35-year-old woman is being examined and the clinician notices the presence of fine twitching movements beneath the surface of the tongue and wasting of one side of the tongue. This finding suggests which of the following?
   (a) Pseudobulbar affect
   (b) Aberrant reinnervation of muscles from CN X
   (c) Denervation of muscles from CN X
   (d) Denervation of muscles from CN XII

9. An 85-year-old man is being evaluated for gait difficulties. He says that he frequently trips walking upstairs or on uneven surfaces. On examination, it is found that joint proprioception is absent in his toes. People with impaired position sense will usually fall if they simultaneously stand with their feet together and do which of the following?
   (a) Flex the neck
   (b) Extend their arms in front of them
   (c) Flex the knees
   (d) Turn the head
   (e) Close their eyes
10. A 60-year-old woman with diabetes awakens with weakness of the right side. On examination upper motor neuron pattern of weakness involving the face, arm, and leg of right side with no sensory abnormalities and language is preserved. A stroke associated with this presentation is most likely with damage to which of the following?
   (a) Internal capsule
   (b) Cerebellum
   (c) Putamen
   (d) Caudate
   (e) Amygdala

Answers: 1. (e), 2. (a), 3. (d), 4. (b), 5. (b), 6. (c), 7. (c), 8. (d), 9. (e), 10. (a).

## References


1. Caplan LC, Hollander J. The effective clinical neurologist. 3rd ed. Shelton: People's Medical Publishing House; 2010.
2. DeGowin RL, Brown DD. DeGowin's diagnostic examination. 9th ed. New York: McGraw-Hill; 2009.
3. Campbell WW, Pridgeon RP. Practical primer of clinical neurology. Philadelphia: Lippincott Williams & Wilkins; 2002.
4. Ross RT. How to examine the nervous system. 3rd ed. Stamford: Appleton & Lange; 1999.
5. Carpenter MB. Core text of neuroanatomy. 4th ed. Baltimore: Williams & Wilkins; 1991. p. 115–223.
6. Gilman S, Winans S. Manter and Gatz's essentials of clinical neuroanatomy and neurophysiology. 10th ed. Philadelphia: F. A. Davis Publishers; 2003. p. 77–118.
7. Wartenberg R. The examination of reflexes: a simplification. Chicago: Year Book Medical Pub; 1945.
8. Marx A, Glass JD, Sutter RW. Differential diagnosis of acute flaccid paralysis and its role in poliomyelitis surveillance. Epidemiol Rev. 2000;22:298–316.
9. Zhovtis Ryerson L, Herbert J, Howard J, Kister I. Adult-onset spastic paraparesis: an approach to diagnostic work-up. J Neurol Sci. 2014;346:43–50.
10. Hachem LD, Ahuja CS, Fehlings MG. Assessment and management of acute spinal cord injury: from point of injury to rehabilitation. J Spinal Cord Med. 2017;40:665–75.

11. Utz M, Khan S, O'Connor D, Meyers S. MDCT and MRI evaluation of cervical spine trauma. Insights Imaging. 2014;5:67–75.
12. Swartz MH. Textbook of physical diagnosis: history and examination. 6th ed. Philadelphia: W. B. Saunders; 2010.
13. Plackett TP, Wright F, Baldea AJ, Mosier MJ, Thomas C, Luchette FA, Ton-That HH, Esposito TJ. Cervical spine clearance when unable to be cleared clinically: a pooled analysis of combined computed tomography and magnetic resonance imaging. Am J Surg. 2016;211:115–21.

# Neuropharmacology

**4**

Swagata Tripathy and Suma Rabab Ahmad

**Key Points**

- Status epilepticus requires prompt management in order to reduce irreversible neurological damage. The drugs commonly used are benzodiazepines, barbiturates, phenytoin, valproic acid, levetiracetam, and propofol.
- Sedatives allay agitation and anxiety and facilitate mechanical ventilation. These include benzodiazepines, propofol, and dexmedetomidine. Opioids are essentially analgesics.
- Neuromuscular blockers are used to facilitate tracheal intubation, provide immobility during surgery, and to prevent refractory shivering during targeted temperature management. They are broadly categorized into depolarizing and non-depolarizing agents.
- Acetylcholinesterase inhibitors like neostigmine and pyridostigmine are used for the treatment of myasthenia gravis.
- Intravenous antihypertensives include beta blockers. Vasodilators are not preferred in traumatic brain injury.
- Thrombolytic agents used for revascularization in acute ischemic stroke may be fibrin specific (alteplase, reteplase) or non-specific (streptokinase).
- Antithrombotic medications include antiplatelets and anticoagulants. These are used at various junctures of management as well as prevention of acute ischemic stroke.

S. Tripathy (✉) · S. R. Ahmad
All India Institute of Medical Sciences, Bhubaneshwar, India


P. U. Bidkar, P. Vanamoorthy (eds.), *Acute Neuro Care*,
https://doi.org/10.1007/978-981-15-4071-4_4

- Intracranial hemorrhage concomitant to antithrombotic agents requires urgent reversal with specific antidotes as well as prothrombin complex concentrate in some cases.
- Nimodipine is a calcium channel blocker used in the management of vasospasm associated with subarachnoid hemorrhage. Milrinone and dobutamine are inotropes used to maintain optimum blood pressure in these patients.
- Hypertonic saline and mannitol are used for reducing intracranial pressure. It is still not established which one is better.

## 4.1 Introduction

Neuro-critical care involves the use of various drugs. Knowledge of these drugs in terms of dose, adverse effects, and use in special populations is essential for good patient care. Medications must be used appropriately during neuro-emergencies and neurological life support. The right choice of medication depends upon the knowledge of the pharmacodynamics and pharmacokinetics of the drug. Medications discussed here include antiepileptic drugs, sedatives, analgesics, neuromuscular blocking drugs, antihypertensive agents, thrombolytic agents, antiplatelets, oral anticoagulants, and hemostatic agents. Drugs used in subarachnoid hemorrhage, for reducing intracranial pressure, managing hyponatremia and myasthenia gravis are also briefly mentioned. Patients presenting with neuro-emergencies are either already consuming these drugs and having certain adverse drug reactions or the physician will have to use these for curtailing the acute episode. The chapter covers salient pearls for using these medications by first responders in the emergency department and neuro-critical care unit.

## 4.2 Antiepileptic Drugs

Status epilepticus (SE) either convulsive or nonconvulsive requires prompt management to reduce the mortality and morbidity associated with it. Continuous electrophysiological monitoring is essential to titrate the drug doses and knowing the treatment endpoints. The antiepileptic drugs (AED) are used at three levels of management [1]. First line AEDs abort seizure activity. These benzodiazepines are GABAa receptor agonists (Table 4.1). Sedation and respiratory depression are dose-dependant adverse effects. Hepatic impairment warrants caution. Second line AEDs prevent seizure recurrence (Tables 4.2 and 4.3). If seizure persists, Third line AEDs are initiated to achieve burst suppression in electroencephalogram (Table 4.4). These cause hypotension and respiratory depression and might require the use of mechanical ventilation and vasopressors. Newer AEDs are increasingly being used as they have a better safety profile and lesser pharmacokinetic interaction profile as compared to the traditional drugs [2–4].

**Table 4.1** First line antiepileptic drugs

| Drug | Lorazepam | Diazepam | Midazolam |
|---|---|---|---|
| Dose | 0.1 mg/kg IV<br>Max. 4 mg/dose<br>Can repeat once in 5 min<br>Rate: 2 mg/min | 0.15–0.2 mg/kg IV/IM<br>Max. 10 mg/dose<br>Can repeat once in 5 min<br>Children: 0.1–1.0 mg/kg<br>Per rectal: 0.2–0.5 mg/kg<br>Rate: 5 mg/min | 0.1–0.2 mg/kg IM once (Maximum IM dose 10 mg for >40 kg, 5 mg for 13–40 kg)<br>RSE: 0.2 mg/kg IV bolus then 0.05–2 mg/kg/h |
| Salient features | BZD of choice for SE<br>Longer onset (2 min): less lipid soluble<br>Longer-acting (>12 h) than diazepam<br>Contains propylene glycol: hypotension and metabolic acidosis with overdosage/ prolonged use | Rapid onset (30 s): high lipid solubility<br>Clinical effectiveness: for 20 min (rapid redistribution-decrease of brain concentrations)<br>Seizure recurrence is high. Second drug is required.<br>100% Oral BA<br>Contains propylene glycol | Buccal, IM, intranasal, sublingual<br>Sudden discontinuation: may lead to withdrawal seizures.<br>Drug tolerance is seen. |

*BZD* Benzodiazepine, *BA* Bioavailability, *RSE* Refractory Status Epilepticus

**Table 4.2** Second line conventional antiepileptic drugs

| Drug | Phenytoin | Valproate sodium | Phenobarbital |
|---|---|---|---|
| Mechanism | Sodium efflux from neurons | Blocks Na channels<br>Increases brain GABA conc.<br>Acts against calcium currents | Barbiturate:<br>Enhances the inhibitory effect of GABAa receptor |
| Dose | Load: 18–20 mg/kg IV<br>Maintenance: 4–6 mg/kg/ day divided in 2–3 doses | Load: 40 mg/kg IV<br>Max: 3000 mg/dose<br>Maintenance: 10–15 mg/kg/day divided into 2–4 doses | 20 mg/kg, additional 10 mg/kg after 10 min<br>Maintenance: 1–5 mg/ kg/h |
| Rate and target serum conc. | 1–3 mg/kg/min or 50 mg/ min—Whichever is slower<br>*Serum conc*: 10–20 μg/mL (normal renal function)<br>Free drug: 1–2 μg/mL<br>In hypoalbuminemia or with highly protein-bound drugs<br>Accurate estimate: 1 h after infusion completes | Up to 6 mg/kg per min<br>*Target conc*: 50–150 μg/mL | 50–100 mg/min<br>*Target conc*: 15–40 μg/mL |

(continued)

**Table 4.2** (continued)

| Drug | Phenytoin | Valproate sodium | Phenobarbital |
|---|---|---|---|
| Adverse effects | Cardiovascular: arrhythmias, hypotension, bradycardia (SA block, AV block)<br>Local: purple glove syndrome, SJS and TEN, DRESS<br>Neurotoxic: Nystagmus (10–20 μg/mL), ataxia, neuropathy, seizures (>50 μg/mL) | Hepatotoxicity<br>Thrombocytopenia<br>Hyperammonemic Encephalopathy (caution: urea cycle disorders)<br>Pancreatitis, insulin resistance | Sedation<br>Respiratory depression<br>Hypotension |
| Salient features | IV: careful cardiac monitoring<br>Propyleneglycol: hypotension<br>Lipid soluble<br>Compatible with saline solutions only.<br>Crystal precipitation in dextrose solutions<br>Clearance decreases with increasing age<br>Highly protein bound<br>STRONG CYP inducer: many potential drug interactions | Less CV side-effects than phenytoin<br>Tightly protein bound<br>CYP enzyme inhibitor: many potential drug interactions<br>Meropenem not to be used with VPA: will reduce VPA levels significantly<br>Avoid in liver derangement | Long acting<br>Requires hemodynamic monitoring<br>Contains propyleneglycol<br>STRONG CYP enzyme inducer: many potential drug interactions |

*Conc.* concentration, *SJS* Steven–Johnson syndrome, *TEN* toxic epidermal necrosis, *DRESS* drug reaction with eosinophilia and systemic symptoms, *SA* sinoatrial, *AV* atrioventricular, *Na* Sodium, *CYP* cytochrome P-450 enzyme system, *GABA* gammaaminobutyric acid, *CV* Cardiovascular, *VPA* valproic acid

**Table 4.3** Second line newer antiepileptic Drugs

| Drug | Fosphenytoin | Levitiracetam | Lacosamide |
|---|---|---|---|
| Mechanism | Prodrug—7–15 min after infusion converts to phenytoin | Exact mech. unknown<br>1. Inhibits burst firing: binds to synaptic vesicular protein 2A—inhibits presynaptic calcium channels and neurotransmitter release [4]<br>2. Indirectly modulates GABA | Inactivation of sodium channels |
| Dose | Load: 20 mg PE/kg<br>Max: 1500 mg PE/dose<br>Maintenance: 4–6 mg/kg/day divided into 2–3 doses | Load: 20–60 mg/kg IV,<br>Max: 4500 mg/dose<br>Maintenance: 1–4 g/day in 2–3<br>divided doses | 200–400 mg IV every 12 h |

**Table 4.3** (continued)

| Drug | Fosphenytoin | Levitiracetam | Lacosamide |
|---|---|---|---|
| Rate and target serum conc. | Up to 150 mg PE/min<br>*Serum conc*: total phenytoin: 10–20 μg/mL<br>Free phenytoin: 1–2 μg/mL<br>Accurate estimate: 1 h after infusion completes | 5 mg/kg/min<br>*Target conc*: 12–46 μg/mL (not typically monitored) | Over 15 min<br>*Target conc*: 2.8–18 μg/mL (not typically monitored) |
| Adverse effects | Paresthesia<br>Hypotension<br>Bradycardia | Neuro psychiatric: Dizziness, behavior disturbances (irritability, agitation, aggression)<br>Anemia | Dizziness, Ataxia<br>PR prolongation, hypotension (rare)<br>Caution: AV block, sick sinus syndrome |
| Salient features | Highly water soluble<br>Easier to administer: less venous irritation than phenytoin<br>Can be given IM<br>Same drug interactions and monitoring parameters | Dose reduction in renal impairment with<br>CrCl < 50 mL/min/1.73 m$^2$<br>CrCl < 30 mL/min/1.73 m$^2$: 250–500 mg PO BID<br>Few drug interactions<br>Safe in liver impairment | Monitor ECG in cardiac diseases<br>Orally: 100% BA<br>Dose reduction in renal impairment<br>Few drug interactions<br>Useful safe adjunct in SE, but further clinical trials required for its efficacy |

*CrCl* creatinine clearance, *PE* phenytoin equivalent

**Table 4.4** Third line antiepileptic drugs

| Drug | Dose | Salient features |
|---|---|---|
| *Propofol*:<br>Decreases the rate of dissociation of GABA from its receptors | Bolus: 1–2 mg/kg IV followed by 2–10 mg/kg/h<br>RSE: 30–250 μg/kg/min | PRIS (severe metabolic acidosis, rhabdomyolysis, cardiovascular collapse) |
| *Thiopentone*:<br>Barbiturate<br>Enhances the inhibitory effect of GABAa receptor | Bolus: 3–5 mg/kg followed by infusion of 3–5 mg/kg/h | Prolonged sedation due to long elimination half-life (up to 26 h), paralytic ileus<br>Increased infection risk<br>Caution: porphyria, liver disease |
| *Ketamine*:<br>NMDA receptor antagonist | RSE: 0.5–4.5 mg/kg IV bolus, then infusion 2.75–10 mg/kg/h (adults) and 10–60 μg/kg/min (children)<br>Oral in NCSE: 1500–2000 mg/d (adults) and 1.5 mg/kg/d in two divided doses (children) | Psychiatric symptoms (more in >16 years of age): can be reduced by 3.75–7.5 mg of midazolam given prophylactically<br>Increased salivation, hypertension, arrhythmias, pheochromocytoma, mental illness, glaucoma<br>Intracranial hypertension is now refuted [2]<br>Neuronal cell necrosis (Olney's Lesions): very high doses in rats (i.e., 40–60 mg/kg, s.c. doses [3] (controversial) |

*PRIS* propofol-related infusion syndrome, *NCSE* nonconvulsive status epilepticus

## 4.3 Sedatives and Analgesics

Sedation is required for allaying agitation and anxiety, facilitation of mechanical ventilation, and suppression of shivering. An ideal agent for neurointensive care sedation should have rapid onset and recovery for prompt neurologic evaluation, cause cerebral vasoconstriction reducing intracranial pressure, maintaining coupling of reduced cerebral blood flow and reduced cerebral metabolic rate of oxygen, seizure suppression, and preserve carbon dioxide reactivity and cerebral autoregulation [5]. Effective analgesia improves patient comfort and diminishes stress response [6]. The various sedatives and analgesics used are described in Table 4.5 [7]. Volatile agents (Isoflurane, Sevoflurane) have become available for use in patients with preserved cerebral blood flow autoregulation through anesthesia conserving device, AnaConDa (sedana Medical AB, Sweden) [8].

**Table 4.5** Sedatives and analgesics

| Drug | Dose | Advantages | Disadvantages |
|---|---|---|---|
| Propofol<br>GABA agonist | 5–200 μg/kg/min | Rapid onset<br>Short duration of action<br>Minimally affected by renal failure | PRIS: higher risk in young people, with >50 μg/kg/min dose for >48 h<br>Hypotension, apnea, pain at injection site<br>Susceptible to bacterial contamination, IV tubing and syringe to be changed 12 hourly<br>Caution: cardiovascular disease, liver dysfunction<br>Contraindications: allergy to egg/soy<br>No amnesia, especially at low doses |
| Dexmedetomidine<br>$A_2$ receptor agonist | Loading: 1 μg/kg<br>Maintenance: 0.2–0.7 μg/kg/h | Fast onset and titration<br>Analgesic and anxiolytic. Patient is arousable for neurological evaluation during infusion<br>Mechanical ventilation not required | Hypotension<br>Bradycardia<br>Caution: cardiovascular disease, severe hepatic dysfunction, hypovolemia |
| Lorazepam<br>GABA agonist | Loading: 0.02–0.04 mg/kg<br>Max IV 2 mg for agitation (rate@ 2 mg/min)<br>Maintenance: 0.01–0.1 mg/kg/h | Anterograde amnesia | Confusion, visual disturbances, dependency, aggressive behavior<br>Infusion not recommended: long context-sensitive half-life, precipitation with obstruction of infusion lines<br>Contraindications: acute narrow-angle glaucoma<br>Caution: deranged liver failure |

**Table 4.5** (continued)

| Drug | Dose | Advantages | Disadvantages |
|---|---|---|---|
| Midazolam<br>GABA agonist | Loading:<br>0.02–0.08 mg/kg<br>Maintenance:<br>0.04–0.3 mg/kg/h | Amnesia<br>Cost-effective | Delirium<br>Tolerance<br>Caution: deranged liver function |
| Morphine<br>μ receptor agonist | Bolus: 2–10 mg IV<br>Intermittent dose: 2–8 mg every 3–4 h<br>Maintenance:<br>0.8–30 mg/h | Analgesic | Itching (histamine release), nausea, vomiting, respiratory depression, hypotension, constipation, urinary retention, dizziness, myoclonus, dependency, miosis<br>May elevate ICP and CBF<br>Caution: renal and liver dysfunction (reduced dose is recommended), asthma |
| Fentanyl<br>μ receptor agonist | Bolus dose:<br>25–125 μg<br>Continuous infusion:<br>10–100 μg/h | More potent<br>Analgesic<br>Acts quickly<br>No direct effect on ICP<br>Liver dysfunction: can be used | Nausea, vomiting, miosis<br>Long context-sensitive half life<br>Respiratory depression, hypotension: not very significant: seen more in hypovolemia, heart failure or with BZD |

*PRIS* propofol-related infusion syndrome, *CBF* cerebral blood flow, *BZD* Benzodiazepine

## 4.4 Neuromuscular Blocking Drugs

Neuromuscular blocking drugs (NMBDs) are used for skeletal muscle relaxation to facilitate tracheal intubation, to prevent coughing reflex in raised intracranial pressure (ICP), for immobility during surgery or for controlling refractory shivering during targeted temperature management.

Myasthenics are less susceptible to depolarizing NMBD (succinylcholine) than to non-depolarizing NMBDs because of fewer functional nicotinic receptors [9]. The efficacy of NMBDs decreases in presence of pyridostigmine and chronic steroid therapy. In Table 4.6 commonly used NMBDs are compared. Hypersensitivity reactions with even life-threatening anaphylaxis and prolonged respiratory depression are the adverse drug effects of non-depolarizing NMBDs. Drug interactions with fluoroquinolones, aminoglycosides, clindamycin, polymyxins, procainamide, and quinidine lead to prolonged muscular weakness.

## 4.5 Intravenous Antihypertensive Agents

These agents are required to decrease blood pressure in stroke and hypertensive patients with traumatic brain injury (TBI). These are also used to decrease the pressor response to tracheal intubation. Comparison of commonly used intravenous

**Table 4.6** Comparison of neuromuscular blocking agents

| Muscle relaxant | Dose | Onset | Duration | Salient features |
|---|---|---|---|---|
| Succinylcholine (depolarizing muscle relaxant) | Adults: IV 0.5–1.5 mg/kg IM 3–4 mg/kg Adolescents: 1 mg/kg Pediatrics: 2 mg/kg | Very rapid IV 30–60 s IM 240 s | Short: 3–5 min Max: 7–10 min | Myalgias Slight increases in ICP (inconclusive data) Bradycardia in children Severe hyperkalemia: with burns, trauma Prolonged effect: with inhibition of plasma cholinesterase Contraindicated: malignant hyperthermia |
| Rocuronium NDMR | IV adults: 0.6 mg/kg (up to 1.2 mg/kg) Pediatrics: 0.45–0.6 mg/kg | Rapid 60–120 s Faster onset with higher dose | Intermediate 20–35 min (up to 60 min) | Refrigeration for storage Anaphylactic reaction |
| Vecuronium NDMR | IV adults and pediatrics 0.1 mg/kg (up to 0.2 mg/kg) Maintenance: 0.01–0.015 mg/kg q20–45 min PRN | Prolonged 180–500 s Faster onset with higher dose (120 s) | Intermediate 20–35 min (up to 60 min) | No significant cardiovascular effects No effect on ICP |
| Atracurium NDMR | 0.4–0.5 mg/kg then 0.08–0.1 mg/kg Maintenance: q25–45 min PRN | Fast 120–180 s | Intermediate 20–35 min | Elimination via enzymatic breakdown-independent of renal or hepatic route Histamine release-bronchospasm, hypotension, tachycardia Laudanosine seizures(rare) |
| Cisatracurium NDMR | IV adults: 0.15 mg/kg (up to 0.2 mg/kg) IV Pediatrics: 0.1 mg/kg IV Infusion: 1–2 μg/kg/min (0.5–10 μg/kg/min reported) | Fast 90–120 s | Prolonged Adults 45–75 min Pediatrics 20–35 min | No histamine release Safely used as a continuous infusion Elimination via enzymatic breakdown |

*Sch* succinylcholine, *ICP* intracranial pressure, *NDMR* non-depolarizing muscle relaxant, *IM* intramuscular, *IV* intravenous

**Table 4.7** Comparison of Intravenous antihypertensive agents

| | Onset (min) | Duration | Half-life | Dosing | Salient features |
|---|---|---|---|---|---|
| Labetalol Nonselective $\beta$ and $\alpha_1$ blockade | 2–5 | 2–4 h | 4–8 h | 20 mg over 2 min. Then 40–80 mg at 10 min intervals until desired BP (maximum dose 300 mg) IV infusion 0.5–2 mg/min | Caution: rapid IV titration prolonged hypotension (dose stacking) Continuous infusion: difficult to titrate due to long half-life. Used only in refractory hypotension Adverse effects: postural hypotension bronchospasm |
| Esmolol Selective $\beta_1$ blocker | 1–2 | 10–30 min | 9 min | 150–400 μg/kg/min | Adverse effects: headache, flushing |

antihypertensives by neurointensivists are given in Table 4.7 [10]. These are contra-indicated in heart block, cardiogenic shock, bradycardia, and decompensated heart failure. Other first-line agents include IV nicardipine or IV clevidipine and if not adequately controlled IV hydralazine and enalapril may be considered [10, 11].

Vasodilators are not preferred in TBI or hemorrhagic stroke as they cause an increase in cerebral vascular volume and intracranial hypertension [11]. They may at times be used in stroke for control of resistant hypertension. However, nitroglycerine is safe in stroke [12]. Sodium nitroprusside has several demerits including unpredictable dose-response and cyanide toxicity [11, 13].

## 4.6 Acetylcholinesterase Inhibitors in Myasthenia Gravis

Acetylcholinesterase inhibitors (AChEIs) are used for the treatment of myasthenia gravis (MG) (neostigmine, pyridostigmine) or in Alzheimer's disease (donepezil, rivastigmine, and galantamine). The breakdown of acetylcholine at the neuromuscular junction (NMJ) is done by acetylcholinesterase. Thereby these drugs increase the concentration of acetylcholine to compete with the acetylcholine receptors antibodies and produce a muscle action potential in MG. MuSK-Ab (antibody) positive MG patients may not respond to AChEIs [14].

Their use is contraindicated in mechanical intestinal or urinary obstruction and should be used with caution in bronchial asthma and with beta-adrenergic receptor blocker (Table 4.8).

**Table 4.8** Comparison of acetylcholinesterase inhibitors used in myasthenia gravis

| Acetylcholinesterase inhibitors | Dose | Pharmacokinetics | Salient features |
|---|---|---|---|
| Neostigmine | IV/IM/SC<br>0.5–2.5 mg every 4–6 h<br>(Total daily dose: 5–20 mg)<br>Oral:<br>15–375 mg/day | Onset:<br>1–20 min (IV)<br>20–30 min (IM)<br>Duration:<br>1–2 h (IV)<br>2.5–4 h (IM) | First-line agent<br>Side-effects<br>Muscarinic effects:<br>Gastrointestinal: diarrhea, nausea, vomiting (30%): commonest (12)<br>Hypersalivation (6%), increased perspiration (4%), urgency (3%), increased bronchial secretion (2%), rash (1%) and miosis (1%)<br>Bradycardia<br>Nicotinic effects (4%): muscle cramps, weakness, fasciculations<br>Hence used along with anticholinergics |
| Pyridostigmine | Oral: 30–90 mg every 4–6 h<br>Sustained release:<br>180–540 mg PO per day or q12 h<br>Max dose: 1.5 g/day<br>Interval between doses: 3–6 h | Oral:<br>BA: 10–20%.<br>Slow onset: Tmax: 2.2 ± 1 h (after 30 mg oral tablet):<br>Hydrolysis: cholinesterases<br>metabolized: Liver<br>Elimination T1/2: 3 h | Not first line due to slow onset<br>CNS manifestations less frequent (does not cross BBB)<br>Extremely high doses: CNS symptoms (confusion, agitation) |

*CNS* central nervous system, *BBB* blood–brain barrier

Overdosage of pyridostigmine can lead to a cholinergic crisis, which must be differentiated, from myasthenic crisis. Overdosage might lead to increasing muscle weakness, respiratory failure, and death. It is treated by giving atropine 1–4 mg IV which can be repeated every 30 min as needed. However, the nicotinic side-effects like skeletal muscle weakness including the respiratory muscles are not reversed by atropine.

For clinical approximation, 15 mg neostigmine orally is equivalent to 500 micrograms neostigmine IV and 1.0–1.5 mg neostigmine IM or SC. Oral pyridostigmine 60 mg is equivalent to 500 μg neostigmine IV and 1–1.5 mg neostigmine IM/SC approximately [15].

## 4.7 Drugs Used in Stroke

Patients presenting with stroke or transient ischemic attack may be on anticoagulants, antiplatelets, antihypertensives, or statins for primary stroke prevention. Majority of the strokes are ischemic in nature: immediate use of thrombolytic agents maybe needed. For secondary prevention of stroke antiplatelets and anticoagulants are used. Both belong to the antithrombotic class of drugs.

### 4.7.1 Drugs Used in Revascularization for Acute Ischemic Stroke

Thrombolytic agents are the intravenous drugs used for revascularization in acute ischemic stroke (AIS). They are of two types: fibrin specific (alteplase, reteplase, and tenecteplase) or non-fibrin specific (streptokinase) drugs (Table 4.9). Fibrin specific drugs facilitate the conversion of plasminogen to plasmin and dissolve the clot by binding to the fibrin surface. Alteplase (tPA), a second-generation thrombolytic is the only Food and Drug Administration (FDA) approved thrombolytic agent for AIS within 3 h or within 3–4.5 h for eligible patients from the time of symptom onset [16]. Tenecteplase might be considered in patients without any major intracranial vessel occlusion [17].

The use of reteplase in clinical practice for AIS is not recommended. It has been used in clinical trials. Streptokinase, having a biphasic half-life (short: 18 min and long: 89 min) is not commonly used now for several reasons. It is antigenic and should not be readministered within 6 months. Some trials on streptokinase have been terminated early because of the increased hemorrhage and mortality [18]. Antiplatelets should be started 24 h after thrombolysis.

**Table 4.9** Comparison of thrombolytic agents (fibrin specific agents)

| | Dose | Half-life | Salient features |
|---|---|---|---|
| Alteplase (tPA) | 0.9 mg/kg IV (maximum 90 mg) infused over 1 h with an initial IV bolus of 10% of the total dose over 1 min | 4–6 min | Dedicated peripheral IV line<br>not antigenic, no allergic manifestations<br>Major risk of treatment: sICH<br>Neurotoxic [19]<br>Do not use antiplatelets and anticoagulants within 24 h of alteplase use |
| Tenecteplase (TNK)<br>527 AA glycoprotein | 0.4 mg/kg IV single bolus dose | 20–24 min to 130 min (for final clearance through liver metabolism) | Equally safe as compared to alteplase [17]<br>Unclear whether it is more effective or as effective as tPA<br>EXTEND-IA TNK trial: showed better outcomes [20] |
| *Reteplase (recombinant plasminogen activator, r-PA)*<br>Nonglycosylated deletion mutein of tPA | Low dose 0.6 mg/kg along with abciximab in trials | 13–16 min | More rapid onset<br>Longer half-life, better penetration into thrombus [21]<br>Lower bleeding risk than alteplase<br>Not antigenic |

*AIS* acute ischemic stroke, *sICH* symptomatic intracranial hemorrhage, *NIH* National Institute of Health

### 4.7.2 Antiplatelet Drugs

Oral antiplatelets are used for after AIS to prevent recurrent ischemic stroke and pulmonary embolism. They inhibit the platelet aggregation and adhesion by various mechanisms. The drugs include cyclo-oxygenase inhibitors (aspirin), adenosine diphosphate inhibitors (thienopyridine derivatives—ticlopidine, clopidogrel), and phosphodiesterase inhibitors (dipyridamole, cilostazol) (Table 4.10). However, there are risks of hemorrhagic complications (hemorrhagic transformation of stroke, gastrointestinal bleeding, etc.) along with irreversible platelet inhibition from 5 to 7 days.

Aspirin is the most commonly used drug. It has been concluded that daily oral therapy with 160–300 mg aspirin, started within 48 h of AIS or TIA onset, improved the long-term outcomes without a major risk of early hemorrhagic complications [24].

Dual antiplatelet treatment with aspirin and clopidogrel started within 24 h in minor AIS for 21 days followed by clopidogrel alone is recommended for secondary prophylaxis [17].

**Table 4.10** Comparison of antiplatelet medications

| Drug | Dose | Salient features |
|---|---|---|
| Aspirin<br>Cox inhibitor | 325 mg: AIS secondary prevention<br>75–100 mg [22, 23]: AIS primary prevention | GI bleed: dose-dependent<br>Risk: not decreased with enteric coated tablets<br>Ibuprofen may inhibit non-enteric coated aspirin effects: so given 8 h before or 30 min after aspirin dose |
| Dipyridamole<br>PDE inhibitor | 200 mg bid | Headache (up to 40% of patients)<br>Tolerance: within 1–2 weeks;<br>Absorption: pH-dependent, affected by proton pump inhibitors |
| Clopidogrel<br>ADP inhibitors | 300–600 mg-loading dose followed by 75 mg daily | Prodrug<br>ADR: diarrhea<br>Hypersensitivity (usually rash)<br>GI bleeding less common<br>TTP rare |
| Ticlopidine<br>ADP inhibitors | 250 mg bid | Prodrug, not used popularly because of the side-effects: GI intolerance, TTP, neutropenia, aplastic anemia |
| Ticagrelor<br>Reversible blocker of ADP P2Y (12) receptor blocker | 180 mg loading followed by 90 mg bid | Does not require conversion to active metabolite<br>>100 mg/day decreases the effectiveness of aspirin<br>ADR: Dyspnea, bleeding (GI, subcutaneous, epistaxis), rash, itching |

*COX* cyclooxygenase, *GI* gastrointestinal, *PDE* phosphodiesterase, *ADP* adenosine diphosphate, *TTP* thrombotic thrombocytopenic purpura, *GI* gastrointestinal, *ADR* adverse drug reactions

The effectiveness of ticagrelor in AIS needs further studies although promising results are expected. Although its use over aspirin is not recommended by the current stroke guidelines [17], it may be used in combination with aspirin. It is useful in *CYP2C19* loss-of-function gene which is very common in the Asian population where clopidogrel is ineffective [25]. It has also been shown to have a lower hazard ratio when compared with aspirin [26]. It has a faster onset and shorter duration of action than clopidogrel. Hence drug adverse effects wear off earlier.

The GpIIb/IIIa inhibitors tirofiban and eptifibatide are safe but efficacy is not established [17]. However, the GpIIb/IIIa inhibitors abciximab has been found to be harmful [17].

### 4.7.3 Oral Anticoagulants

Oral anticoagulants are used for the prevention of recurrent ischemic stroke (cardioembolic) in moderate to high-risk patients with atrial fibrillation (AF). They are also used for the treatment of deep vein thrombosis and venous thromboembolism (Table 4.11).

Commonly used vitamin K antagonists include warfarin and acenocoumarol. Acenocoumarol (1 mg, 2 mg, and 4 mg tablets) has a shorter half-life (10 h) and lesser drug interactions than warfarin.

Non-vitamin K antagonist oral anticoagulants are the novel oral anticoagulants (NOACs). They are used in cardioembolic stroke of non-valvular origin although their role is not well established. There are two classes of NOACs: The direct thrombin inhibitors—dabigatran and direct factor Xa inhibitors—rivaroxaban, apixaban, and edoxaban.

NOACs are becoming popular as they have several advantages over warfarin. NOACs do not require frequent INR monitoring as in the case of warfarin. They have a faster and predictable onset of action, shorter half-life (5–15 h), and fewer drug and food interactions. Genetic polymorphism does not affect their metabolism as in warfarin. NOACs have a significantly lower risk for intracranial bleeding, [27] but are associated with a greater risk of gastrointestinal bleeding than warfarin. The dose of NOACs should be titrated as per the renal function. NOACs administration within the last 48 h of stroke or any abnormal coagulation tests for these specific agents is a contraindication for receiving tPA in a patient with an AIS. If a patient on NOACs requires ASA for AIS, there is an increased risk of bleeding and one must consider the risk to benefit ratio until the NOACs have had time to be cleared from the body (i.e. approximately 3–5 half-lives).

Current guidelines do not provide the best time to start anticoagulants because of the risk of hemorrhagic conversion. However, this varies from 4 to 14 days from stroke onset [28] (Table 4.11).

**Table 4.11** Comparison of oral anticoagulant agents [29]

| Drug | Dose | Onset and half-life | Contraindications |
|---|---|---|---|
| Warfarin<br>Vitamin K antagonist | Variable (Oral:2–10 mg once daily)<br>INR goal: 2–3<br>With mechanical valves goal: 2.5–3.5 | Onset:<br>48–120+ h<br>Half-life:<br>20–60 h<br>(variable) | Large Esophageal Varices<br>Platelet <50 x $10^9$/$mm^3$<br>Pregnancy<br>Child-Pugh C<br>Within 72 h of surgery |
| Dabigatran<br>Direct thrombin Inhibitor | *VTE treatment/ nonvalvularafib*:<br>150 mg BID (CrCl>30 mL/min)<br>75 mg BID (CrCl 15–30 mL/min)<br>*DVT prophylaxis*:<br>150 mg PO BID1–4 h after surgery (CrCl>30 mL/min) | Onset: 1–2 h<br>Half life:<br>12–17 h | CrCl ≤15 mL/min: not recommended |
| Rivaroxaban<br>Direct Xa inhibitor | *VTE treatment*:<br>15 mg BID with food for 21 days followed by 20 mg OD<br>*DVT prophylaxis*:<br>10 mg OD<br>*Nonvalvularafib*:<br>20 mg OD with food;<br>15 mg OD: CrCl 15–50 mL/min | Onset: 2–4 h<br>Half-life: 5–9 h<br>11–13 (elderly) | Severe hepatic dysfunction (Child-Pugh C)<br>CrCl ≤ 15 mL/min |
| Apixaban<br>Direct Xa inhibitor | *VTE treatment*:<br>10 mg BID for 7 days followed by 5 mg BID for 6 months<br>*DVT prophylaxis*:<br>2.5 mg BID<br>*Nonvalvularafib*:<br>2.5 mg BID if ≥2 of the following:<br>≥80 yo, ≤60 kg, Cr ≥1.5 mg/dL | Onset: 3–4 h<br>Half-life:<br>8–12 h | Severe hepatic dysfunction (Child-Pugh C)<br>CrCl ≤ 15–25 mL/min |

*Nonvalvularafib* nonvalvular atrial fibrillation, *DVT* deep venous thrombosis, *VTE* venous thromboembolism

## 4.8 Drugs Used in Intracranial Hemorrhage

Patients on antiplatelet or oral anticoagulants may present with intracranial hemorrhage (ICH), which might need drug reversal. At times immediate reversal for emergency surgery is required. These patients may also present with life-threatening gastrointestinal bleed and bleed from other areas, which might require urgent reversal.

When reversing an anticoagulant, the risk of continued bleeding to the risk of thrombosis should be individualized in each case. Cerebral venous sinus

**Table 4.12** Reversal of vitamin K antagonist [29]

| | |
|---|---|
| *First-line* | *4F-PCC IV*: if available<br>Vitamin K 2.5 mg oral or 1-2 mg IV |
| *INR* | *4F-PCC IV DOSE* |
| <4.5 | 25 units/kg IV |
| 4.5–10 | 35 IU/kg IV |
| >10 | 50 IU/kg IV |
| Any INR and serious or life-threatening bleeding | Urgent reversal required<br>Vitamin K 10 mg IV over 30 min<br>2000 IU 4F-PCC<br>If INR still elevated after 30 min and bleeding is continuing: second dose of PCC can be given |
| *Second-line* | 15–20 mL/kg *FFP* recheck INR after FFP is given |

*ICH* intracranial bleed

thrombosis-associated ICH reversal is to be avoided. To determine if the reversal is needed, timing of the last dose of anticoagulant administered should be enquired. It takes 3–5 half-lives from the last intake for a drug to be eliminated.

If an oral anticoagulant has been ingested within 2 h of presentation, 50 g oral activated charcoal may be administered. The drug should be discontinued. Thrombotic agents like tranexamic acid and resuscitation with blood products may be required.

Warfarin reversal is done by IV or oral vitamin K (1–10 mg), prothrombin complex concentrates (PCC), and fresh frozen plasma (FFP) (Table 4.12). Higher doses of vitamin K achieve quicker reversal with the risk of anaphylaxis being low. PCCs are of three types:

- 3 factor PCC: contains factor II, IX, and X
- 4 factor PCC: contains factor II, VII, IX, and X
- FEIBA (factor VIII inhibitor bypassing activity)/activated PCC (aPCC): contain four coagulation factors (inactive and activated forms).

However, PCCs are not commonly available in our subcontinent. Risk of transfusion-related lung injury (TRALI) and circulatory overload is lesser with PCC than FFP. PCC is preferred over FFP for warfarin reversal. Although few low quality studies have shown more rapid correction of INR with vitamin K and PCC than vitamin K and FFP, an improvement in patient clinical outcome with PCC has not been demonstrated [31].

Reversal of the effect of NOACs has specific antidotes (Table 4.13); however, they are not available widely. Renal dysfunction may delay elimination half-life of NOACs.

For reversal of thrombolytics (Alteplase) cryoprecipitate 10 U or antifibrinolytics are used. In patients taking antiplatelet drugs (aspirin, clopidogrel) and requiring urgent reversal for neurosurgical procedures or aneurysmal SAH reversal with platelet transfusions are done, although its efficacy is questionable [32, 33]. Desmopressin 0.4 µg/kg IV single doses can be used; platelet function tests should be done [30].

**Table 4.13** Reversal of novel oral anticoagulants [30]

| | |
|---|---|
| Direct thrombin inhibitors: Dabigatran | Idarucizumab 5 g IV (in two 2.5 g/50 ml vials)<br>If bleeding continues: hemodialysis or idarucizumab redosing |
| For other DTIs: Argatroban Bivalirudin, Desirudin, Lepirudin | Activated PCC (FEIBA) 50 units/kg IV<br>OR<br>4 factor PCC 50 units/kg IV |
| Direct factor Xa inhibitors<br>Rivaroxaban<br>Apixaban<br>Edoxaban | Andexanet alfa<br>*Low dose*: (≥8 h or rivaroxaban≤10 mg, Apixaban≤5 mg)<br>Bolus: 400 mg at a target rate of 30 mg/min followed by<br>Infusion: 4 mg/min for up to 120 min<br>*High dose*: (other cases)<br>Bolus: 800 mg at a target rate of 30 mg/min followed by<br>Infusion: 8 mg/min for up to 120 min<br>Activated PCC (FEIBA) 50 units/kg IV<br>OR<br>4 factor PCC 50 units/kg IV |

For every 100 units of heparin administered in the previous 2–3 h, 1 mg IV protamine is used: up to 50 mg can be given in a single dose. For fondaparinux reversal activated PCC (FEIBA) 20 units/kg IV is used. For each 1 mg enoxaparin, 1 mg IV protamine (up to 50 mg in a single dose) is used for reversal within 8 h and 0.5 mg IV protamine per 1 mg enoxaparin 8–12 h. For >12 h utility is questionable. For each 100 U dalteparin reversal, protamine 1 mg IV is used for reversal [30].

## 4.9 Drugs Used in Subarachnoid Hemorrhage

Delayed ischemic neurological deficits (DIND) caused by arterial vasospasm is a major cause for poor outcome in subarachnoid hemorrhage (SAH). Randomized trials have shown that prophylactic treatment with nimodipine has decreased the proportion of patients with DIND and is cost-effective [34]. This is based on the hypothesis that vasospasm caused by vascular smooth muscle contraction is dependent on calcium influx. Dihydropyridine calcium antagonist nimodipine blocks this influx. Nimodipine is routinely given per orally in a dose of 60 mg. Some centers routinely administer nimodipine intravenously. Parenteral route by continuous IV infusion of nimodipine at the rate of 0.2 mg/ml at 10 ml/h is more reliable and will have stable plasma concentrations. If there is hypotension (SBP <110 mmHg), a temporary reduction in the infusion rate is done to 5 ml/h. Although oral and intravenous routes have similar efficacy, the oral route is safer and cost-effective. Hence the parenteral route can be reserved for patients with deranged enteral absorption or metabolism [35]. Intraarterial nimodipine can be given by angiography. It can lead to bradycardia and hypotension during instillation.

Inotropes like IV dobutamine are often used in SAH to maintain a high cardiac output with cardiac output monitoring and preventing vasospasm (Table 4.14). Intraarterial milrinone infusion followed by intravenous administration (up to 14 days after initial bleeding) can be effective for cerebral vasospasm treatment

**Table 4.14** Comparison of inotropes in subarachnoid hemorrhage

| Inotropes | Action | Dose | Cautions |
|---|---|---|---|
| Dobutamine<br>α, $\beta_1$, $\beta_2$ agonist | Increases cardiac contractility | 2.5–15 μg/kg/min<br>Max 40 μg/kg/min IV | Decrease in SVR-hypotension<br>Tolerance: with prolonged administration |
| Milrinone<br>Phosphodiesterase 3 inhibitor | Increases cardiac contractility, vasodilator | 50 μg/kg × 10 min loading then 0.5 μg/kg/min to 1.5 μg/kg/min IV | Elimination reduced in renal dysfunction<br>CrCl < 50 mL/min reduce dose<br>Adverse effects:<br>Hypotension<br>Arrhythmias<br>Thrombocytopenia |

*SVR* systemic vascular resistance, *CO* cardiac output, *CrCl* creatinine clearance

[36]. However, supporting randomized control trials are lacking and concomitant hypotension might decrease cerebral perfusion pressure.

Tranexamic acid was being used earlier to decrease the rebleeding risk in SAH. However, after reports that it increased the risk of DIND and venous thrombosis it is now not routinely used as doesnot outcome [37]. Recent reports that short term antifibrinolytic treatment should be continued until the aneurysm is repaired needs further randomized trials [38].

## 4.10 Hyperosmolar Therapy: Drugs Used to Reduce the Intracranial Pressure

Mannitol and hypertonic saline are agents used commonly and in equal preference to decrease raised ICP [39]. It is unclear which one is superior. Both the agents act by creating osmotic fluid shifts and are equipotent in equiosmolar dosages. Dosage, concentration, and administration protocols need to be as per institution protocols.

The common dosing and adverse effects for both these agents are presented in Table 4.15. Hypertonic saline may be given in continuous infusion. Central line access is recommended. Frequent serum sodium levels will need to be monitored 4–6 hourly. The duration of effect is 90 min to 4 h. It remains within the vascular compartment longer than mannitol and so is useful in hypovolemic patients. This enables better cardiac output and hence better cerebral perfusion. It also has a better reflection coefficient than mannitol. Agents with lower reflection coefficients have a greater risk of accumulating inside the brain. It tends to cross the blood–brain barrier lesser than mannitol. There is some anecdotal evidence of better results as compared to mannitol in terms of reduction of intracranial pressure but further randomized controlled trials are needed.

Mannitol maybe administered via a peripheral vein. Duration of the effect is 90 min to 6 h. An osmolar gap >20 mmol/dL marks inadequate clearance of

**Table 4.15** Hyperosmolar therapy

| Agent | Dosing | Adverse reactions |
|---|---|---|
| Mannitol | 0.5–1 g/kg over 5–15 min; every 4–6 h | Sudden discontinuation of high doses may cause rebound rise in ICP<br>Dehydration<br>Hypotension<br>Dyselectrolytemia—hypokalemia, hyponatremia, etc.<br>Acute kidney injury<br>Fluid overload/pulmonary edema |
| Hypertonic saline | Bolus dosing<br>3%: 2.5–5 mL/kg over 5–20 min<br>5%: 2.5–5 mL/kg over 5–20 min<br>7.5%: 1.5–2.5 mL/kg over 5–20<br>23.4%: 30 mL over 10–20 min<br>Continuous infusion titrated to a goal Na range (155–160 meq/dL) | Hypernatremia, hyperchloremia<br>Congestive heart failure<br>Acute kidney injury<br>Coagulation abnormality<br>Preexisting hypernatremia<br>Hyperchloremic metabolic acidosis<br>Thrombophlebitis<br>Osmotic demyelination syndrome (rapid correction in chronic hyponatremia) |

mannitol and will increase the risk of rebound rise in ICP. Mannitol maybe warmed to dissolve crystals, which precipitate in the bottle [40].

## 4.11 Management of Symptomatic Hyponatremia

Hypertonic saline may also be used in the treatment of symptomatic hyponatremia.

The European Society of Intensive Care Medicine and the European Society of Endocrinology recommend the treatment of hyponatremia as follows [41]:

- *Symptomatic hyponatremia*: Maybe acute, or acute on chronic in nature. *Management will include* intravenous infusion of hypertonic saline, aiming to increase 6 mmol/L over 24 h (maximum 12 mmol/L) and 8 mmol/L next 24 h till the serum sodium reaches 130 mmol/L.
- *Hyponatremia due to SIADH*: Should be treated with fluid restriction. Oral supplementation of sodium chloride and loop diuretics may be added as needed.
- *For patients dehydrated patients*, intravenous infusion of 0.9% saline or a balanced crystalloid solution at 0.5–1.0 mL/kg/h will correct the serum sodium levels.
- Lithium, demeclocycline, and vaptans are not recommended for patients with moderate or profound hyponatremia.

## 4.12 Summary

Pharmacological management of neuro-critical patients is challenging and should be individualized after assessing the risk-benefit ratio. We should aim to achieve neuroprotection, maintaining the cognitive and functional status of the patient.

Knowledge of pharmacokinetics and pharmacodynamics of drugs used in these patients is essential to achieve these goals.

## Multiple Choice Questions

1. The drug of choice for partial seizures is:
   (a) Carbamazepine
   (b) Diazepam
   (c) Ethosuximide
   (d) Phenytoin
2. The mechanism of action of antiepileptic drugs is:
   (a) Enhancement of GABA-ergic (inhibitory) transmission
   (b) Inhibition of excitatory (usually glutamate-ergic) transmission
   (c) Modification of ionic conductance
   (d) All of the above
3. Osmolality of Hypertonic saline is about
   (a) 900 mosm/dL
   (b) 1100 mosm/dL
   (c) 557 mosm/dL
   (d) 630 mosm/dL
4. All are true about Nimodipine except—Nimodipine
   (a) Has low oral bioavailability (2.7–27.9%),
   (b) Has a short half-life (2 h),
   (c) Is highly protein bound (98–99%),
   (d) Is renally metabolized.
5. Regarding dose of thrombolytic in acute ischemic stroke which is correct
   (a) Alteplase—0.9 mg/kg IV (Maximum 90 mg) infused over 1 h with an initial IV bolus of 10% of the total dose over 1 min
   (b) Tenecteplase—0.4 mg/kg IV single bolus dose
   (c) Both a and b
   (d) Neither a and b
6. *Clopidogrel* is a prodrug: the major enzyme involved in the conversion of *clopidogrel* into an active metabolite is
   (a) *CYP2C19*
   (b) ABCB1
   (c) P2Y12
   (d) GPIIIA
7. Only test necessary prior to initiating alteplase thrombolysis
   (a) Blood glucose
   (b) International normalized ratio,
   (c) Activated partial thromboplastin time
   (d) Platelet count

8. Alteplase should not be administered if
   (a) Patient has got treatment dose of LMWH within last 24 h
   (b) Patient has got abciximab
   (c) Both a and b
   (d) Neither a or b
9. All are true about Mannitol except:
   (a) Mannitol is secreted and reabsorbed by the tubules.
   (b) It retains water and causes an "osmotic diuresis."
   (c) It is useful clinically in management of rhabdomyolysis.
   (d) It is used in medical management of raised ICP.
10. Management of DIND
   (a) Pharmacologically induced hypertension
   (b) Intravascular volume optimization
   (c) Intraarterial Papaverine
   (d) All the above

Answers: 1. (a), 2. (d), 3. (a), 4. (d), 5. (c), 6. (a), 7. (a), 8. (c), 9. (a), 10. (d)

## References

1. Glauser T, et al. Evidence-based guideline: treatment of convulsive status epilepticus in children and adults: report of the guideline committee of the American Epilepsy Society. Epilepsy Curr. 2016;16(1):48–61.
2. Himmelseher S, Durieux ME. Revising a dogma: ketamine for patients with neurological injury? Anesth Analg. 2005;101(02):524–34.
3. Zanos P, Moaddel R, Morris PJ, Riggs LM, Highland JN, Georgiou P, Pereira EFR, Albuquerque EX, Thomas CJ, Zarate CA Jr, Gould TD. Ketamine and ketamine metabolite pharmacology: insights into therapeutic mechanisms. Pharmacol Rev. 2018;70(3):621–60.
4. Abou-Khalil B. Levetiracetam in the treatment of epilepsy. Neuropsychiatr Dis Treat. 2008;4(3):507–23.
5. Villa FA, Citerio G. Sedation and analgesia in neurointensive care. In: Layon AJ, Gabrielli A, Friedman WA, editors. Textbook of neurointensive care, vol. 1. 2nd ed. New York: Springer; 2014.
6. Hughes CG, McGrane S, Pandharipande PP. Sedation in the intensive care setting. Clin Pharmacol. 2012;4:53–63.
7. Oddo M, Crippa IA, Mehta S, Menon D, Payen JF, Taccone FS, Citerio G. Optimizing sedation in patients with acute brain injury. Crit Care. 2016;20(1):128.
8. Vanaclocha N, Chisbert V, Quilis V, Bilotta F, Badenes R. Sedation during neurocritical care. J Neuroanaesthesiol Crit Care. 2019;06(02):056–61.
9. Baraka A. Anaesthesia and myasthenia gravis. Can J Anaesth. 1992;39(5 Pt 1):476–86.
10. Appleton JP, Sprigg N, Bath PM. Blood pressure management in acute stroke. Stroke Vasc Neurol. 2016;1:e000020.
11. Bowry R, Navalkele DD, Gonzales NR. Blood pressure management in stroke: five new things. Neurol Clin Pract. 2014;4(5):419–26.
12. Krishnan K, Scutt P, Woodhouse L, Adami A, Becker JL, Berge E, Cala LA, et al. Glyceryl trinitrate for acute intracerebral hemorrhage: results from the efficacy of nitric oxide in stroke (ENOS) trial, a subgroup analysis. Stroke. 2016;47:44–52.

13. Zaidi G, Chichra A, Weitzen M, Narasimhan M. Blood pressure control in neurological ICU patients: what is too high and what is too low? Open Crit Care Med J. 2013;6(1: M3):46–55.
14. Mehndiratta MM, Pandey S, Kuntzer T. Acetylcholinesterase inhibitor treatment for myasthenia gravis. Cochrane Database Syst Rev. 2014;(10):CD006986.
15. Ismail A. How do you convert an oral pyridostigmine dose to a parenteral neostigmine dose? [Internet]. London: UK Medicines Information Pharmacist for NHS Healthcare Professionals; 2017. https://www.sps.nhs.uk/.
16. Hacke W, Kaste M, Bluhmki E, Brosman M. Thrombolysis with alteplase 3 to 4.5 hours after acute ischemic stroke. N Engl J Med. 2008;359:1317–29.
17. Powers WJ, Rabinstein AA, Ackerson T, Adeoye OM, Bambakidis NC, Becker K, Biller J, Brown M, Demaerschalk BM, Hoh B, Jauch EC, Kidwell CS, Leslie-Mazwi TM, Ovbiagele B, Scott PA, Sheth KN, Southerland AM, Summers DV, Tirschwell DL, on behalf of the American Heart Association Stroke Council. 2018 guidelines for the early management of patients with acute ischemic stroke: a guideline for healthcare professionals from the American Heart Association/American Stroke Association. Stroke. 2018;49:e46–99.
18. Multicenter Acute Stroke Trial--Europe Study Group, Hommel M, Cornu C, Boutitie F, Boissel JP. Thrombolytic therapy with streptokinase in acute ischemic stroke. N Engl J Med. 1996;335:145–50.
19. Kaur J, Zhao Z, Klein GM, Lo EH, Buchan AM. The neurotoxicity of tissue plasminogen activator? J Cereb Blood Flow Metab. 2004;24(9):945–63.
20. Campbell BCV, et al. Tenecteplase versus alteplase before thrombectomy for ischemic stroke. N Engl J Med. 2018;378:1573–82.
21. Verstraete M. Third generation thrombolytic drugs. Am J Med. 2000;109(1):52–8.
22. Singh VP, Yadav P, Malhotra M, Theengh DP, Malhotra R, Patnaik SS. Role of aspirin in the primary prevention of artherosclerotic vascular disease: a reappraisal. JIACM. 2013;14(2):143–8.
23. Arnett DK, Blumenthal RS, Albert MA, Michos ED, Buroker AB, Miedema MD, et al. 2019 ACC/AHA guideline on the primary prevention of cardiovascular disease. Circulation. 2019;140(11):e596–646.
24. Sandercock PAG, Counsell C, Tseng MC, Cecconi E. Oral antiplatelet therapy for acute ischaemic stroke. Cochrane Database Syst Rev. 2014;(3):CD000029.
25. Han Y, et al. Influence of genetic polymorphism on clopidogrel response and clinical outcome in patients with acute ischemic stroke CYP2C19 genotype on clopidogrel response. CNS Neurosci Ther. 2015;21(9):692–7.
26. Wang Y, Minematsu K, Wong KSL, Amarenco P, Albers GW, Denison H, et al. Ticagrelor in acute stroke or transient ischemic attack in Asian patients. Stroke. 2017;48:167–73.
27. Paciaroni M, Agnelli G, Falocci N, Caso V, Becatti C, Marchesilli S, et al. Early recurrence and cerebral bleeding in patients with acute ischemic stroke and atrial fibrillation: effect of anticoagulation and its timing: the RAF study. Stroke. 2015;46:2175–82.
28. Seiffge DJ, Werring DJ, Paciaroni M, Dawson J, Warach S, Milling TJ, Engelter ST, Fischer U, Norrving B. Timing of anticoagulation after recent ischaemic stroke in patients with atrial fibrillation. Lancet Neurol. 2019;18(1):117–26.
29. Brophy GM, Human T. Pharmacotherapy pearls for emergency neurological life support. Neurocrit Care. 2017;27(1):51–73.
30. Sarma AK, Ghoshal S, Craven SJ, Sarwal A. Intracerebral hemorrhage: a brief evidence-based review of common etiologies, mechanisms of secondary injury, and medical and surgical management. J Neuroanaesthesiol Crit Care. 2019;06(02):119–30.
31. Hemphill JC 3rd, Greenberg SM, Anderson CS, Becker K, Bendok BR, Cushman M, Fung GL, Goldstein JN, Macdonald RL, Mitchell PH, Scott PA, Selim MH, Woo D, on behalf of the American Heart Association Stroke Council, Council on Cardiovascular and Stroke Nursing, and Council on Clinical Cardiology. Guidelines for the management of spontaneous intracerebral hemorrhage: a guideline for healthcare professionals from the American Heart Association/American Stroke Association. Stroke. 2015;46:2032–60.

32. Jehan F, Zeeshan M, Kulvatunyou N, Khan M, O'Keeffe T, Tang A, Gries L, Joseph B. Is there a need for platelet transfusion after traumatic brain injury in patients on P2Y12 inhibitors? J Surg Res. 2019;236:224–9.
33. Holzmacher JL, Reynolds C, Patel M, Maluso P, Holland S, Gamsky N, et al. Platelet transfusion does not improve outcomes in patients with brain injury on antiplatelet therapy. Brain Inj. 2018;32(3):325–30.
34. Barker FG, Ogilvy CS. Efficacy of prophylactic nimodipine for delayed ischemic deficit after subarachnoid hemorrhage: a metaanalysis. J Neurosurg. 1996;84:405–14.
35. Kronvall E, Undren P, Romner B, Saveland H, Cronqvist M, Nilsson OG. Nimodipine in aneurysmal subarachnoid hemorrhage: a randomized study of intravenous or peroral administration. J Neurosurg. 2008;110(1):58–63.
36. Fraticelli AT, Cholley BP, Losser MR, Saint Maurice JP, Payen D. Milrinone for the treatment of cerebral vasospasm after aneurysmal subarachnoid hemorrhage. Stroke. 2008;39:893–8.
37. Roos T. Antifibrinolytic treatment in subarachnoid hemorrhage: a randomized placebo- controlled trial. STAR Study Group. Neurology. 2000;54:77–82.
38. Hillman J, Fridriksson S, Nilsson O, et al. Immediate administration of tranexamic acid and reduced incidence of early rebleeding after aneurismal subarachnoid hemorrhage: a prospective randomized study. J Neurosurg. 2002;97:771–8.
39. Hays AN, Lazaridis C, Neyens R, Nicholas J, Gay S, Chalela JA. Osmotherapy: use among neurointensivists. Neurocrit Care. 2011;14(2):222–8.
40. Kheirbek T, Pascual JL. Hypertonic saline for the treatment of intracranial hypertension. Curr Neurol Neurosci Rep. 2014;14(9):482.
41. Simon EE. Hyponatremia treatment & management. Medscape; 2018.

# 5 Role of Ultrasound in Neuroemergencies

Saurabh Anand, Nitin Manohar, and Astha Palan

**Key Points**

- Ultrasound has a wide variety of applications in neurologically ill patients
- There are a wide variety of ultrasound probes available for clinical use
- Measurement of optic nerve sheath diameter using ultrasound is a non-invasive method to detect the presence of intracranial hypertension. Optic nerve sheath diameter more than 5 mm is believed to correlate positively with the presence of intracranial hypertension
- Transcranial Doppler uses low-frequency ultrasound probes to measure cerebral blood flow and vessel pulsatility over extended time periods with high temporal resolution. It can also be used for prognostication of stroke
- Cardiac dysfunction is commonly associated with subarachnoid hemorrhage and a screening echocardiography may facilitate detection of the same.
- Ultrasound may be useful for pupillary examination, evaluation of the thorax and abdomen in the setting of trauma

S. Anand (✉)
Department of Neuroanaesthesia and Neurocritical Care, Artemis Hospitals, Gurugram, Haryana, India

N. Manohar · A. Palan
Department of Neuroanaesthesia and Neurocritical Care, Yashoda Hospitals, Secunderabad, Telangana, India



P. U. Bidkar, P. Vanamoorthy (eds.), *Acute Neuro Care*,
https://doi.org/10.1007/978-981-15-4071-4_5

**Case Scenario**

55 years old, 80 kg male, is a known case of hypertension. He had complaints of severe headache and loss of consciousness. NCCT head was done which shows SAH aneurysmal bleed (Fisher grade III). Patient shifted into the emergency on ventilator support. GCS on arrival was E2VTM5. On admission his BP was 85/60 mm of Hg. His sodium was 119 mg/dL and Hb 8.0 g/dL. DSA was done which showed irregular wide neck saccular aneurysm measuring approximately 3 mm at the right ICA bifurcation. His chest X-ray showed signs of pulmonary edema. Cardiac enzymes were raised.

How POCUS and TCD will help us in managing this patient is what we are going to learn in this chapter.

## 5.1 Introduction: USG as a Point of Care

Point of care ultrasound has been described as the third hand of emergency physician [1]· USG involves exposing desired body parts to high-frequency sound waves to produce images. As ultrasound images are captured in real-time, the structure and movement of organs and blood flowing through vessels can also be seen. USG is easily available, portable and gives real-time information that has expanded its use outside the radiology suite.

## 5.2 Common Modes Used

- *A mode*: It is the simplest mode used. A single transducer scans a line through body with echoes plotted on screen as a function of depth. It allows for accurate focus of the destructive wave energy.
- *B mode*: In this mode, a linear array of transducers simultaneously scans a plane through the body that can be seen as a two-dimensional picture on the screen.
- *M mode*: M means motion in this mode. A rapid sequence of B mode scans whose images follow each other on the screen enables us to see and measure a range of motion as organ boundaries that produce reflections.
- *Doppler mode*: This mode uses the Doppler effect for measuring and visualizing blood flow. It is used to assess whether blood is moving toward or away from the probe and its relative velocity. This information is displayed graphically using spectral Doppler or as an image either as color Doppler or power Doppler. This Doppler shift produces a very distinct and pulsing sound that is presented audibly [2]. Table 5.1 and Fig. 5.1 [3] show the types of probes most commonly used.

**Table 5.1** Types of probes commonly used

| Probe type | Frequency (MHz) | Applications |
|---|---|---|
| Curvilinear | 2–5 | FAST, renal, aorta, IVC, pelvic, bladder, bowel |
| Linear | 6–15 | Ocular, trachea, thyroid, thoracic, vascular access, DVT, MSK, soft tissue |
| Phased array/ sector | 1–5 | Cardiac, abdominal, renal, pediatric abdomen, bladder, bowel, IVC |

Abbreviations: *DVT* deep venous thrombosis, *FAST* focused assessment with sonography in trauma, *IVC* inferior vena cava, *MSK* musculoskeletal, *POCUS* point of care ultrasound

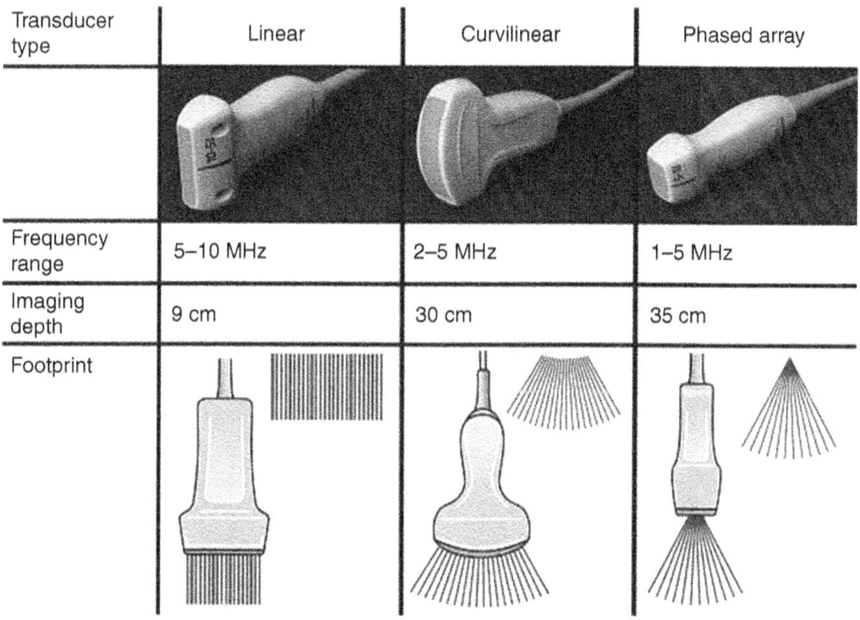


**Fig. 5.1** Types of USG probes commonly used

## 5.3 USG in Intracranial Hypertension

### 5.3.1 Optic Nerve Measurement (ONSD) and Correlation with Intracranial Hypertension

Raised intracranial pressure is a life-threatening situation. It can be measured with invasive devices like EVD, intracranial probes but this is associated with complications like infection or bleeding [4]. This led to the use of non-invasive methods like CT, MRI, and transcranial Doppler to measure ICP, but there is a limited correlation between these methods and intracranial pressure values. The use of ocular ultrasound was first reported in 1965 [5]. It has been proposed that measurement of the optic nerve sheath diameter through the ocular window may be a non-invasive method for the detection of intracranial hypertension. Moreover, good intra- and inter-observer reproducibility has been demonstrated [6]. The most distal part of the optic nerve has a dural covering known as optic nerve sheath and when the ICP rises it becomes dilated, this is the basis for the relation between ICP and ONSD measurement [7]. These changes are more in the anterior portion of the nerve sheath, an area that is easily accessible by ultrasound. Because of the late onset of clinical signs in cases of intracranial hypertension, early ultrasound detection allows for immediate therapeutic action leading to improved outcomes. Ultrasound is less time consuming and can be performed bedside so there is no need of transferring the critically ill patients to radiology suite. ONSD can only act as a screening tool for raised ICP, it cannot give absolute values of ICP. A learning curve of ten measurements with three abnormal scans is proposed for physicians with experience in USG and 25 scans may be adequate for a non-experienced person [8, 9]. Serial measurement of ONSD can also be used to access the response to the treatment of raised ICP.

### 5.3.2 Optic Nerve Sheath Diameter Measurement

A high frequency (7–10 MHz) linear transducer is used with power reduced. The depth is set to 5–6 cm. The transducer is placed over closed eyelid after generously applying gel (Fig. 5.2). The optic nerve is identified as hypoechoic structure traversing along a regular course behind the eyeball. To measure ONSD, a vertical line measuring 3 mm is drawn from junction between the optic nerve and the eyeball. Once the 3 mm line is

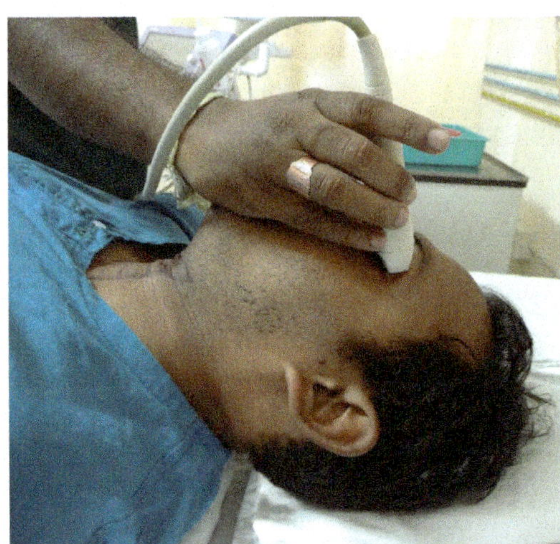

**Fig. 5.2** Probe position for ONSD

made, a horizontal line across the optic nerve is drawn perpendicular to the previous line. This second line gives the diameter of the optic nerve sheath in millimeters (Fig. 5.3). It is recommended to take an average of three measurements of ONSD.

For most of the authors included in the review, 5 mm is the cut-off point for determining that the scan is positive for intracranial hypertension, other authors proposed different values (Table 5.2).

### 5.3.3 Transcranial Doppler (TCD) in Raised ICP

TCD derived parameters change during an increase of ICP, such as the shape of the FV pulse waveform or the pulsatility index (PI). In patients with raised ICP, mean and diastolic blood flow velocities decrease, and PI increases as PI = PSV − EDV/MFV. The normal value of PI is between 0.6 and 1.1.

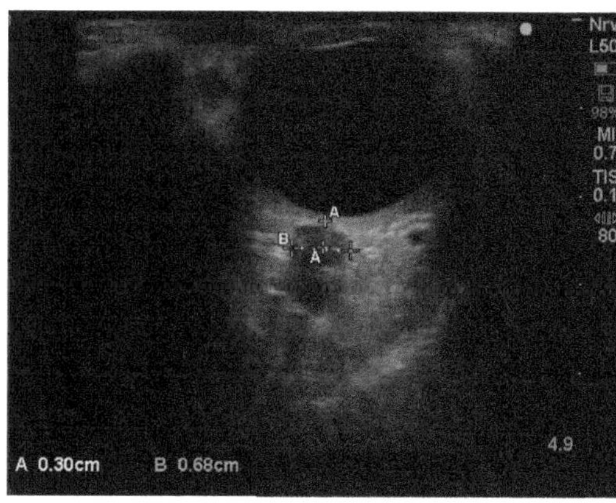


**Fig. 5.3** ONSD measurement by USG

**Table 5.2** Cut-off values for ONSD

| Study | Optic nerve diameter (mm) | % Sensitivity | % Specificity |
|---|---|---|---|
| Blaivas et al. | 5.0 | 100 | 95 |
| Goel et al. | 5.0 | 98.6 | 92.8 |
| Tayal et al. | 5.0 | 100 | 63 |
| Kimberly et al. | 5.0 | 88 | 93 |
| Moretti et al. | 5.2 | 93.1 | 73.8 |
| Moretti et al. | 5.2 | 94 | 76 |
| Geeraerts et al. | 5.9 | 95 | 79 |
| Geeraerts et al. | 5.9 | 87 | 94 |
| Soldatos et al. | 5.9 | 74.1 | 100 |
| Major et al. | 5.0 | 100 | 86 |

The relationship between ICP and PI is complex and beyond the scope of this chapter. Though, various authors show the relationship between ICP and PI like—Bellner et al. [10]: ICP = (10.972 × PI) − 1.284.

PI positively correlates with ICP; a change of 2.4% is reflected by a 1 mm change in ICP. TCD has been demonstrated to screen patients with mild or moderate TBI (traumatic brain injury) at risk of secondary neurological deterioration [11].

## 5.4 Subarachnoid Hemorrhage

### 5.4.1 Transcranial Doppler

Transcranial Dopper (TCD) study involves the use of a low-frequency (≤2 MHz) transducer probes to insonate the basal cerebral arteries through relatively thin bone windows. It allows dynamic monitoring of cerebral blood flow velocity (CBF-V) and vessel pulsatility over extended periods with a high temporal resolution. It can be used bedside and allows continuous monitoring of CBF-V. The factor limiting its utility is that it is operator dependent. TCD uses pulsed wave Doppler to image vessels at various depths. The received echoes generate an electrical impulse in the USG probe and are processed to calculate the Doppler shift and velocity, to produce a spectral waveform with peak systolic velocity (PSV) and end-diastolic velocity (EDV) values [12] (Fig. 5.5). There are four acoustic windows—transtemporal, suboccipital, transorbital, and submandibular (Fig. 5.4). The transtemporal window is located above the zygomatic ridge between the lateral canthus of the eye and auricular pinna is the most frequently used window and can insonate the middle (MCA), anterior (ACA), posterior cerebral arteries (PCA), and terminal internal carotid artery (ICA) [13, 14].

**TCD indices**

- Mean flow velocity (MFV) is a central parameter in TCD and is equal to (PSV + (EDV × 2))/3
- Gosling's pulsatility index (PI) provides information on downstream cerebral vascular resistance and is equal to (PSV-EDV)/MFV
- The Lindegaard ratio (LR) allows differentiation between hyperdynamic flow and vasospasm and is defined as MCA MFV/Extracranial ICA MFV [12] (Table 5.3)
- Modified LR or Sviri Ratio: BA MFV/Extracranial VA MFV [12] (Table 5.4)

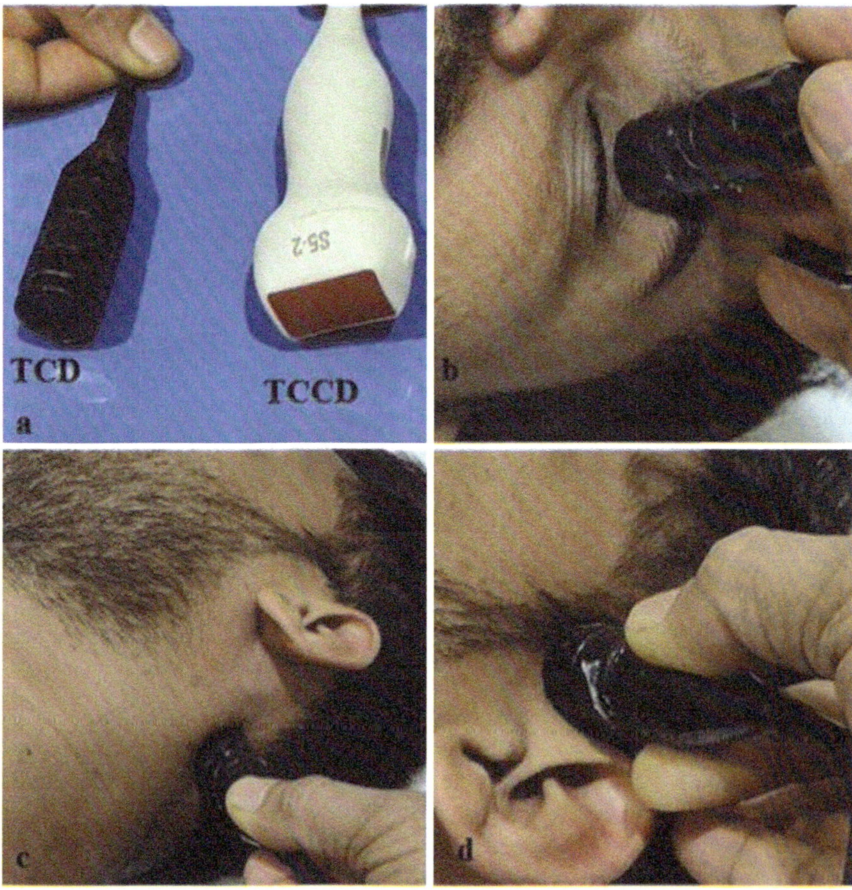


**Fig. 5.4** (**a**) Probes for TCD and TCCD, (**b**) Transorbital window, (**c**) Transforaminal window, (**d**) Transtemporal window

**Table 5.3** Grading of MCA vasospasm severity

| Degree of MCA or ICA vasospasm | MFV (cm/s) | LR |
|---|---|---|
| Mild (<25%) | 120–149 | 3–6 |
| Moderate (25–50%) | 150–199 | 3–6 |
| Severe (>50%) | >200 | >6 |

**Table 5.4** Grading of BA vasospasm severity

| Degree of BA vasospasm | MFV (cm/s) | Modified LR |
|---|---|---|
| May represent vasospasm | 70–85 | 2–2.49 |
| Moderate (25–50%) | >85 | 2.5–2.99 |
| Severe (>50%) | >85 | >3 |

### 5.4.2 Transcranial Color-Coded Duplex (TCCD)

A 2-MHz transducer can be used in the ultrasound systems, to perform transcranial color-coded duplex (TCCD) sonography of the skull [15]. For TCCD, a phased array transducer is used. TCCD has an added advantage of providing parenchymal imaging with a structural flow map of cerebral vessels, but, only few successful examinations can be done, because of lack of good temporal bone windows [15]. Figures 5.5 and 5.6 show MCA waveform on TCD and TCCD, respectively.

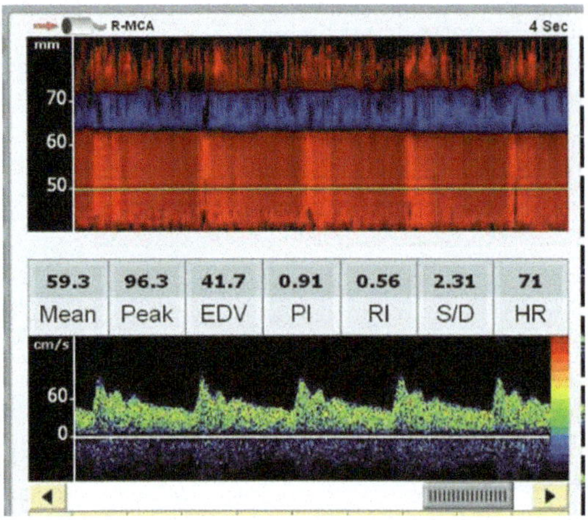


**Fig. 5.5** MCA waveform on TCD

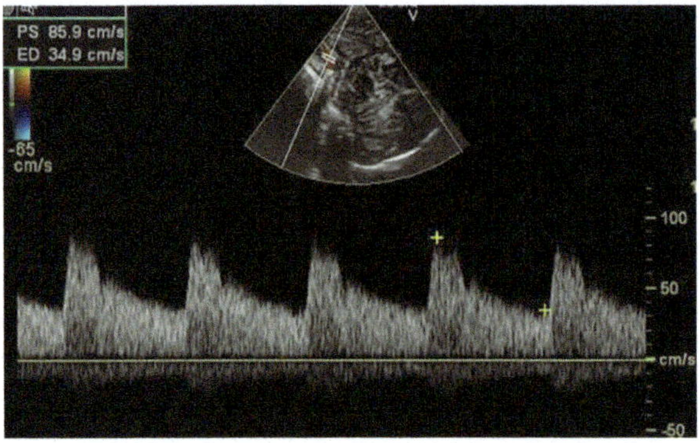


**Fig. 5.6** MCA waveform on TCCD

### 5.4.3 TCD or TCCD Guided Protocol in Vasospasm [16]

#### 5.4.3.1 Algorithm for Vasospasm

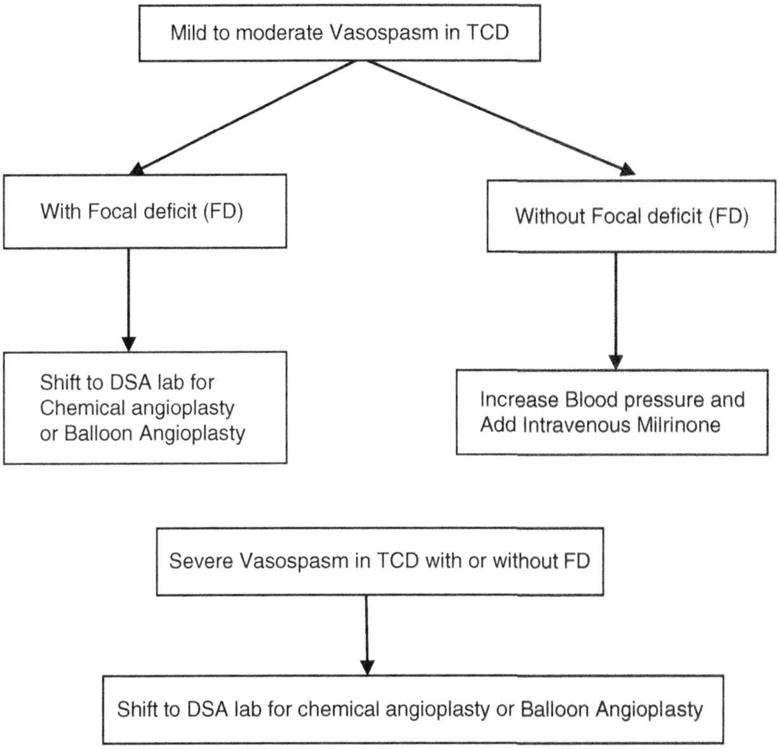


## 5.5 Screening Echocardiography (ECHO) in SAH

Cardiac dysfunction and regional wall motion abnormalities (RWMA) are common with diffuse SAH and screening ECHO helps to detect the left ventricular systolic function and presence of any RWMA (Fig. 5.7). Figure 5.8 shows probe placement for different views for screening ECHO.

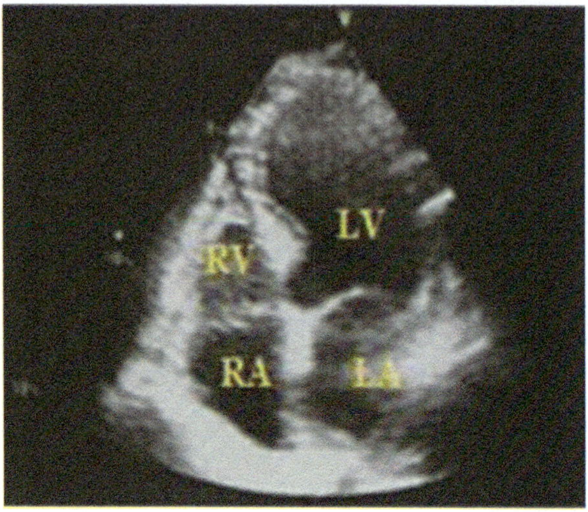


**Fig. 5.7** Apical four-chamber view 2D ECHO showing LV apical ballooning and normal contracting base

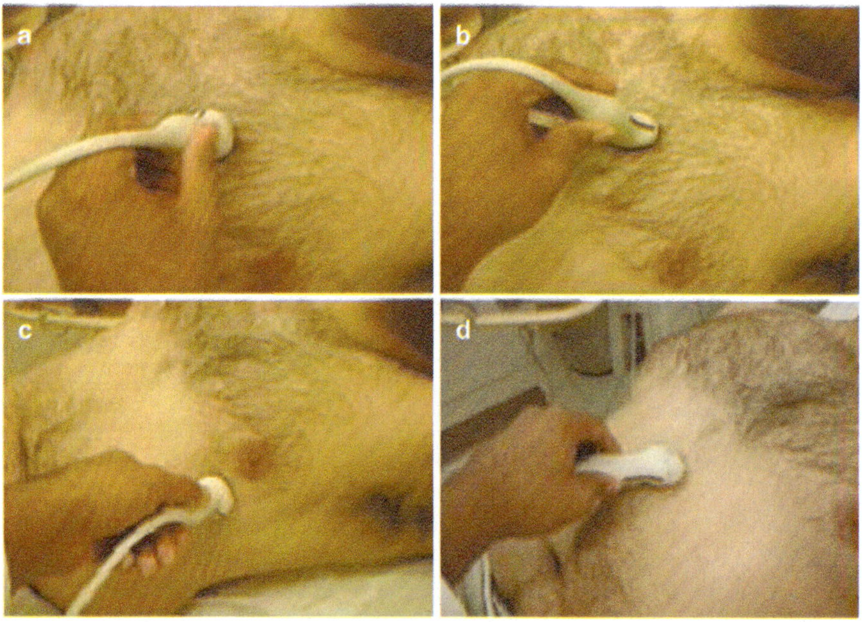


**Fig. 5.8** Probe position for screening ECHO. (**a**) Parasternal long axis view; (**b**) Short axis view; (**c**) Apical four-chamber view; (**d**) Subcostal view

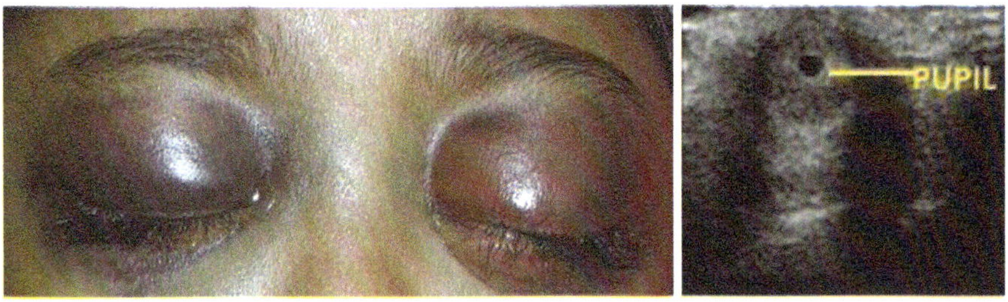


**Fig. 5.9** Pupillary examination by USG in case of swollen eye

### 5.5.1 Trauma

**Pupils** When clinical examination of the pupil is not possible (e.g raccoon eyes), accurate determination of pupillary diameter and consensual light reflex can be elicited using USG (Fig. 5.9).

## 5.6 Focused Assessment with Sonography for Trauma (FAST) and EFAST (Extended FAST)

Ultrasonographic examination of thorax allows in rapid assessment of a patient with polytrauma having pneumothorax/hemothorax, respiratory failure with normal oxygenation, pleural effusion, or consolidation. Thoracic USG is superior to chest radiography and can be used as a screening tool for the characterization of respiratory abnormalities in critically ill patients in the emergency room and the ICU. Lung ultrasonography has 94% sensitivity and 96% specificity for pneumonia [17] and has 91% sensitivity and 98% specificity for pneumothorax [18, 19].

The FAST scan uses USG to identify any intra-abdominal source of hemorrhage. The advantages are it can be done rapidly bedside if initially negative can be repeated as and when clinically required. The extended FAST includes the FAST scan with the subcostal view of the heart along with anterior and lateral chest examination. It can be performed in cases with thoracic trauma.

It can diagnose pericardial effusion in thoracic trauma cases which may require immediate decompression if hemodynamic instability is present. Figure 5.10 shows probe placement for FAST and E FAST scan. Ultrasonography provides rapid identification of life-threatening injuries which may require immediate intervention.

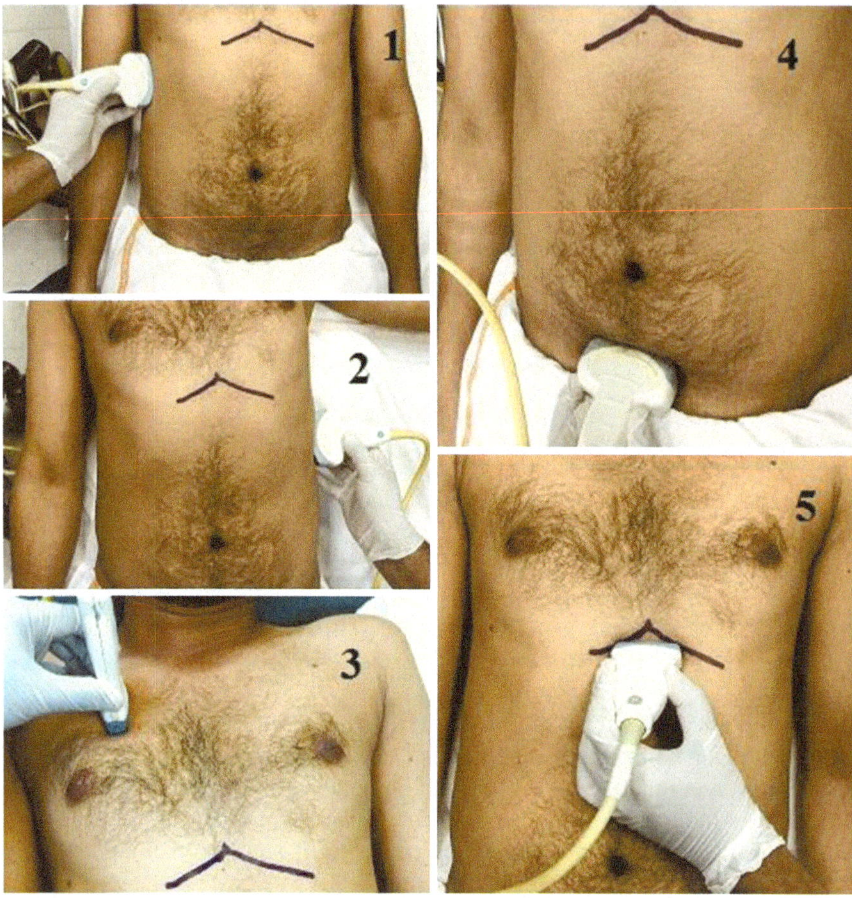


**Fig. 5.10** Probe Position for FAST and E-FAST. (1) The hepatorenal angle (Morrison's pouch) and the right diaphragm; (2) The spleno-renal interface and left diaphragm; (3) Pleura Bilateral: The fifth view is the pleura (bilaterally); (4) Pelvis in both planes—transverse and longitudinal; (5) Pericardial: Subxiphoid or intercostal views of the pericardium

Ultrasonography is superior to standard supine radiography for the detection of hemothorax [20]. CT whole body is the most commonly used imaging modality in trauma patients; POCUS remains the best primary tool for the emergency evaluation of abdominal and thoracic trauma. Bedside ultrasonography in trauma is performed more rapidly than a CT scan and is recommended for patients with thoracic or abdominal trauma [21].

### 5.6.1 Algorithm for Trauma

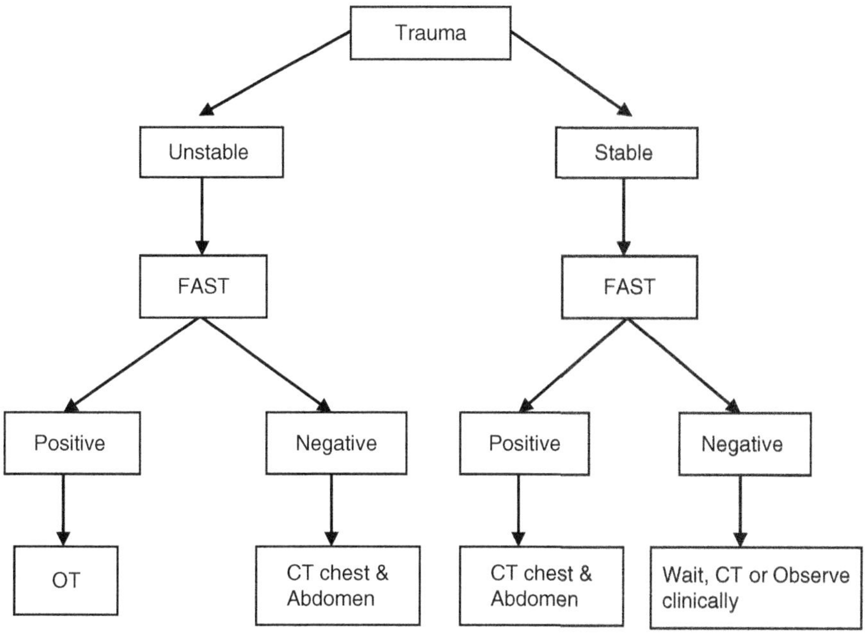


### 5.6.2 IVC Assessment for Fluid Responsiveness in Trauma

The patient is positioned supine. A subcostal view of the heart is obtained, then the USG pointer should be directed toward the patient's left flank. Once the right atrium is identified, turn the probe 90 degrees counterclockwise. The pointer should be now directed toward the patient's head (Fig. 5.11). The IVC is identified as it enters the right atrium. Put ultrasound on M mode (Fig. 5.12). Place the M mode cursor across the IVC approximately 2 cm inferior to the junction with the right atrium and measure the IVC diameter.

In spontaneously breathing patients, the patient is likely to be fluid responsive if:

- IVC measuring <2 cm in diameter coupled with IVC collapse>50% with each breath or
- IVC collapsibility >12%
- IVC collapsibility = (max diameter − min diameter)/(max diameter) × 100
- In mechanically ventilated patients who are passive on the ventilator, if the IVC distensibility>18%, the patient is likely to be fluid responsive.
- IVC distensibility = (max diameter − min diameter)/(min diameter) × 100

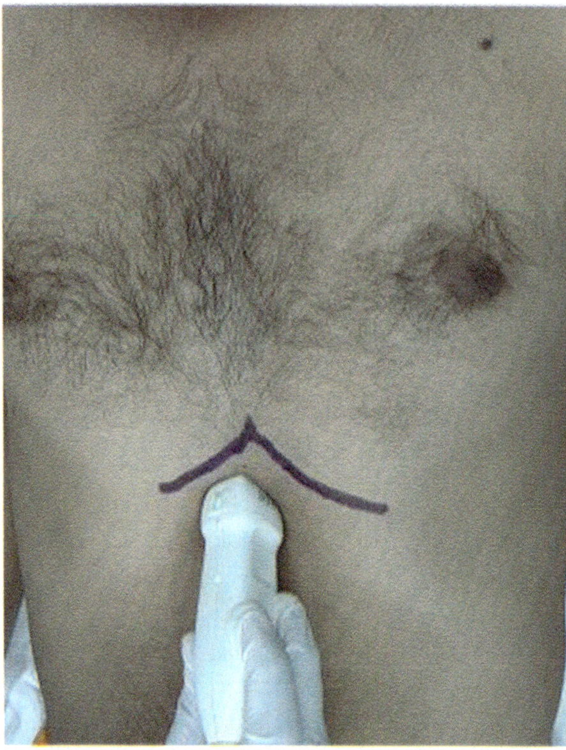

**Fig. 5.11** Probe position for IVC

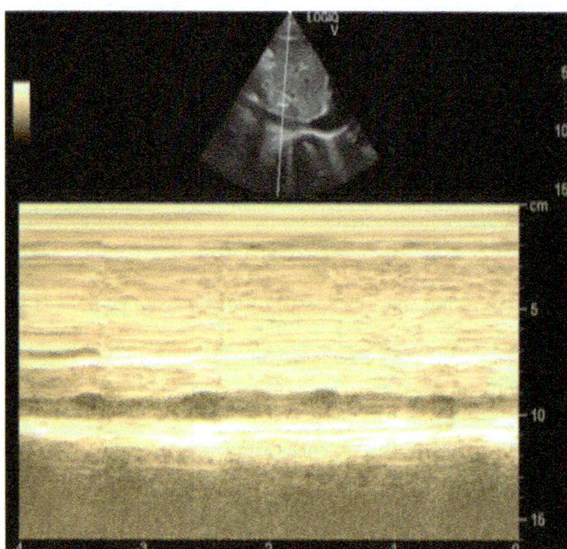


**Fig. 5.12** IVC measurement on M mode

## 5.7 Lung USG in Neurogenic Pulmonary Edema

**Neurogenic Pulmonary Edema (NPE)** It is an acute life-threatening condition seen in central nervous system injury. It usually appears within minutes to hours after injury and has a high mortality rate if not treated appropriately [22]. Bedside lung ultrasound can give information on lung status in neurocritically ill patients with acute respiratory failure. In normally aerated lungs, the ultrasound beam finds the lung air and no image is seen because no acoustic mismatch occurs to reflect the beam [23]. Figure 5.13 shows the probe placement for lung ultrasound. The only detectable structure is the pleura, seen as a hyperechoic horizontal line which moves synchronously with respiration (Fig. 5.14). When the air content decreases, as in pulmonary edema, the acoustic mismatch needed to reflect the ultrasound beam is created, and some images are seen. In the presence of extravascular lung water as in pulmonary edema, the ultrasound beam finds thickened subpleural interlobular septa. This reflected beam creates some comet-tail reverberation artifacts called B lines or comet tails (Fig. 5.15). Lung ultrasound has the potential to become a reference tool for bedside dynamic respiratory monitoring in ICU.

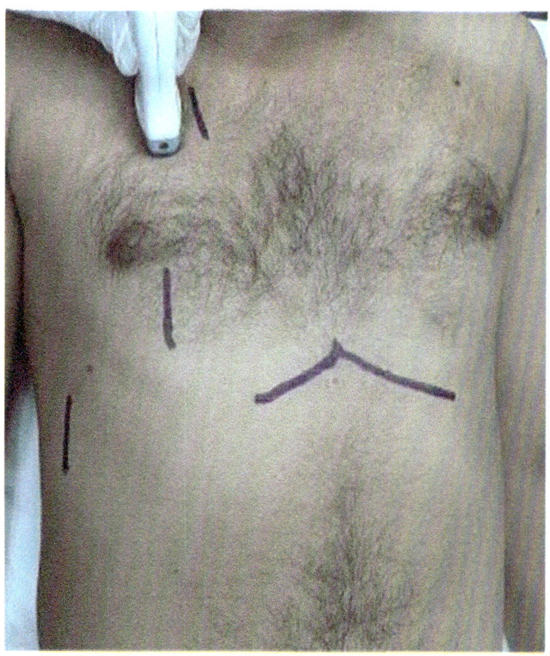

**Fig. 5.13** Probe position for lung USG

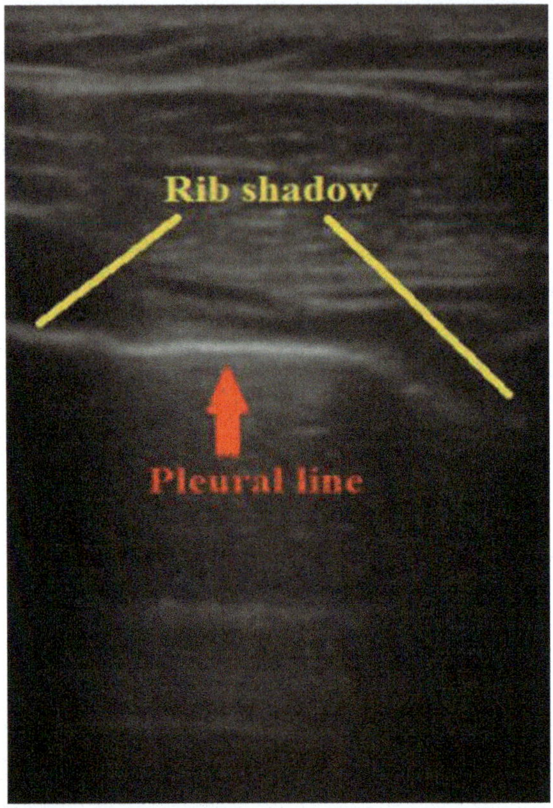


**Fig. 5.14** Normal lung USG showing rib shadow and pleural line

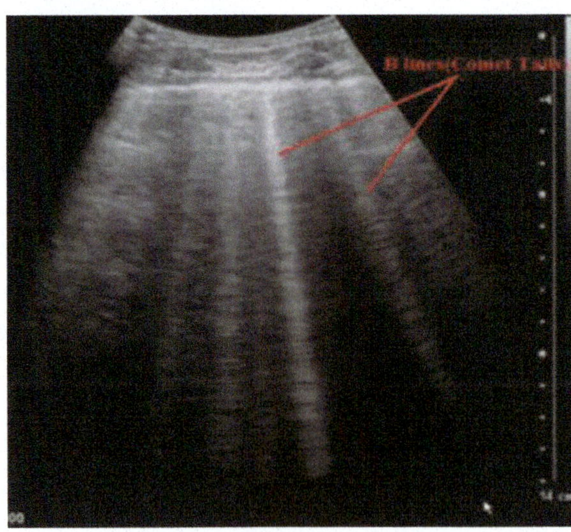

**Fig. 5.15** Lung USG showing B lines in neurogenic pulmonary edema

## 5.8 Role of USG in Stroke

Transcranial ultrasound Doppler can be used for assessment of cerebral vasculature. The use of transcranial Doppler ultrasound in stroke are—detection of site and degree of occlusion of cerebral vasculature, monitoring of recanalization of vessels with thrombolysis, detection of micro emboli, right to left shunts, monitoring during carotid revascularization procedures, and detection of degree of vasospasm after subarachnoid hemorrhage.

### 5.8.1 TCD in Acute Ischemic Stroke

TCD has a specificity of 90% in demonstrating MCA occlusions in patients with acute MCA stroke within 5 h. Alexandrov et al. [24] have shown major arterial occlusions in 69% of patients with acute hemispheric stroke, who may be eligible for thrombolytic treatment. TCD can diagnose vessel occlusion and can also be used for assessment of recanalization following thrombolytic treatment (Table 5.5

**Table 5.5** Thrombolysis in Brain Ischemia (TIBI) grading in stroke on TCD

| TIBI flow grade | Definition | Example |
|---|---|---|
| Grade 0 Absent flow | Absent flow signals are defined by the lack of regular pulsatile flow signal despite varying degrees of background noise | 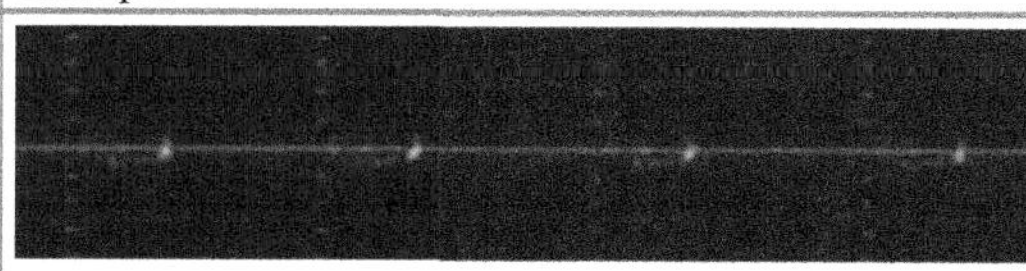 |
| Grade 1 Minimal flow | – Systolic spikes of variable velocity and duration<br>– Absent diastolic flow during all cardiac cycles<br>– Reverberating flow | 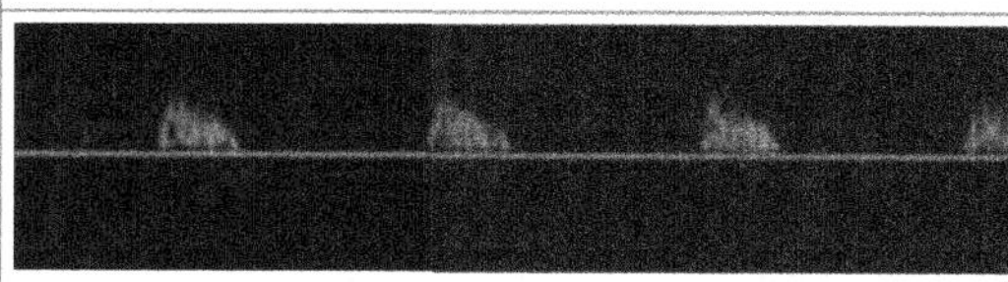 |
| Grade 2 Blunted flow | – Flattened systolic flow acceleration of variable duration compared to control<br>– Positive end diastolic velocity and pulsatility index <1.2 | 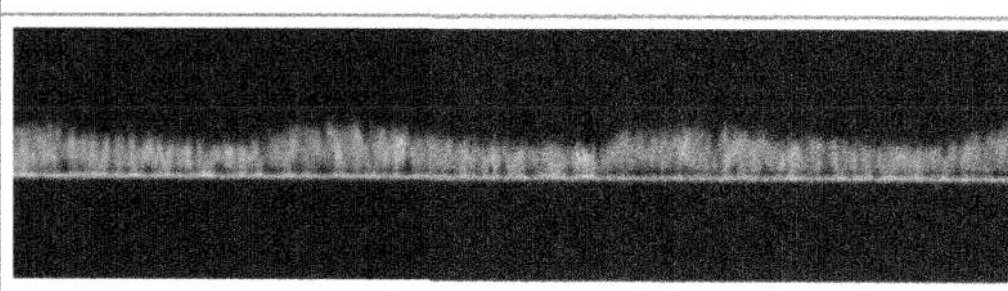 |

(continued)

**Table 5.5** (continued)

| TIBI flow grade | Definition | Example |
|---|---|---|
| Grade 3 Dampened flow | – Normal systolic flow acceleration<br>– Positive end diastolic velocity<br>– Decreased mean flow velocities by 30% compared to control | 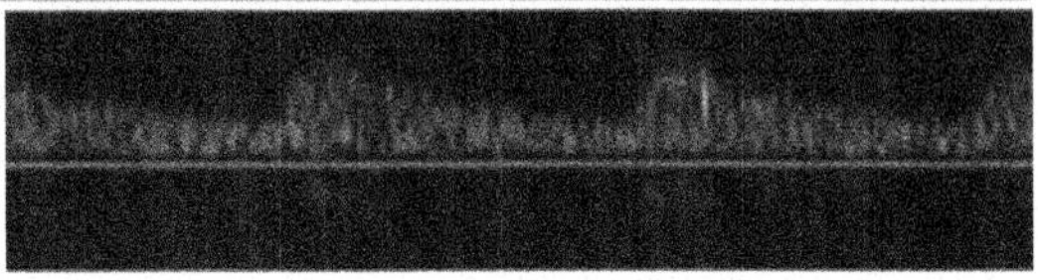 |
| Grade 4 Stenotic flow | – MFV of >80 cm/s and velocity difference of > 30% compared to the control side or<br>– If both affected and comparison sides have MFV <80 cm/s due to low end diastolic velocity, MFV >30% compared to the control side and signs turbulence |  |
| Grade 5 Normal flow | – <30% mean velocity difference compared to control<br>– Similar waveform shapes compared to control | 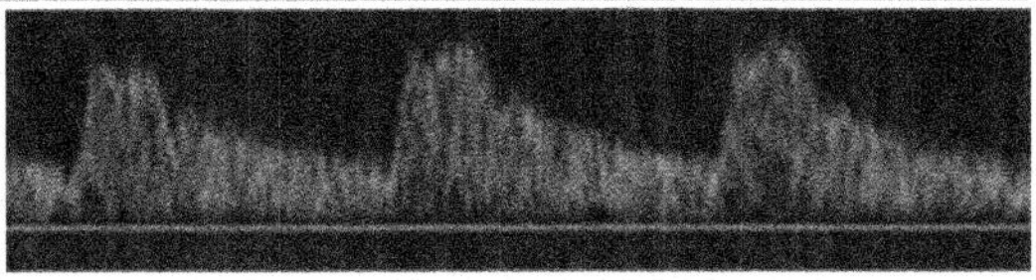 |

[25]). TCD can also be used for risk stratification and prognostication in stroke patients. A normal TCD at 6 h post ischemic stroke is an independent predictor of early improvement [26, 27]. In acute MCA stroke, blood flow velocity on TCD of <30 cm/s within 12 h after stroke correlated with poor recovery [28]. In patients with stroke of arterial origin micro emboli are predictors of early recurrence [29].

TCD can be used for diagnosis of cerebral hyperperfusion syndrome which can occur after carotid endarterectomy or stenting. An increase in peak blood flow velocity or pulsatility index of 100% in the ipsilateral middle cerebral artery detected by TCD is an early way to predict intracerebral hemorrhage [30]. Immediate corrective measures can be taken to prevent further damage.

## 5.9 Summary

- USG has successfully moved from radiology department to Emergency and Intensive Care Units and has become part and parcel of Neurocritical care.

- It has a wide variety of applications in neurologically ill patients with real-time point of care information at the bedside.
- USG has developed into an invaluable tool providing valuable clinical information having a major impact on patient care providing immediate diagnostic information not assessable by clinical examination alone.

## Multiple Choice Questions

1. The linear probe used has the frequency in range of:
   (a) 2–5 HZ
   (b) 6–15 HZ
   (c) 1–5 HZ
   (d) 10–15 HZ
2. PI is defined as:
   (a) PSV-EDV/PSV
   (b) PSV-EDV/MFV
   (c) MFV-EDV/MFV
   (d) PSV-MFV/EDV
3. Severe vasospasm in TCD is defined as:
   (a) LR > 3
   (b) LR > 4
   (c) LR > 5
   (d) LR > 6
4. FAST and EFAST can identify all of the following except:
   (a) Hemothorax
   (b) Hemoperitoneum
   (c) Urinary bladder injury
   (d) Cervical spine injury
5. Cut-off value generally taken for raised ICP in ONSD examination is:
   (a) 3 mm
   (b) 4 mm
   (c) 5 mm
   (d) 7 mm
6. In spontaneously breathing patients, the patient is likely to be fluid responsive if—IVC measuring ---------- cm in diameter coupled with IVC collapse >--------% with each breath
   (a) 1.5, 35%
   (b) 2, 50%
   (c) 2.5, 50%
   (d) 2, 40%
7. TCD can be used to monitor all except?
   (a) Vasospasm after SAH
   (b) Non-invasive ICP monitoring
   (c) Stenosis or occlusion of intracranial vessels
   (d) Midline shift

8. All are windows used for insonation of intracranial blood circulation except?
   (a) Transtemporal
   (b) Transorbital
   (c) Transforaminal
   (d) Submandibular
9. All are indicators of raised ICP except?
   (a) Pulsatility index >1.2
   (b) Optic nerve sheath diameter >5 mm
   (c) High end systolic velocity and low end diastolic velocity on TCD
   (d) Lindegaard ratio = 1
10. Uses of USG in a trauma patient include all except?
   (a) Diagnosing pneumothorax
   (b) Diagnosing cardiac tamponade
   (c) Diagnosing pupillary asymmetry in a swollen raccoon eye
   (d) Measuring intracranial hematoma volume

Answers: 1. (b), 2. (b), 3. (d), 4. (d), 5. (c), 6. (b), 7. (d), 8. (d), 9. (d), 10. (d)

## References


1. Frazzetta G, Faraci C, Mancuso SI, Fragati G, DiGiovani S, Costanzo L. Emergency ultrasound in critical patients: the "bedside ultrasonography" as the "third hand" of emergency surgeon. Austin J Emerg Crit Care Med. 2015;2:1–4.
2. Carovac A, Smajlovic F, Junuzovic D. Application of ultrasound in medicine. Acta Inform Med. 2011;19:168.
3. Ramsingh D, Gatling J. Teaching point-of-care ultrasound (POCUS) to the perioperative physician. In: Bowe EA, Schell RM, DiLorenzo AN, editors. Education in anesthesia: how to deliver the best learning experience. Cambridge: Cambridge University Press; 2018. p. 131–50.
4. Tayal VS, Neulander M, Norton HJ, Foster T, Saunders T, Blaivas M. Emergency department sonographic measurement of optic nerve sheath diameter to detect findings of increased intracranial pressure in adult head injury patients. Ann Emerg Med. 2007;49:508–14.
5. Ochoa-Pérez L, Cardozo-Ocampo A. Ultrasound applications in the central nervous system for neuroanaesthesia and neurocritical care. Rev Colomb Anestesiol. 2015;43:314–20.
6. Bäuerle J, Lochner P, Kaps M, Nedelmann M. Intra-and interobsever reliability of sonographic assessment of the optic nerve sheath diameter in healthy adults. J Neuroimaging. 2012;22:42–5.
7. Fledelius HC. Ultrasound in ophthalmology. Ultrasound Med Biol. 1997;23:365–75.
8. Dubourg J, Javouhey E, Geeraerts T, Messerer M, Kassai B. Ultrasonography of optic nerve sheath diameter for detection of raised intracranial pressure: a systematic review and meta-analysis. Intensive Care Med. 2011;37:1059–68.
9. Qayyum H, Ramlakhan S. Can ocular ultrasound predict intracranial hypertension? A pilot diagnostic accuracy evaluation in a UK emergency department. Eur J Emerg Med. 2013;20:91–7.
10. Bellner J, Romner B, Reinstrup P, Kristiansson KA, Ryding E, Brandt L. Transcranial Doppler sonography pulsatility index (PI) reflects intracranial pressure (ICP). Surg Neurol. 2004;62:45–51.
11. Bouzat P, Francony G, Declety P, Genty C, Kaddour A, Bessou P, Brun J, Jacquot C, Chabardes S, Bosson JL, Payen JF. Transcranial Doppler to screen on admission patients with mild to moderate traumatic brain injury. Neurosurgery. 2011;68:1603–10.

12. Naqvi J, Yap KH, Ahmad G, Ghosh J. Transcranial Doppler ultrasound: a review of the physical principles and major applications in critical care. J Vasc Med. 2013;2013:629378.
13. Moppett IK, Mahajan RP. Transcranial Doppler ultrasonography in anaesthesia and intensive care. Br J Anaesth. 2004;93:710–24.
14. Nicoletto HA, Burkman MH. Transcranial Doppler series part II: performing a transcranial Doppler. Am J Electroneurodiagnostic Technol. 2009;49:14–27.
15. Bathala L, Mehndiratta MM, Sharma VK. Transcranial Doppler: technique and common findings (part 1). Ann Indian Acad Neurol. 2013;16:174.
16. Anand S, Goel G, Gupta V. Continuous intra-arterial dilatation with nimodipine and milrinone for refractory cerebral vasospasm. J Neurosurg Anesthesiol. 2014;26:92–3.
17. Chavez MA, Shams N, Ellington LE, Naithani N, Gilman RH, Steinhoff MC, Santosham M, Black RE, Price C, Gross M, Checkley W. Lung ultrasound for the diagnosis of pneumonia in adults: a systematic review and meta-analysis. Respir Res. 2014;15:50.
18. Alrajhi K, Woo MY, Vaillancourt C. Test characteristics of ultrasonography for the detection of pneumothorax: a systematic review and meta-analysis. Chest. 2012;141:703–8.
19. Soult MC, Weireter LJ, Britt RC, Collins JN, Novosel TJ, Reed SF, Britt LD. Can routine trauma bay chest x-ray be bypassed with an extended focused assessment with sonography for trauma examination? Am Surg. 2015;81:336–40.
20. Zanobetti M, Coppa A, Nazerian P, Grifoni S, Scorpiniti M, Innocenti F, Conti A, Bigiarini S, Gualtieri S, Casula C, Ticali PF. Chest abdominal-focused assessment sonography for trauma during the primary survey in the emergency department: the CA-FAST protocol. Eur J Trauma Emerg Surg. 2018;44:805–10.
21. Cohen HL, Langer J, McGahan JP, Bahner D, Blaivas M, Fox J, American Institute of Ultrasound in Medicine, et al. AIUM practice guideline for the performance of the focused assessment with sonography for trauma (FAST) examination. J Ultrasound Med. 2014;33:2047.
22. Merenkov VV, Kovalev AN, Gorbunov VV. Bedside lung ultrasound: a case of neurogenic pulmonary edema. Neurocrit Care. 2013;18:391–4.
23. Via G, Storti E, Gulati G, Neri L, Mojoli F, Braschi A. Lung ultrasound in the ICU: from diagnostic instrument to respiratory monitoring tool. Minerva Anestesiol. 2012;78:1282–96.
24. Alexandrov AV, Bladin CF, Norris JW. Intracranial blood flow velocities in acute ischemic stroke. Stroke. 1994;25:1378–83.
25. Malferrari G, Zedde M. Neurosonological evaluation of the acute stroke patients. In: Neuroimaging for clinicians-combining research and practice, vol. 14. London: Intech; 2011. p. 259–98.
26. Toni D, Fiorelli M, Zanette EM, Sacchetti ML, Salerno A, Argentino C, Solaro M, Fieschi C. Early spontaneous improvement and deterioration of ischemic stroke patients: a serial study with transcranial Doppler ultrasonography. Stroke. 1998;29:1144–8.
27. Alexandrov AV, Black SE, Ehrlich LE, Caldwell CB, Norris JW. Predictors of hemorrhagic transformation occurring spontaneously and on anticoagulants in patients with acute ischemic stroke. Stroke. 1997;28:1198–202.
28. Halsey JH Jr. Prognosis of acute hemiplegia estimated by transcranial Doppler ultrasonography. Stroke. 1988;19:648–9.
29. Valton L, Larrue V, le Traon AP, Massabuau P, Géraud G. Microembolic signals and risk of early recurrence in patients with stroke or transient ischemic attack. Stroke. 1998;29:2125–8.
30. Jansen C, Sprengers AM, Moll FL, Vermeulen FE, Hamerlijnck RP, Van Gijn J, Ackerstaff RG. Prediction of intracerebral haemorrhage after carotid endarterectomy by clinical criteria and intraoperative transcranial Doppler monitoring: results of 233 operations. Eur J Vasc Surg. 1994;8:220–5.

# Basics of Neuroradiology

# 6

Zulfiqar Ali and Nidhi Gupta

**Key Points**

- CT and MRI are the most widely used investigations to confirm or refute a neurological diagnosis
- An image on a CT is produced when a highly collimated X-ray beam passes through a patient
- The degree to which photons are absorbed or scattered depends on the density of the tissue
- Contrast agents may be used to enhance attenuation of the X-ray beams
- Renal function should be assessed before administration of contrast agents because they are excreted by kidneys
- CT calculates tissue density in terms of voxels. The density of a voxel is expressed in Hounsefield units
- Water has been assigned a Hounsefield unit of zero whereas air has been assigned a Hounsefield unit of −1000
- Acute clotted blood is hyperdense while chronic clotted blood is hypodense

Z. Ali (✉)
Sheri Kashmir Institute of Medical Sciences (SKIMS), Srinagar, Jammu and Kashmir, India

N. Gupta
Indraprastha Apollo Hospitals, New Delhi, India


P. U. Bidkar, P. Vanamoorthy (eds.), *Acute Neuro Care*,
https://doi.org/10.1007/978-981-15-4071-4_6

## 6.1 Introduction

Neuroradiology is an essential tool in the management of patients with neurological and neurosurgical disorders. This chapter will aim to acquaint the reader to understand how images are formed on computed tomography (CT) and magnetic resonance imaging (MRI) along with a review of the relevant neuroanatomy. This understanding will be helpful to the reader in the interpretation of images and diagnosis of various neurological disorders.

## 6.2 Basic Principles of CT Imaging

An image on a CT is produced when a highly collimated X-ray beam passes through a patient. In a CT scan, the image is produced by firing of X-rays at a moving object. This image is then detected by an array of rotating detectors and processed on a computer to produce a series of cross-sectional images. The different types of tissues absorb or scatter the photons depending upon the tissue density. Dense structures as bone absorb more photons and appear white, while less-dense structures appear black as they absorb a smaller number of photons [1]. The tissues in the body are made of minute millions and millions of small cubes. CT calculates the density of these tissues in terms of voxels (voxel constitutes a notional three-dimensional space and is a 3-dimensional equivalent of a pixel) [2]. The density of a voxel (or a cube) in the body can be determined by a scale termed as the Hounsfield unit scale. Practically Hounsfield units range from −1000 (least dense) to +1000 (most dense). By convention pure water has been assigned a value of Zero Hounsfield units and air has been assigned a value of −1000 [3]. The Hounsfield units of various tissues are summarised in Table 6.1.

**CT Contrast Agents:** The iodinated intravenous contrast agents increase the attenuation of X-ray beams and thus contrast-enhancing structures have a higher density on images. The newer non-ionic intravenous contrasts have a lower osmolality and fewer idiosyncratic reactions [4]. As the contrast agents are excreted by the kidneys, renal function should be assessed before giving the contrast agent to prevent acute renal injury.

**Table 6.1** Hounsfield units of various tissues, air and pure water

| | |
|---|---|
| Air | −1000 |
| Fat | −70 |
| Pure water | 0 |
| Cerebrospinal fluid | +8 |
| White matter | +30 |
| Grey matter | +45 |
| Blood | +70 |
| Bone/calcification | +1000 |

**CT Angiography:** In CT angiography a thin-section CT imaging of cranium is done after intravenous administration of a contrast agent. These images are processed to visualize CT angiographic images, for the detection of aneurysms, vascular malformations, vascular stenosis, and dissections.

**CT Perfusion:** After administration of intravenous contrast injection, imaging of the brain is done sequentially over time to determine the density of each voxel of the brain as the contrast enters and leaves the brain. The various maps that are created by CT perfusion are a) time to peak (TTP), b) mean transit time (MTT), c) cerebral blood flow (CBF), d) and cerebral blood volume (CBV) [5]. A simple way to analyze the data in the setting of acute stroke is to look at the TTP and MTT maps first. If TTP and MTP are symmetric and normal, there are no infarctions or no tissue is at risk. However, if there is a vascular territory that has delayed TTP or prolonged MTT, with an area of significantly decreased CBV, this corresponds to dead tissue in the infarcted core. However, if there is a normal CBV with a decreased CBF, this tissue is oligaemic and at risk for infarction but is potentially salvageable. The data from CT perfusion may act as a guide for thrombolysis in acute cerebral infarction [5].

**Windowing:** Windowing is a technique used to enhance contrast for a particular tissue or an abnormality that is being evaluated. Window settings are described mainly by two terms, (a) window width (WW) (b) and window level (WL) [6]. WW shows the range of HU displayed and WL denotes the HU in the center of the window width. Altering the window settings helps to maximize the pickup rate of different pathologies.

**Normal CT Scan:** A modern helical CT scanning technique comprises a rotating X-ray tube and an array of detectors. The detected X-rays are then converted into a computerized signal which is used to produce a series of cross-sectional images on a grey-white scale. The raw data can be reconstructed into different imaging planes, i.e. axial, sagittal, and coronal planes. Head CTs are performed at an angle parallel to the base of the skull. Slice thickness may vary, but in general, it is between 5 and 10 mm for a routine Head CT. Once we are interpreting the CT image, the right side of the image is the left side of the patient's anatomy and vice versa.

**Basic CT Anatomy:** The *orbitomeatal line (canthomeatal line)* was traditionally used to obtain the initial axial plane for CT of the brain. It was defined as a plane running from the outer canthus of the eye to the midpoint of the external auditory meatus [7]. With the introduction of volumetric scans, the whole head is scanned and then axial images are reconstructed at any desired angle. Many centers have now switched over to AC-PC line which is defined as a line passing through the superior edge of the anterior commissure (AC) and the inferior edge of the posterior commissure (PC).

On an axial CT scan (Fig. 6.1) we can see the right and left hemispheres separated by the falx—an invagination of the dura. The supratentorial and infratentorial compartments are separated by the tentorium. The main areas of interest are at the level of lateral ventricles, at the level of the third ventricle, at the level of the fourth ventricle, and at the level of the spinal cord. (Fig. 6.2) Supratentorial cuts (in an axial section) show the lateral ventricles (Fig. 6.2) (anterior and posterior horns) and the slit-shaped third ventricle (Fig. 6.2). The anterior (Fig. 6.3) and posterior limb (Fig. 6.3) of the internal capsule help in delineation of the caudate nucleus (Fig. 6.3) (which appears embedded in the anterior horns of lateral ventricles), globus pallidus (Fig. 6.3) and putamen (Fig. 6.3) (which lies lateral to the limbs of the internal capsule) [8].

Infratentorial cuts are visualized above the level of the foramen magnum and at the level of the fourth ventricle. In the infratentorial cuts the right and left cerebellum

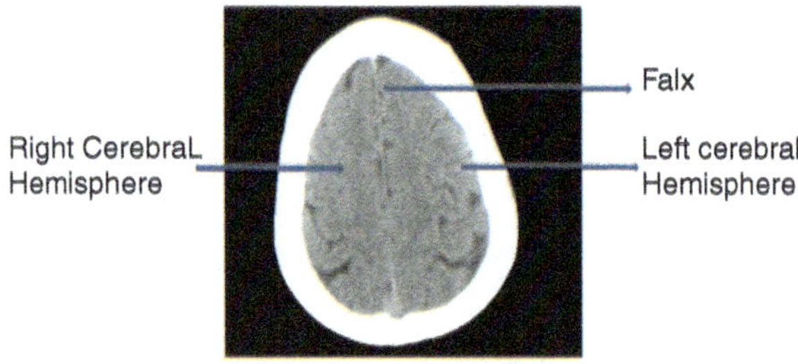


**Fig. 6.1** Right and left cerebral hemisphere along with falx in the midline

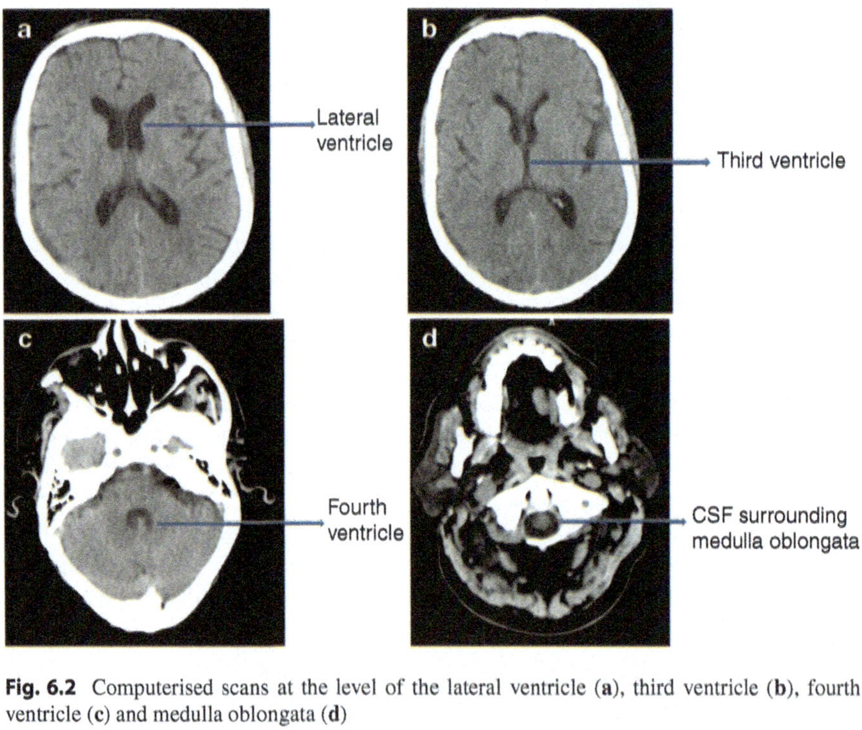


**Fig. 6.2** Computerised scans at the level of the lateral ventricle (**a**), third ventricle (**b**), fourth ventricle (**c**) and medulla oblongata (**d**)

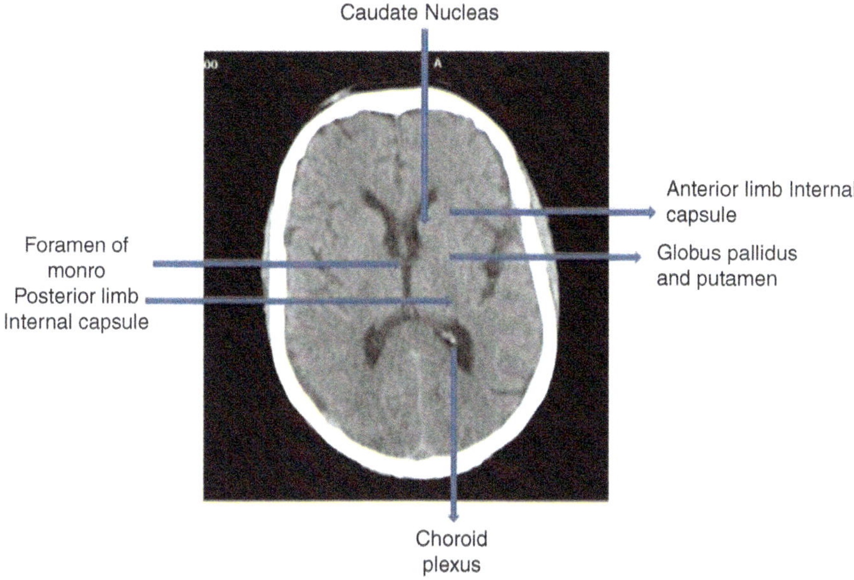


**Fig. 6.3** Computerised scans showing the internal capsule along with other associated anatomical structures

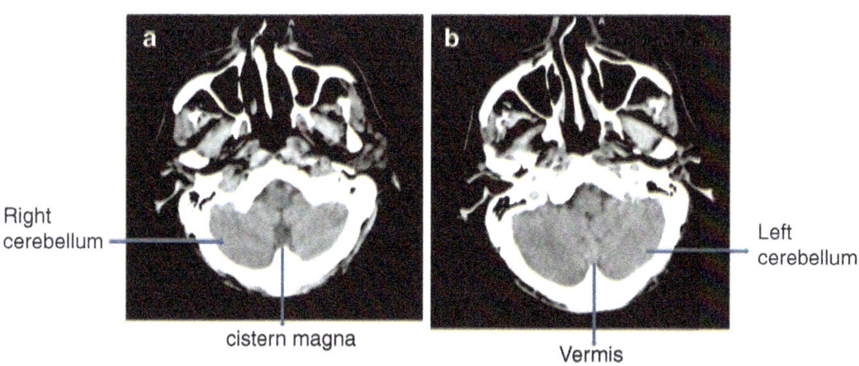


**Fig. 6.4** (a) Right cerebellum along with cisterna magna. (b) Left cerebellum along with vermis

with vermis (Fig. 6.4) (in the midline) pons (Fig. 6.4) and cisterna magna are infratentorial. The cerebellar tonsils are seen inferiorly. The brain stem is separated superiorly to inferiorly into midbrain, pons, and medulla. On an axial CT scan of the brain, the midbrain resembles a Mickey-Mouse—where ears of Mickey-Mouse represent the cerebral peduncles. As we move inferiorly, we see the pons, medulla, spinal cord, and the foramen magnum. In a normal axial image, the cerebrospinal fluid spaces can be seen around the spinal cord (Fig. 6.2d), with no crowding of the cerebral tonsils.

The Sylvian fissure (Fig. 6.5) separates the frontal and parietal lobes (Fig. 6.5) above from the temporal lobe below. Similarly, the central sulcus (Fig. 6.6) separates the anterior frontal lobe from the posterior parietal lobe. The central sulcus looks like

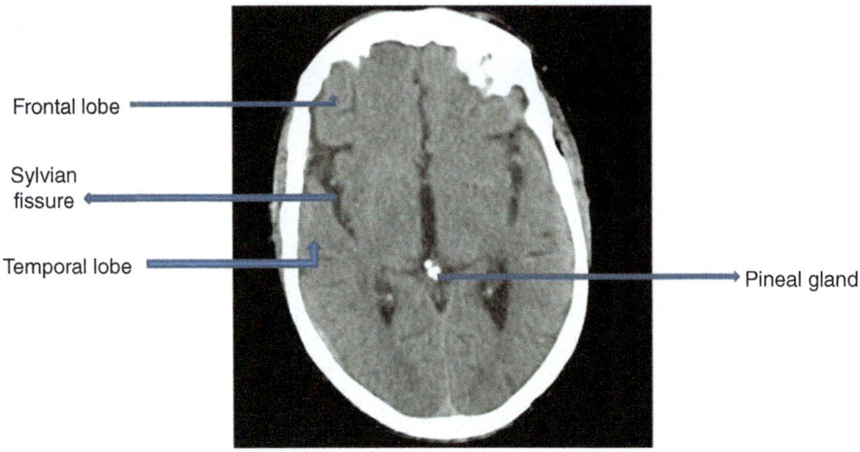


**Fig. 6.5** Computerised scans showing frontal lobe and temporal lobe separated by Sylvian fissure. Pineal gland is the central hyperdense structure in the middle

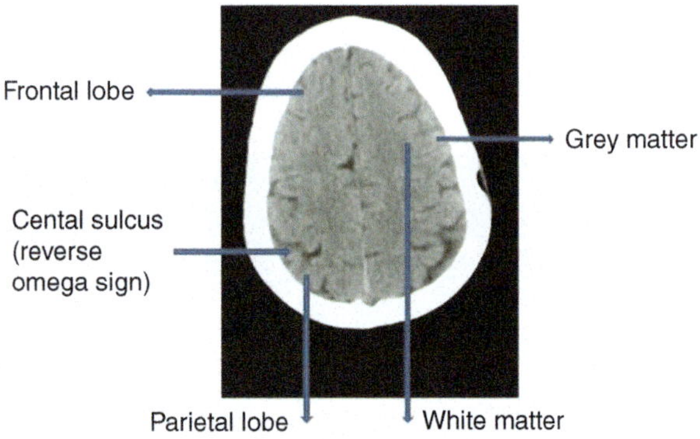


**Fig. 6.6** Supratentorial cut of a computerised scan showing the frontal and parietal lobe separated by a central sulcus. Grey white matter differentiation can be clearly seen

a reverse omega sign. (Fig. 6.6) Within the notch of the omega sign lies the motor control area of the hand. The area in front of central sulcus forms the precentral gyrus (motor area) and the area behind is the postcentral gyrus (sensory control).

**Grey and White Matter Structures:** Each of the lobes has an outer portion made of grey matter (Fig. 6.6) called cortex. The deep grey matter (Fig. 6.3) structures of importance are the caudate nucleus, the globus pallidus, and putamen and the thalamus. The white matter structures (Fig. 6.8) that are of importance are the internal capsule, the external capsule, the corona radiate, and the centrum semiovale [9].

**Cerebrospinal Spaces:** Cerebrospinal fluid is formed in the choroid plexus in the lateral ventricles. It flows from lateral ventricles into the third ventricle by foramen of Monro (Fig. 6.3), through cerebral aqueduct into the fourth ventricle, flows into the subarachnoid spaces through the foramen of Luschka and foramen of Magendie.

On an axial section of a computerized scan the third ventricle looks like a median cleft between the two thalami and the hypothalamus. Its anterior wall is formed by the lamina terminalis, and posteriorly there is the pineal recess (Fig. 6.5). Any blockage of the cerebrospinal fluid system will cause dilatation of the ventricular system-hydrocephalus. In a normal brain, the ventricles and subarachnoid spaces are seen clearly. The ventricles or subarachnoid spaces are neither dilated nor effaced. In brain atrophy, both ventricles and subarachnoid spaces are dilated. In brain edema all cerebrospinal fluid spaces are effaced while in hydrocephalus the ventricles are dilated but the subarachnoid spaces are effaced (Fig. 6.9).

**Basal Cisterns:** Basal cisterns are the cerebrospinal fluid pools that sit at the bottom of the brain. The important cisterns are in front of the pons (prepontine cisterns), above the sella turcica (suprasellar cistern), on the sides of midbrain lies the ambient cistern (Fig. 6.7) and posteriorly the quadrigeminal cistern (behind the mid brain) is seen (Figs. 6.8 and 6.9).

The basic conceptual approach to identify the main pathologies in neurocritical care involves (a) to rule out bleed, (b) rule out stroke, (c) soft tissues or fractures and) to identify mass effect or herniation pattern.

Acutely clotted blood once present on the brain appears to be denser (high Hounsfield unit) than other structures like brain parenchyma. Hence it appears hyperdense (bright in color). An epidural hematoma (Fig. 6.10) appears as a biconvex structure [10] (as a lens). It does not cross the suture lines. A subdural hematoma (Fig. 6.10) is cresenteric. It may cross the sutures but generally, it may not cross the midline. A subarachnoid hemorrhage (Fig. 6.11) appears as a hyperdensity in the subarachnoid spaces. CT has a very high (>95%) sensitivity for identifying a subarachnoid hemorrhage within the first 12 h. This sensitivity declines progressively with time. An intraparenchymal hemorrhage (Fig. 6.11) may appear as hyperdense blood in the parenchyma itself. An acutely clotted blood has a high density. It has a Hounsfield value of +80. However, as the age of blood progresses over time, its density decreases

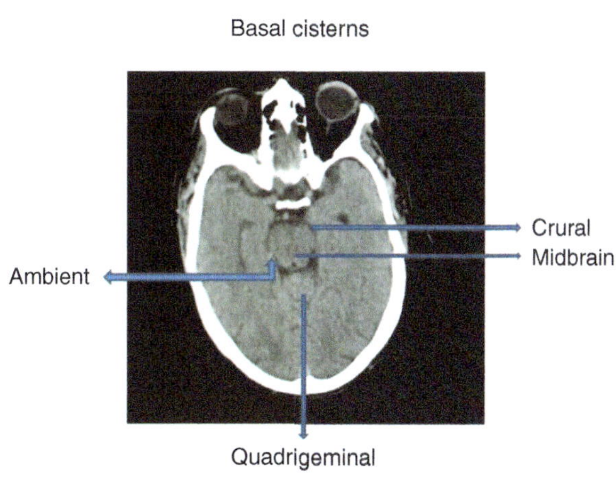


**Fig. 6.7** Computerised scan showing the midbrain and the surrounding crural ambient and quadrigeminal cisterns

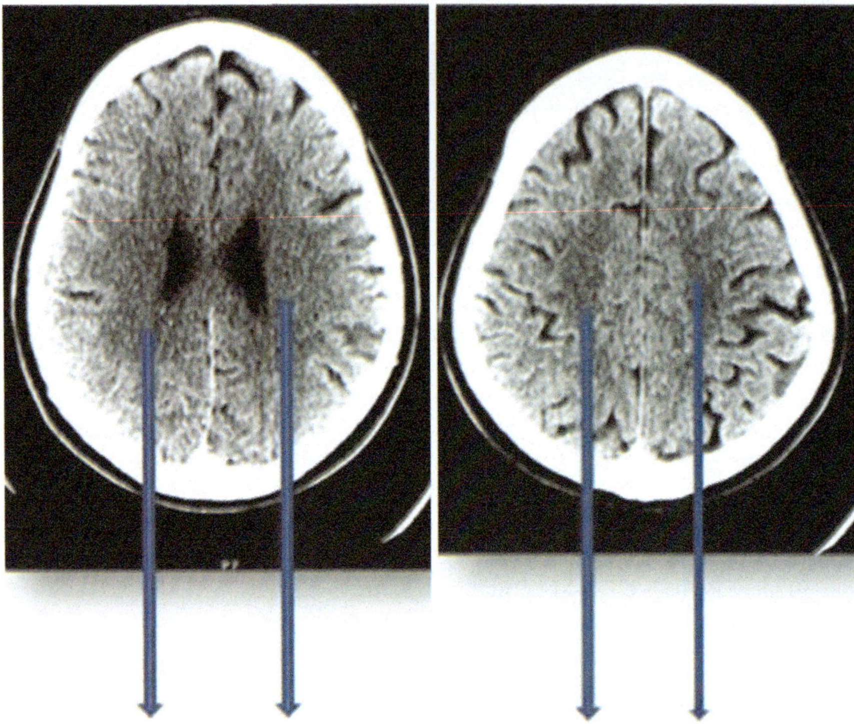


**Fig. 6.8** Computerised scan showing the deep grey matter structures: Corona radiate and centrum semiovale

over time, as the blood products break down. An acute SDH may be hyperdense to the brain up to 1 week, and subacute SDH (Fig. 6.12) may be isodense to brain in around 1–3 weeks while a chronic SDH (Fig. 6.12) may be hypodense beyond 3–4 weeks [11]. Hyperacute blood has a lower density when compared to acutely clotted blood. Hence, in an ongoing bleed with an extradural hematoma, the hyperdense bleed may have multiple hypodense spots that signify the ongoing hemorrhage (hyperacute blood). There are other structures which are hyperdense in the brain. There a Choroid plexus (Fig. 6.3) is often calcified in the lateral ventricles. The pineal gland (Fig. 6.5) in midline may be commonly calcified. Globus pallidus and dentate nucleus may be calcified with a hyperdense appearance on CT. In trauma, a skull vault fracture (Fig. 6.13) is reviewed on bone windows. A locule of air within the subcutaneous tissue may be a clue to the overlying bony discontinuity.

**Ischaemic Stroke:** The *first thing* to look for in stroke is the hyperdense vessel sign [12]. As acute clot is white in appearance on computerized tomography, called hyperdense sign (Fig. 6.14) in the vascular territory involved. In the hyperacute phase (i.e. <3 h from symptom onset), changes occurring within the brain parenchyma at the cellular level may not be depicted on a CT scan [13, 14].

The *second thing* that develops is the loss of grey-white matter differentiation (Fig. 6.14) "loss of the insular ribbon sign" [15]. This implies the loss of the normal grey white matter differentiation in the insular cortex of the affected side. Normally the grey-white is slightly denser than the white matter. In an acute ischemic stroke the cells distal to occlusion are deprived of the blood supply. As a result, they cannot function normally. They do not make ATP and their sodium-potassium ATPase stops working. This results in the swelling of the cells distal to the occlusion with an increase in water content—cytotoxic edema. As water is less dense so that density of the grey matter in the infarcted area reduces and looks similar to the white matter. In the *third stage*, the infarcted tissue decreases in density over time. The mass effect is maximum 3–5 days over time. Lastly in the chronic phase, all strokes will result in a negative mass effect often resulting in a dilatation of the ipsilateral ventricle-ex-vacuo dilatation (Fig. 6.14). The various types of vascular territory infarcts are shown in Fig. 6.15. The anterior cerebral artery infarct is seen in the form of a strip pattern while the middle cerebral artery infarct covers a wider area as middle cerebral artery supplies blood to more than eighty percent of the brain.

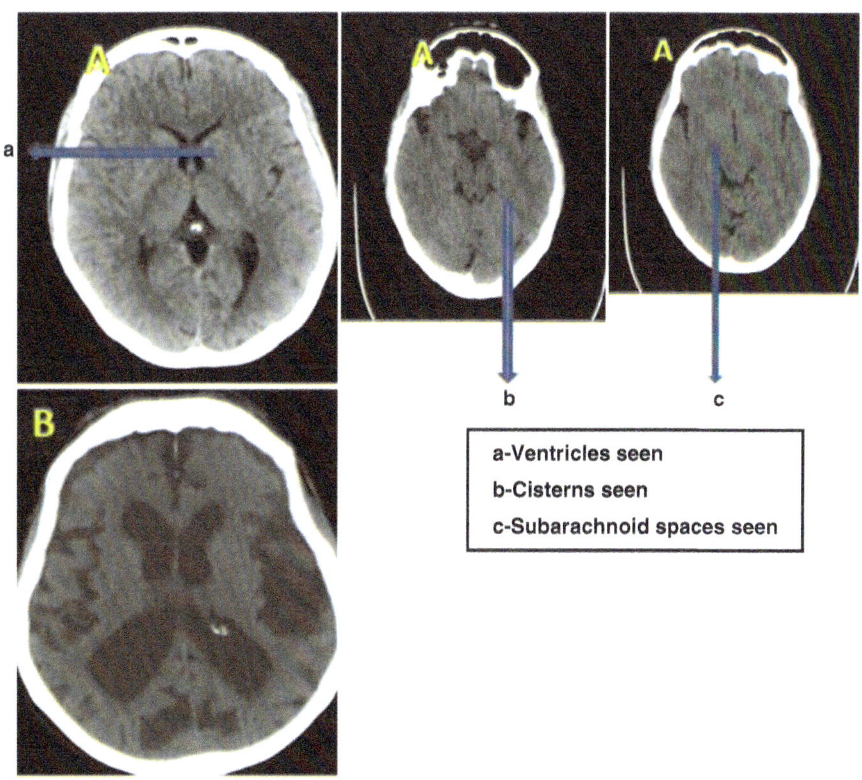


**Fig. 6.9** Computerised scan showing the cerebrospinal fluid system in a normal scan and various pathologies. (**a**) Normal: All CSF spaces are visible neither effaced nor dilated. (**b**) Atrophy: All CSF spaces are dilated. (**c**) Hydrocephalus: The ventricles are dilated while the subarachnoid spaces are effaced. (**d**) Edema: All CSF spaces are effaced

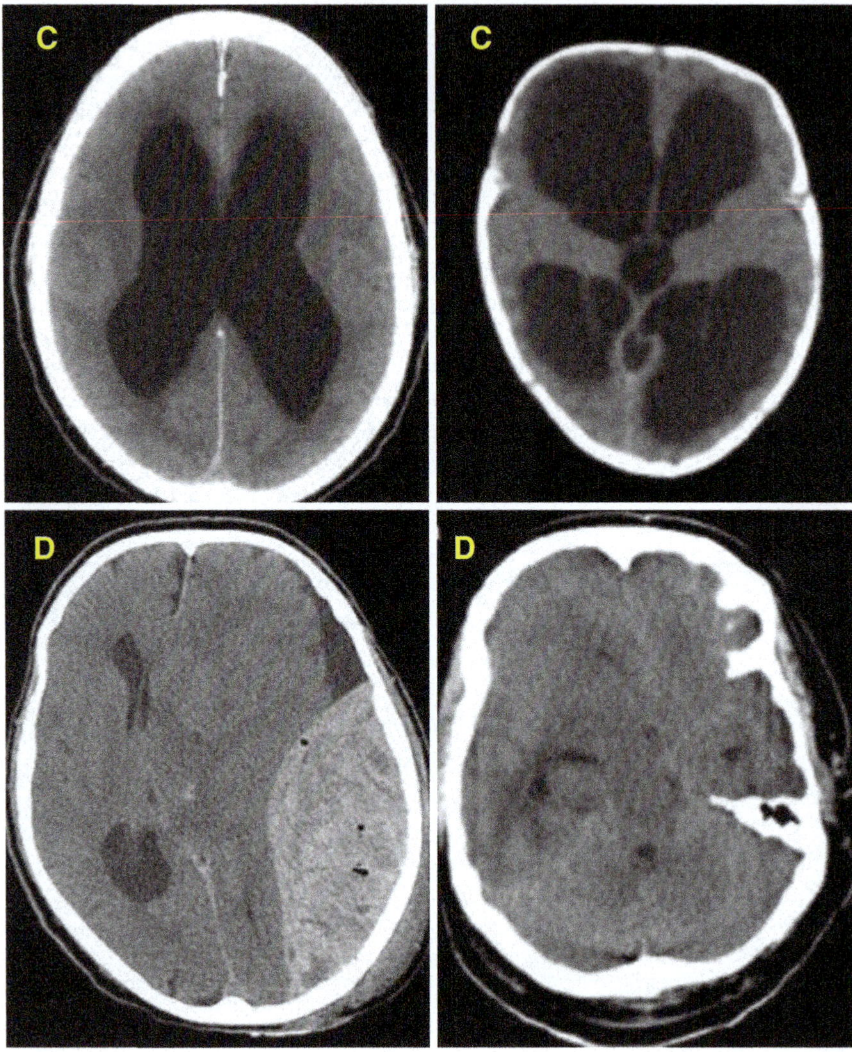


**Fig. 6.9** (continued)

**Mass Effect and Herniation Patterns:** The *first step* to detect the mass effect is to look for sulcal effacement. If we find that sulcal effacement is present, this signifies that something is causing the mass effect. *Secondly*, we look for the midline shift. We look for the midline shift by drawing a line from the falx anteriorly to the falx posteriorly (line a). Then we measure the distance from that line to a midline structure, most commonly the septum pellucidum (line b) (Fig. 6.16).

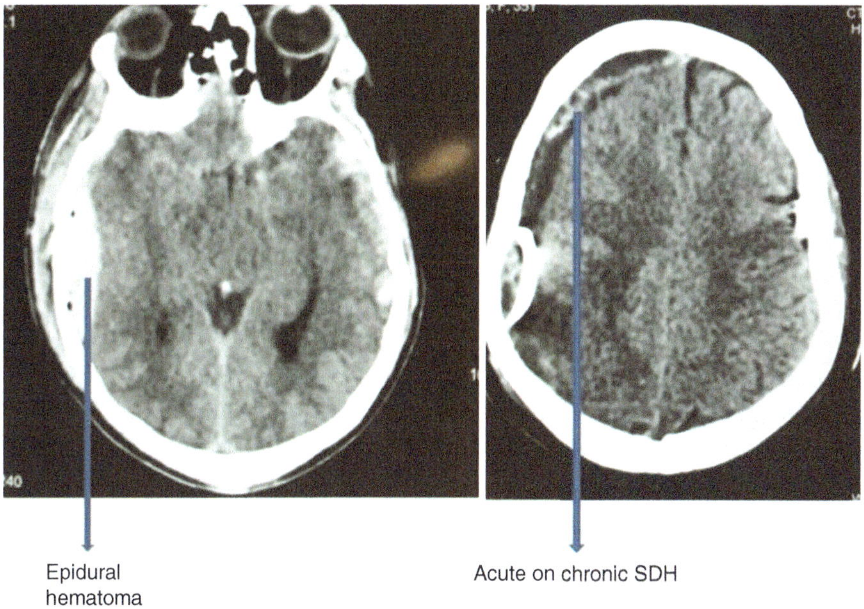


**Fig. 6.10** A computerised scan with (left) hyperdense biconvex opacity showing an extradural haematoma and (right) hypodense and hyperdense lesion (acute on chronic) SDH in the frontoparietal region

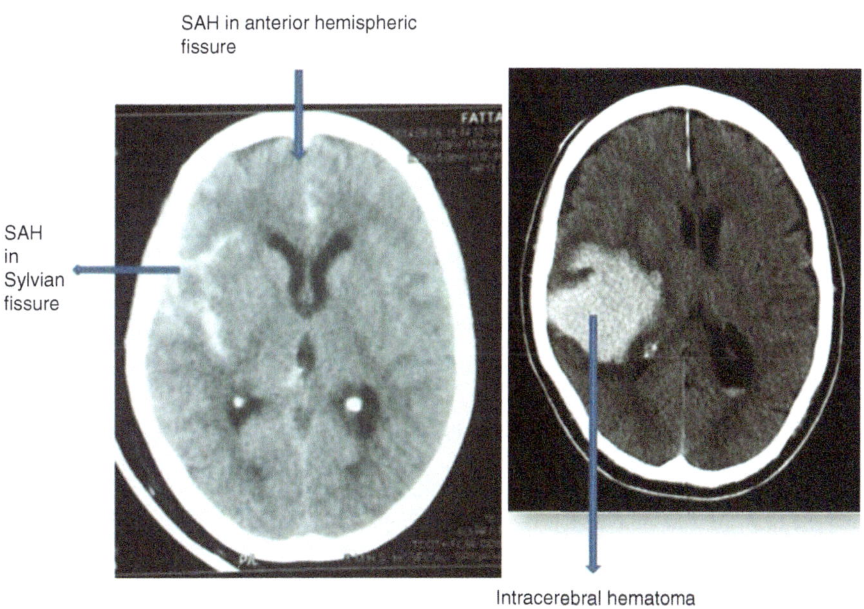


**Fig. 6.11** A computerised scan with (left) hyperdense opacity in the anterior hemispheric fissure and the Sylvian fissure—(SAH) and (right) hyperdense lesion (intracerebral haematoma)

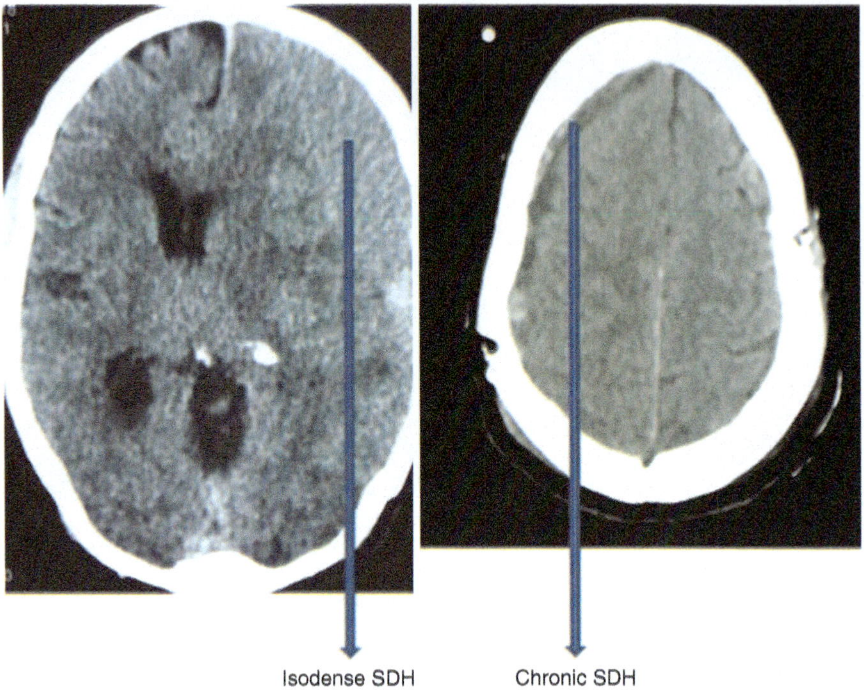


**Fig. 6.12** A computerised scan with (left) isodense opacity (subacute SDH) in the left frontal region and (right) hypodense opacity in the right frontoparietal region (chronic SDH)

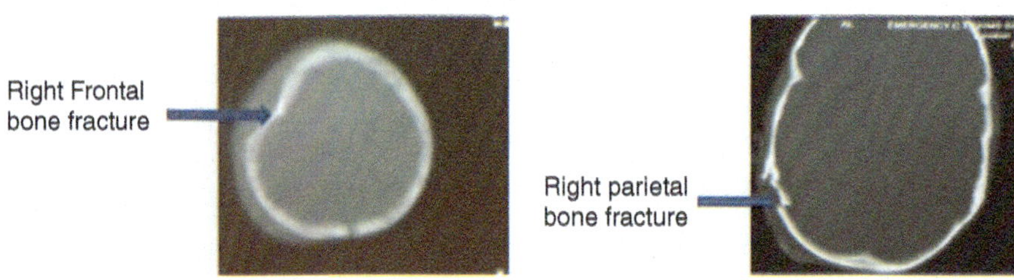


**Fig. 6.13** A computerised scan (bone window) with (left) right frontal bone fracture and (right) right parietal bone fracture

The basic *herniation syndromes* to be detected are as follows [16]:

(a) **Subfalcine herniation:** It is the displacement of the brain under the free edge of the falx. Whenever we have a midline shift a subfalcine herniation will be present (Fig. 6.16).
(b) **Uncal herniation:** Is identified by suprasellar cistern. After identifying the suprasellar cistern we identify the uncus. In uncal herniation, there is displacement of the uncus towards the contralateral side with effacement of the suprasellar cistern (Fig. 6.17).

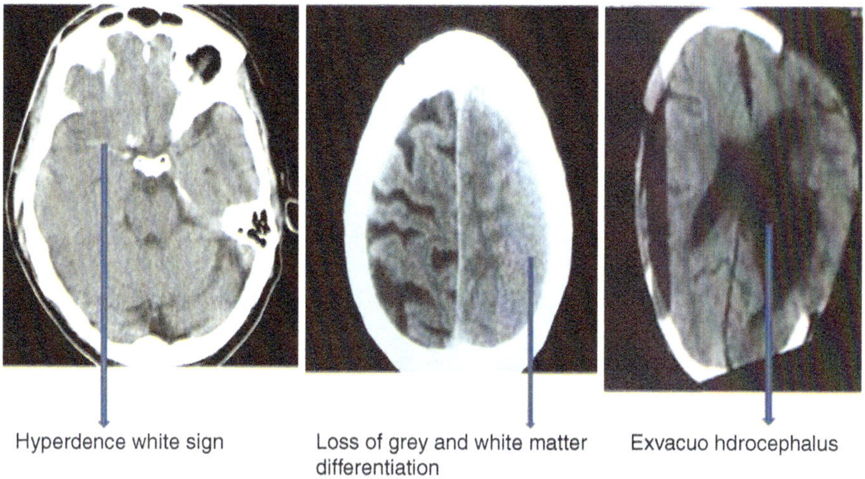


**Fig. 6.14** A computerised scan showing (left panel) a clot in the middle cerebral artery in Sylvian fissure, loss of grey white differentiation (in middle panel) and ex vacuo hydrocephalus (in the right panel)

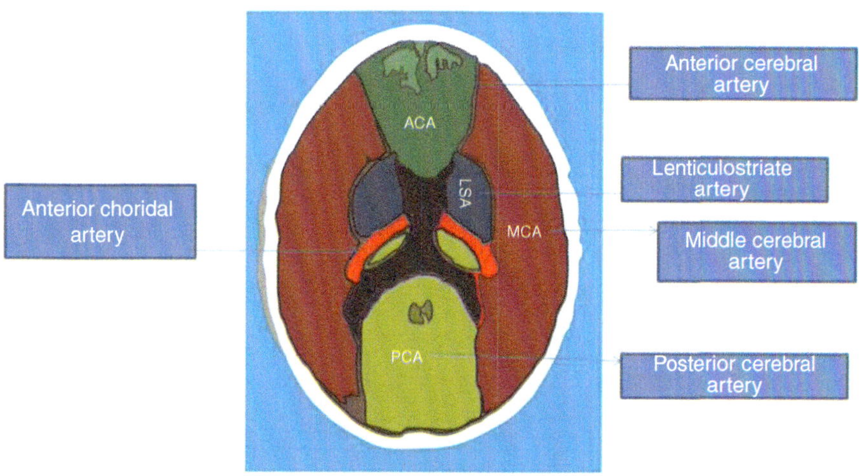


**Fig. 6.15** demonstrates cerebral vascular territories. *ACA* anterior cerebral artery, *MCA* middle cerebral artery, *PCA* posterior cerebral artery, *LSA* lenticulostriate arteries, *ACHA* anterior choroidal artery

(c) **Descending supratentorial herniation:** We have a descent of the supratentorial contents through the tent into the infratentorial space.

(d) **Tonsillar herniation:** This is detected by overcrowding of the contents in the foramen magnum and needs urgent decompression. In ascending transtentorial herniation the quadrigeminal cisterns are obliterated by compression from the infratentorial compartment.

**Fig. 6.16** demonstrates (line a) vertical line connecting the falx anteriorly to the falx posteriorly. The horizontal line (line b) measures the distance from the septum pellucidum to the midline (line a)

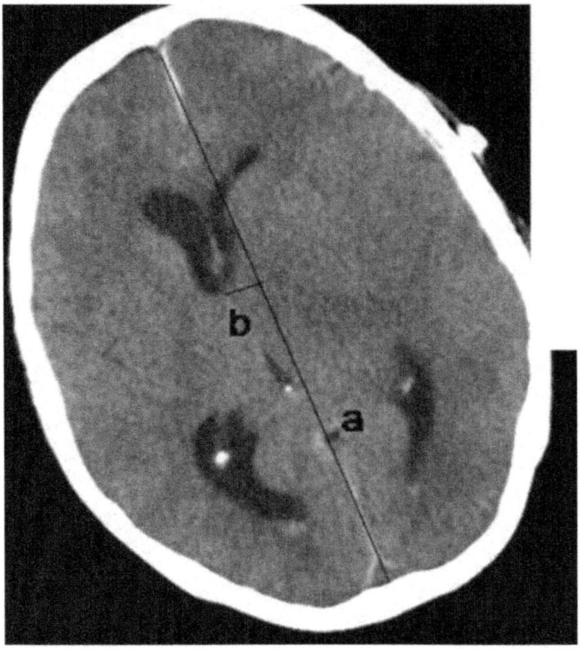


**Fig. 6.17** Computerised tomography scan with obliteration of suprasellar cistern due to bilateral uncal herniation

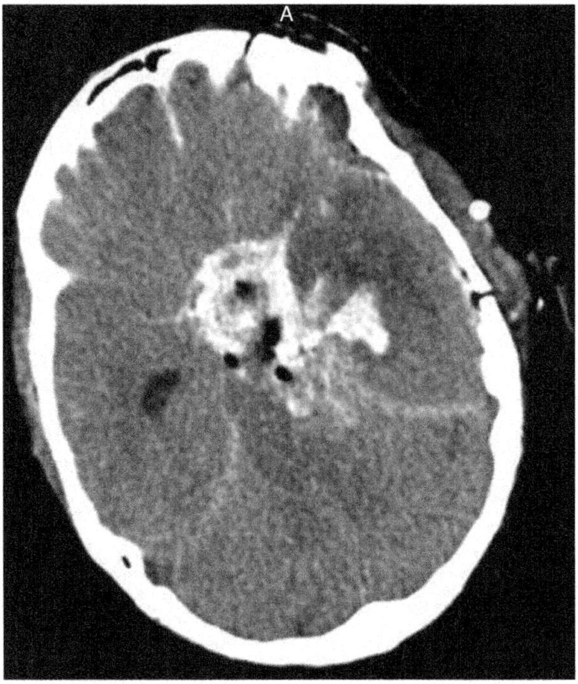


Bilateral uncal hemiation – suprasellar cisterns absent on both sides

## Multiple Choice Questions

1. Hounsfield units of pure water is:
   (a) 0
   (b) −1000
   (c) +1000
   (d) +30
2. CT features of epidural haematoma include:
   (a) Hyperdense image of collected blood
   (b) Biconvex opacity
   (c) does not cross suture lines
   (d) all the above
3. Radiological feature of hydrocephalus in CT brain is:
   (a) Ventricles dilated but subarachnoid spaces effaced.
   (b) both ventricles and subarachnoid spaces dilated.
   (c) effacement of both ventricles and subarachnoid spaces.
   (d) none of the above.
4. Pick out the correct statement:
   (a) An acute SDH is hyperdense to brain up to 1 week.
   (b) A subacute SDH may be isodense to brain in 1–3 weeks.
   (c) A chronic SDH may appear hypodense beyond 3–4 weeks.
   (d) All of the above.
5. CT brain features of ischaemic stroke include:
   (a) Hyperdense vessel sign
   (b) loss of grey white matter differentiation.
   (c) Ex vacuo hydrocephalus.
   (d) All of the above.

Answers: 1. (a), 2. (d), 3. (a), 4. (d), 5. (d).

## References


1. Allisy-Roberts PJ, Williams J. Farr's physics for medical imaging. 2nd ed. Philadelphia: Saunders; 2007. p. 108–13.
2. Hacking C, Jones J. CT head (an approach). Radiopaedia. http://radiopaedia.org/articles/ct-head-an-approach. Accessed 25 Dec 2018.
3. Bell DJ, Greenwayl K. Hounsfield unit. https://radiopaedia.org/articles/hounsfield-unit. Accessed 25 Dec 2018.
4. Singh J, Daftary A. Iodinated contrast media and their adverse reactions. J Nucl Med Technol. 2008;36:69–74.
5. Lui YW, Tang ER, Allmendinger AM, Spektor V. Evaluation of CT perfusion in the setting of cerebral ischemia: patterns and pitfalls. Am J Neuroradiol. 2010;31:1552–63.
6. Xue Z, Antani S, Long LR, Demner-Fushman D, Thoma GR. Window classification of brain CT images in biomedical articles. AMIA Annu Symp Proc. 2012;2012:1023–9.
7. Gaillard F. https://radiopaedia.org/articles/orbitomeatal-line. Accessed 25 Dec 2018.

8. Osborne T, Tang C, Sabarwal K, et al. Part 1: basic principles of computed tomography and relevant neuroanatomy. http://www.southsudanmedicaljournal.com/archive/august-2016/how-to-interpret-an-unenhanced-ct-brain-scan.-part-1-basic-principles-of-computed-tomography-and-relevant-neuroanatomy.html. Accessed 25 Dec 2018.
9. Parizel PM, Makkat S, Van Miert E, Van Goethem JW, van den Hauwe L, De Schepper AM. Intracranial hemorrhage: principles of CT and MRI interpretation. Eur Radiol. 2001;11:1770–83.
10. Toyama Y, Kobayashi T, Nishiyama Y, Satoh K, Ohkawa M, Seki K. CT for acute stage of closed head injury. Radiat Med. 2005;23:309–16.
11. Rao MG, Singh D, Khandelwal N, Sharma SK. Dating of early subdural haematoma: a correlative clinico-radiological study. J Clin Diagn Res. 2016;10:HC01–5.
12. Chavhan GB, Shroff MM. Twenty classic signs in neuroradiology: a pictorial essay. Indian J Radiol Imaging. 2009;19:135–45.
13. El-Koussy M, Schroth G, Brekenfeld C, Arnold M. Imaging of acute ischemic stroke. Eur Neurol. 2014;72:309–16.
14. Beauchamp NJ Jr, Bryan RN. Acute cerebral ishemic infarction: a pathophysiologic review and radiologic perspective. AJR. 1998;171:73–84.
15. Truwit CL, Barkovich AJ, Gean-Marton A, Hibri N, Norman D. Loss of the insular ribbon: another early CT sign of acute middle cerebral artery infarction. Radiology. 1990;176:801–6.
16. Skalski M. CT head (an approach). Radiopaedia. https://radiopaedia.org/cases/brain-herniation-types. Accessed 25 Dec 2018.

# 7 Raised ICP and Brain Herniation

Kiran Jangra, Hemant Bhagat, and Nidhi Panda

**Key Points**

- Raised ICP and brain herniation are potentially life-threatening condition
- Recognition of patient with raised ICP and brain herniation needs good clinical skills
- Prompt resuscitation of the brain is the key to the management
- The initial management consists of AB-5C protocol followed by CT scanning
- Subsequently a Four Tier algorithm should be followed for the management of the patients

**Case Scenario**

A 28 years, male, presented in emergency room with a severe traumatic head injury after being in a motorcycle accident without wearing a helmet. The physical examination revealed a Glasgow Coma Scale of 6, decerebrate posturing, pupils bilaterally fixed and 4 mm in size, and cerebral spinal fluid otorrhea on the right side. Computed tomography of the head showed left frontal and temporal subdural haemorrhage and underlying contusion with 8-mm midline shift, effacement of the suprasellar cisterns and effacement of the 3rdand 4th ventricles. Systemic examination revealed bradycardia, and hypertension with an initial blood pressure of 221/105 mmHg.

K. Jangra · H. Bhagat (✉) · N. Panda
Postgraduate Medical Education and Research, Chandigarh, India



P. U. Bidkar, P. Vanamoorthy (eds.), *Acute Neuro Care*,
https://doi.org/10.1007/978-981-15-4071-4_7

## 7.1 Introduction

Intracranial pressure (ICP) is the pressure exerted by intracranial contents (brain parenchyma, Cerebrospinal fluid, and blood) on the walls of the cranial vault. Normal values of ICP range from 10 to 15 mmHg in adults and older children, 3–7 mmHg in young children, and 1.5–6 mmHg in full-term infants [1]. The values higher than 20–25 mmHg needs to be treated, and values more than 40 mmHg can be immediate life-threatening [2].

The rise in ICP occurs due to the increase in the volume of intracranial contents, and it can occur in various neurological injuries and medical conditions enumerated in Table 7.1. It can cause severe damage to the brain that is consistently associated

**Table 7.1** Causes of raised intracranial pressure

| |
|---|
| 1. Intracranial space-occupying lesions<br>Blood (Epidural, Subdural, Intracranial, Intraventricular)<br>Tumour<br>Abscess |
| 2. Increased brain parenchyma volume (cerebral oedema)<br>Ischaemic Stroke<br>Hypoxic injury<br>Reye's Syndrome<br>Acute Hyponatraemia<br>Hepatic encephalopathy<br>Post dialysis (Disequilibrium syndrome)<br>Eclampsia<br>Certain toxin and medications (such as lead, retinoic acid)<br>Posterior Reversible encephalopathy syndrome<br>*Breakdown of blood brain barrier leading to vasogenic oedema*<br>Hypertensive encephalopathy<br>Post carotid endarterectomy/stenting<br>Oedema surrounding the tumour<br>High Altitude cerebral oedema<br>Hypoxia<br>Hypercarbia<br>Hyperpyrexia<br>Seizures |
| 3. Increased CSF volume<br>Hydrocephalus<br>Choroid plexus papilloma<br>Decreased CSF absorption due to destruction/obstruction of arachnoid villi (meningitis, post traumatic, after subarachnoid haemorrhage, post venous sinus thrombosis) |
| 4. Increased blood volume<br>Vascular malformations<br>Traumatic brain injury<br>Subarachnoid haemorrhage<br>Dural sinus thrombosis<br>Jugular venous obstruction |

with a poor outcome and may even prove to be fatal [3]. So, intensive monitoring, prompt diagnosis and timely management of raised ICP are essential to save brain from secondary damage. It is vital to understand the mechanism and pathophysiology of ICP elevation in order to effectively manage it before irreversible neuronal damage occurs.

## 7.2 Pathophysiology

Brain, blood, and cerebrospinal fluid (CSF) form the intracranial contents and as per Monroe-Kellie hypothesis, the sum of volumes of intracranial contents is constant. If there is an increase in volume of any one of these, it must be compensated by equal decrease in another to keep intracranial pressure constant (Fig. 7.1). Once these compensations are exhausted, ICP starts rising [4].

Initially, volume expansion of intracranial contents leads to only mild increase in ICP. It is compensated by the shift of cerebrospinal fluid (CSF) into the paraspinal space followed by displacement of blood from the intracranial to extracranial venous system. There is a very little compensation by compression of the brain parenchyma. Once these compensations are exhausted, there is a sharp increase in ICP with even a slight increase in intracranial volume. This is represented by compliance curve (Fig. 7.2) which is non-linear for cranial cavity [5, 6].

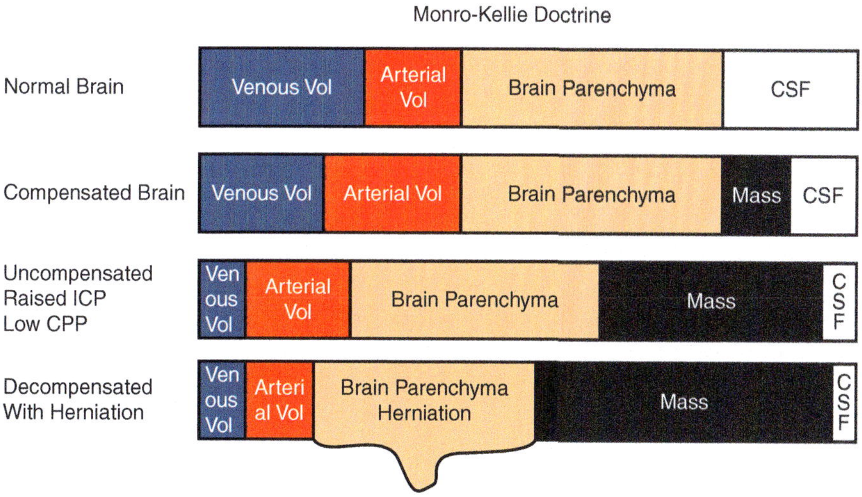


**Fig. 7.1** Monro-Kellie doctrine

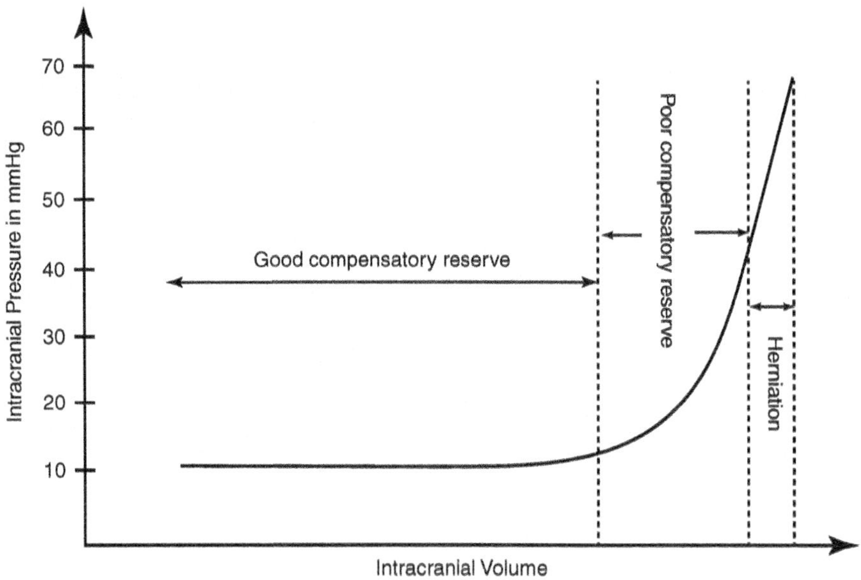


**Fig. 7.2** Intracranial pressure-volume curve. In this curve the initial flat part represents a good compensatory reserve, and exponential part representing reduced compensatory reserve or poor intracranial compliance

## 7.3 Consequences of Raised ICP

There are two major consequences of raised ICP including hypoxic-ischaemic injury secondary to reduction in cerebral perfusion pressure (CPP), and compression and herniation of brain parenchyma leading to brain damage or death. Cerebral perfusion pressure is defined as mean arterial pressure minus ICP. Increased ICP causes cerebral ischaemia by decreasing cerebral perfusion pressure unless there is a proportionate increase in MAP. However, this strategy is only partially efficacious in increasing CPP during raised ICP. If ICP increases above diastolic blood pressure, cerebral perfusion during diastole stops, and it is detected as reverberating flow or short systolic peaks on transcranial Doppler. A further rise in ICP above systolic blood pressure, there is a complete caseation of blood flow on TCD. These events are usually terminal and are seen in brain death. Hence it is vital to timely reduce ICP and to maintain MAP to adequately perfuse the brain [7, 8].

The cranial cavity is compartmentalised by the reflections of dura known as falx cerebri and tentorium cerebelli. Raise in ICP creates pressure gradients between compartments and causes a shift of brain parenchyma across these reflections and through skull openings leading to herniations. Various sites of brain herniation are depicted in Fig. 7.3.

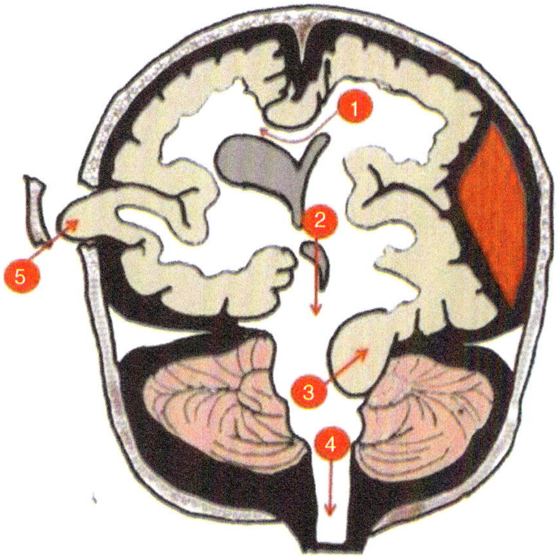


**Fig. 7.3** Herniation sites. 1. Cingulate/Subfalcine; 2. Central transtentorial; 3. Lateral transtentorial (Uncal); 4. Tonsillar; 5. Transcalvarial

## 7.4 Signs and Symptoms

Symptoms of raised ICP are mostly nonspecific, such as headache, vomiting, blurring of vision, disorientation, and lethargy. The signs include hypertension, depressed consciousness, papilledema, VI$^{th}$ cranial nerve palsy and Cushing's triad (hypertension, bradycardia, and irregular respiration). The symptoms and signs of various cerebral herniation syndromes are enumerated in Table 7.2. As the signs and symptoms of raised ICP are nonspecific, there is a need for further evaluation by direct measurement or imaging studies [9].

## 7.5 Diagnosis

The management of raised ICP should be based on patient's medical history, clinical findings, results of computed tomography (CT) scan and values of ICP.

### 7.5.1 Computed Tomography (CT) Scanning

In the emergent scenarios of suspected intracranial lesions (brain code), a head CT scan should be obtained to identify any lesion that may need a surgical intervention. After initial resuscitative measures (airway, breathing, circulation; ABC) and stabilisation, and/or initial hyperosmolar therapy (if indicated, must be started prior to transport), the patients should be shifted to radiological suite. CT is a preferred

**Table 7.2** Herniation syndromes

| Herniation sites | Mechanism/pathophysiology | Signs and symptoms |
|---|---|---|
| Uncal herniation | 1. Displacement of medial temporal lobe (uncus) in suprasellar cistern. Compression on parasympathetic followed by somatic component of oculomotor nerve<br>2. Infarction of ipsilateral visual cortex<br>3. Cerebral peduncle of midbrain of opposite side is pushed against the edge of tentorium. Lateral displacement of brain stem to compress the contralateral corticospinal track<br>4. Distortion of the ascending arousal system<br>5. Duret haemorrhage | 1. Dilated pupils and lack of pupillary reaction to light. Ptosis and "down and out position" of the ipsilateral eye<br>2. Contralateral homonymous hemianopia<br>3. Ipsilateral hemiparesis or hemiplegia<br>4. Unconsciousness<br>5. Decorticate posture, respiratory depression and death |
| Central transtentorial herniation | 1. Early stage<br>Phase of central herniation, the diencephalon (the thalamus and hypothalamus) and the medial parts of both temporal lobes are forced through a notch in the tentorium cerebelli<br>There is a stretching of the small penetrating vessels of the posterior cerebral and communicating arteries which supply the hypothalamus and thalamus<br>2. Late stage-oculomotor failure<br>3. Compression of pituitary stalk | 1. Agitation and drowsiness; pupils are small but reactive, planter responses are flexor<br>Respiration contain deep sighs, yawns and occasional pauses then progress to Cheyne-Stokes<br>Oculocephalic reflexes are intact<br>2. Difficult to arouse, decorticate, decerebrate posture. Pupils become irregular and then fixed at mid-position<br>Oculocephalic movements are difficult to elicit<br>Motor tone increases and planter responses are extensor<br>3. Diabetes insipidus |
| Subfalcine herniation | Compression of cingulate gyrus and intracranial hypertension<br>Characterised by shift of septum pellucidum, effacement of anterior horn of lateral ventricle, compression of anterior cerebral artery against falx | Nonspecific signs of raised ICP such as neurological headache and deterioration in GCS<br>In severe cases, contralateral leg weakness |
| Tonsillar herniation | Cerebellar tonsils move downwards through foramen magnum<br>Compression of medulla oblongata and upper spinal cord against external wound | Unconsciousness<br>Cardiac and respiratory dysfunction<br>Cushing triad (hypertension, bradycardia, irregular respiration) |
| Transcalvarial herniation | Compression against external defect | Physical signs depend on the part and extent of brain herniation |

technique in emergency situations over magnetic resonance imaging (MRI) due to its wide-spread availability and speed of imaging.

CT scanning may reveal any space-occupying lesion, ventriculomegaly or cerebral oedema, and diffuse brain swelling, but initial CT may be normal in approximately 10–15% of patients with raised ICP [9]. Other signs suggestive of increased ICP include loss of sulci-gyri and grey-white matter distinction, effacement of lateral ventricles, compressed 3rd ventricle, obliteration of perimesencephalic cisterns and midline shift.

### 7.5.2 ICP Monitoring

There are various modalities available for the determination of ICP, including both non-invasive and invasive (Table 7.3). The empirical treatment of suspected elevated ICP is often started immediately without delay. However, these therapies may not be fully satisfying if instituted without ICP monitoring because most of these therapies are targeted to optimise CPP, and that can be calculated only if we know ICP.

There is a conflicting evidence in the literature regarding use of intracranial pressure monitors. One of the well-designed randomised controlled trial by chestnut et al. studied the management of patients with traumatic brain injury based on ICP monitoring (target ICP <20 mmHg) versus based on clinical and radiological findings. They concluded that management based on ICP monitoring was not superior to that based on clinical and radiological findings. Still, there is insufficient data to abandon the utility of ICP monitoring. Hence, it is recommended that the ICP monitoring should be used during multi-modal monitoring in patients with severe neurological injuries [10–12].

There are various modalities available for measuring the ICP. Most of these modalities may lose their efficacy after a certain time in case of prolonged monitoring. The advantages and disadvantages of these techniques are summarised in Table 7.3. The non-invasive techniques are not as robust as invasive techniques, and hence, their use should be limited to the screening and as an adjunct but not as replacements of invasive ICP modalities.

## 7.6 Management of Raised ICP/Herniation

The stepwise management of raised ICP is depicted in Fig. 7.4. Management in emergency department of patients with acutely raised ICP should follow initial AB—5Cs protocol [13]. This protocol includes, securing the airway (A), breathing of the patient (B), check for circulation (C1), correct physiological factors (blood sugar, arterial blood gases and serum electrolytes (C2), cerebral resuscitation (decrease ICP and maintain CPP, C3), cerebral decongestant (mannitol/ hypertonic saline/intravenous anaesthetics [thiopentone/propofol] (C4), and catheterize (C5) as diuretics are being used. Following this, shift the patient for CT scanning of brain.

**Table 7.3** Monitors for measuring intracranial pressure

| Monitor | Description | Advantages | Disadvantages |
|---|---|---|---|
| *Invasive monitors* | | | |
| Intraventricular (EVD, external ventricular drain) | • Intraventricular catheter is placed in lateral ventricle and is connected via saline-filled tubing to the external transducer<br>• Zeroed at the level of external auditory meatus/circle of Willis | • "Gold standard" modality for monitoring<br>• Allows re-zeroing<br>• Has a therapeutic role also with the ability to drain CSF and administer drugs Measures global ICP | • Most invasive modality<br>• High rate of infection<br>• Placement is technically demanding and can be difficult in case of effaced ventricles<br>• Fluid leaks, air bubbles, blood clots and brain tissue can all lead to erroneous ICP readings by interfering with pressure wave conduction<br>• Must be re-zeroed each time the level of the patient's head is altered |
| Intraparenchymal (microtransducer and fibreoptic) | • Introduced into the brain parenchyma via a hollow screw inserted into the skull | • Low rate of infection and haemorrhage<br>• Easy to placement<br>• very little zero drift | • Lower accuracy compared to ventriculostomy<br>• Inability to drain CSF<br>• Re-zeroing cannot be done in case of zero drift |
| Subarachnoid (subarachnoid bolt) | • Small bolt is threaded through a burr hole with the tip placed 1 mm under the dura<br>• Screw is connected to a stopcock assembly via a saline-filled extension tube connected to an external transducer<br>• Zero-balanced at the level of the screw in the subarachnoid space | • Low rate of infection and haemorrhage<br>• Ability to drain CSF | • Unreliable accuracy<br>• Arachnoid can bock the bolt |
| Epidural | Transducer/catheter are placed in epidural space | Low rate of infection and haemorrhage | • Unreliable accuracy<br>• System malfunction, misplacement and baseline drift<br>• Inability to drain CSF |

| | | | |
|---|---|---|---|
| *Non-invasive monitoring* | | | |
| Tympanic membrane displacement | • ICP waves are transmitted via cochlear duct to the inner ear then via the oval window to the auditory ossicles of the middle ear which are firmly attached to the tympanic membrane<br>• The degree of displacement tympanic membrane can be recorded using a probe placed into the external auditory meatus | Non-invasive may prove valuable as a screening tool in patients suspected of having intracranial hypertension | unreliable |
| Optic nerve sheath diameter (ONSD) | Optic nerve sheath diameter is measured using high frequency rectilinear probe over closed eyelids | Non-invasive modality relatively low cost and wide availability | Inaccurate and unreliable |
| Transcranial Doppler | 2 MHz probe is used to measure pulsatility index | Strong correlation exists between pulsatility index (PI) and ICP in patients | Inaccurate and unreliable, making it a poor replacement for invasive monitoring |

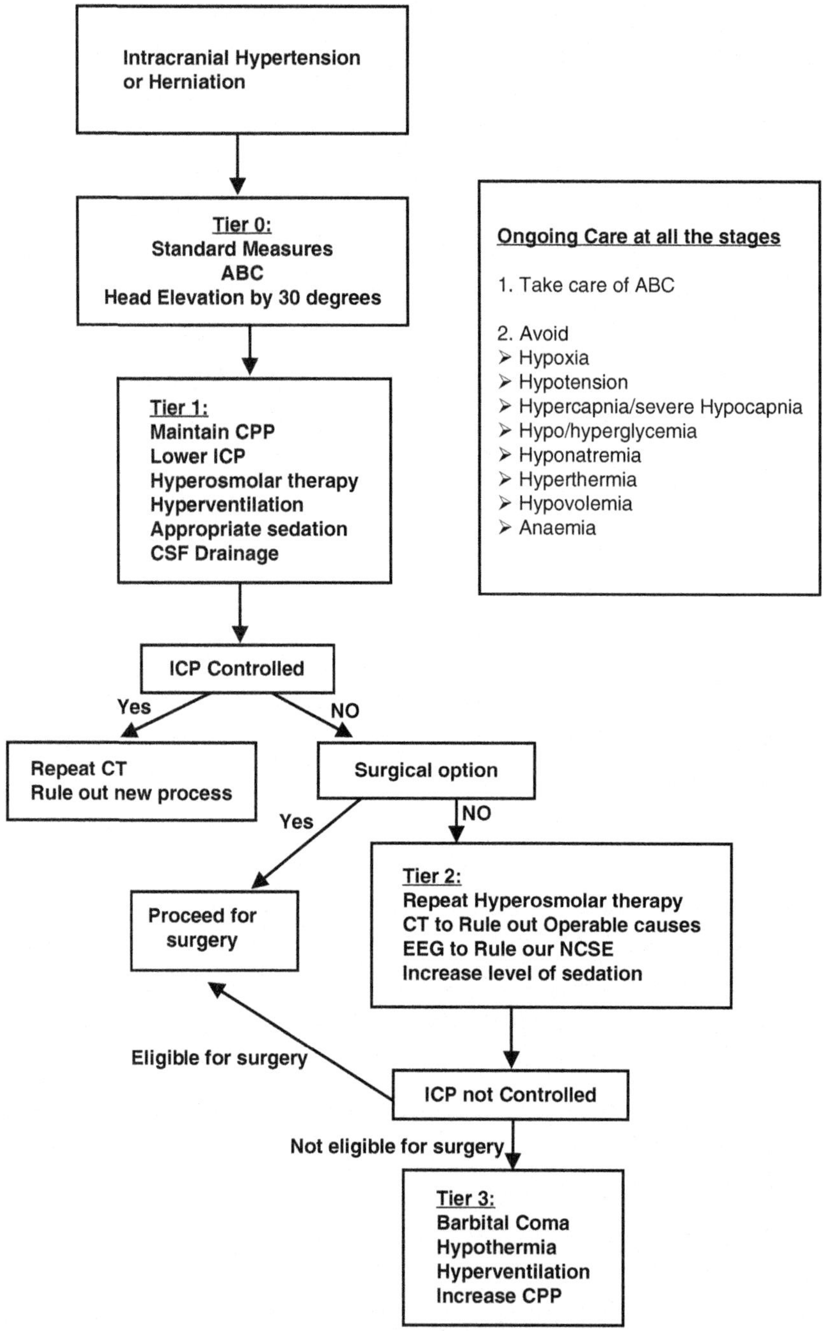


**Fig. 7.4** Flow diagram of management of raised intracranial pressure/herniation. *ABC* airway breathing circulation, *CPP* cerebral perfusion pressure, *ICP* intracranial pressure, *CSF* cerebrospinal fluid

### 7.6.1 **Initial Resuscitation: Tier Zero** (Summarised in Table 7.4)

#### 7.6.1.1 ABCs

A primary aim of the management of patients with raised ICP is to prevent secondary brain damage. The assessment of airway, breathing, and circulation must be performed in all the patients to prevent hypotension and hypoxemia, which not only causes secondary brain insults but also can be life-threatening, if left untreated. Patients having a Glasgow Coma Scale (GCS) score of less than 8, signs of herniation, and irregular respiration or apnoea need a definitive airway. Oxygenation should be appropriately maintained. Mechanical ventilation and positive end-expiratory pressure have adverse effects on ICP as these impedes the venous drainage. To impede venous return PEEP should be higher than ICP. Hence, patients with raised ICP can tolerate higher PEEP. Transmission of PEEP to ICP also depends on lung compliance, and in patients with stiffer lungs where PEEP is needed to improve oxygenation, PEEP is not transmitted to ICP. PEEP in these patients actually decreases ICP by correcting hypoxia [14]. If there is evidence of circulatory failure, adequate volume resuscitation should be done.

#### 7.6.1.2 Facilitate CSF Drainage

Elevation of the headend of the patient's bed and maintaining head in neutral position helps in the facilitation of cerebral venous outflow and promotes the displacement of CSF from intracranial to the spinal compartment. With a 30° headend elevation, there is a reduction in ICP without any effect on either CPP or CBF in

**Table 7.4** Management of intracranial hypertension: tier zero

| |
|---|
| • *ABCs* |
| – Intubate patient if GCS ≤ 8 or inadequate respiratory effort and as needed to protect the airway |
| – Administer supplemental oxygen to maintain $SpO_2$ >92% |
| – Maintain $PaCO_2$ 35–40 mmHg |
| – Maintain euvolemia |
| – Maintain target MAP ≥80 mmHg/SBP >100 mmHg |
| – Avoid Anaemia |
| • Elevate head of bed to 30° |
| • Maintain head in neutral position to avoid jugular vein constriction |
| – Loosen the neck ties |
| – Remove tight neck collars |
| – Take care of the pressure (airway, intrathoracic, intra-abdominal) |
| • Avoid/treat hyponatraemia |
| – Maintain serum sodium ≥140 mEq/L with isotonic intravenous fluids (no dextrose) |
| • Avoid hyperthermia (temperature 36–37 °C) |
| • Maintain normoglycaemia |
| • Minimise external stimuli that can increase ICP such as tracheal suctioning. Ensure adequate sedation |
| • Consider systemic steroids in case of vasogenic oedema (tumours/abscess) |
| • Stop ongoing seizures using antiepileptics |

most of the cases. Sudden and steep head-up positions can compromise CPP. Hence the ICP and arterial transducers should be zeroed at the same level (the level of external auditory meatus). Increased intra-abdominal or intrathoracic pressures can also exacerbate ICP by interfering with the cerebral venous outflow. Even in the absence of abdominal compartment syndrome, the release of abdominal fascial can effectively reduce the ICP [15]. Ties of ETT and tight cervical collars that impede cerebral venous outflow should be loosened.

#### 7.6.1.3 Manage Agitation/Temperature

Patients should be sedated and stimuli that may elevate ICP, such as tracheal suctioning, should be minimised. Hyperthermia increases the cerebral metabolism and can lead to ischaemic damage if CBF is not increased proportionately. In patients with raised ICP, CBF is already compromised, hyperthermia can aggravate secondary brain insults. All measures should be instituted to prevent and treat hyperthermia.

#### 7.6.1.4 Hyperosmolar Solutions

The use of hypo-osmolar fluids can increase brain water content and results in increased ICP. So, only iso- or hyperosmotic fluids should be used for resuscitation. If hyponatraemia is present due to other associated conditions, it should be promptly corrected. In patients with vasogenic oedema secondary to brain tumours or abscesses, corticosteroid therapy should be initiated [16, 17]. If the head CT scan is not done previously, it should be performed when the patient is stable for the transport to the radiology suite.

### 7.6.2 Tier One (Summarised in Table 7.5)

For treating acutely raised ICP any effect on both mannitol and hypertonic saline (HTS) are found to be equally efficacious [18–21]. Mannitol is administered intravenously in a dosage of 0.5–1 g/kg and may be repeated every 4–6 h under the monitoring of serum osmolality [19]. There is no additional therapeutic benefit once serum osmolality exceeds 320 mOsm/kg. HTS is available in various strengths ranging from 2 to 23.4%. HTS (23.4%) has been shown to decrease ICP and also reverse the transtentorial herniation [22]. While using HTS, serum sodium concentration should be monitored every 4–6 h, and if it increases to >160 mEq/L, HTS should be stopped. HTS can be administered alone or in combination with the mannitol.

In cases of acute obstructive hydrocephalus, a external ventricular drainage (EVD) should be placed urgently. EVD can be used to monitor ICP and If ICP is high, CSF can be drained in the boluses of 5–10 mL at one time [23].

In addition to these, hyperventilation to achieve a $PaCO_2$ of 30–35 mmHg may be considered for a brief period (<2 h) during impending herniation [24, 25]. If still ICP remains high, and/or clinical signs of herniation persist, review the patient for decompressive surgical options [26, 27]. If surgery is not an option in a given scenario and ICP is persistently high, then one should move to Tier Two therapies. If ICP is controlled, then a head CT scan is considered to rule out new processes.

**Table 7.5** Management of intracranial hypertension: tier one

| • Ensure all physiologic goals from *Tier Zero* are met |
|---|
| • *Airway/breathing/Circulation* |
| • Consider ICP monitoring (if available and indicated) GCS ≤8 after resuscitation |
| • Maintain cerebral perfusion pressure (CPP) ≥60 mmHg if ICP is available |
| – Ensure adequate volume resuscitation |
| – Consider adding ionotropic /vasopressor support after adequate volume resuscitation—titrate to keep CPP >60 mmHg |
| • Treat sustained ICP >22 mmHg for 10 min |
| – Verify correct ICP waveform and appropriate level EVD transducer |
| – When acute obstructive hydrocephalus is present as determined by neuroimaging, an external ventricular drainage (EVD) system should be placed emergently |
| – If EVD is in place-Drain 5–10 mL of CSF for acute rise |
| – Consider hyperosmolar therapy |
| First line therapy for ICP >22 mmHg for ≥10 min |
| Mannitol 0.25–1.0 g/kg IV-push × 1 if serum sodium <160 and/or serum osmolality <320 mOsm/L |
| Monitor serum osmolality every 4–6 h if using mannitol |
| Hold mannitol therapy for serum sodium ≥160 mEq/L and/or serum osmolality ≥320 mOsm/L |
| 7.5% Hypertonic Saline 250 mL IV bolus over 15 min × 1 if serum sodium <160 mmol/L |
| Measure serum sodium every 4–6 h |
| Notify intensivist if serum sodium changes by >2 mEq/L/4 h from previous measurement |
| Hold hypertonic saline therapy for serum sodium ≥160 mEq/L |
| Bolus 23.4% NaCl has been associated with ICP reduction and reversal of transtentorial herniation |
| – As a temporising measure (impending herniation), consider short-term (<2 h) hyperventilation ($PaCO_2$ 30–34 mmHg) to acutely reduce ICP, while definitive treatment is provided [23, 24] |
| – There is no role prophylactic hyperventilation and should be avoided in the first 24 h after traumatic brain injury |
| • If ICP is not controlled, and/or clinical signs of herniation do not resolve with Tier One interventions, consider decompressive surgical options [25, 26] |
| • If surgery is not appropriate or not undertaken, move to Tier Two. If ICP is controlled with Tier One interventions, consider repeating the head CT scan to rule out new processes |

If brain imaging study was not performed earlier, then once the patient is stable to be shifted to radiological suite, a head CT scan should be obtained, to determine the cause of intracranial hypertension and herniation.

### 7.6.3 Tier Two (Summarised in Table 7.6)

Tier Two should be initiated if Tier one interventions fail to control ICP. If HTS has been used previously and serum sodium level >160 mmol/L is achieved, target serum sodium can be raised, but it is unlikely to provide an additional benefit. The absolute value of the target for serum sodium depends on the pathophysiological state of the patient. Serum sodium should be maintained at the level where ICP has

**Table 7.6** Management of intracranial hypertension: tier two

| *The following interventions should be considered if ICP is persistently >22 mmHg for more than 60 min after discussion with neurosurgeons and intensivists*: |
|---|
| • Ensure all physiologic goals from *Tier One* are met |
| • Repeat hyperosmolar therapy as long as serum sodium <160 mEq/L—recommend: |
| – 23.4% sodium chloride 30 mL IV-syringe × 1 over 15 min |
| – Use 7.5% sodium chloride 250 mL IV bolus × 1 when volume resuscitation also needed |
| Continue serum sodium checks every 4 h |
| • Consider head CT scan to rule out space-occupying lesion |
| • Consider continuous EEG monitoring to rule out non-convulsive status epilepticus (if not already present) |
| • Consider bolus dosage of sedative/hypnotics over the infusion and then increasing sedative and analgesic therapy |
| • Paralysis |
| – Ensure RASS -5 before initiation of paralytic |
| – Start muscle relaxants and adjust dose according to Train of Four 1/4 |
| • Early (within 2.5 h), short-term (48 h post-injury), prophylactic hypothermia is not recommended to improve outcomes in patients with diffuse brain injury |
| • Begin mild hyperventilation with goal $PaCO_2$ 30–34 mmHg |
| • If all these measures fail move on to tier 3 |

stabilised until brain oedema starts waning. Along with hyperosmolar therapy, sedation should also be increased as agitation can compromise ICP. The addition of, sedative-hypnotics, such as propofol, reduces $CMRO_2$ and CBF volume resulting in reduced ICP [28]. These agents may cause cardiovascular depression that can be managed with maintaining euvolemia, and/or vasopressors to achieve CPP goals.

If ICP is still not responsive, consider rescue decompressive surgery. If medical management fails to lower the ICP, then decompressive surgery may be considered for reducing ICP. Various decompressive surgical interventions include placement of a ventricular drain, evacuation of space-occupying lesions and uni- or bilateral craniectomies.

Patients with acute deterioration in neurological status due to space-occupying lesions benefit the most by surgical decompression [29, 30]. Decompressive craniectomy may also have mortality benefits in various conditions, including diffuse brain swelling due to diffuse brain injury [31–34] various conditions, including ischaemic stroke with oedema surrounding the infarct [35, 36], meningoencephalitis and other non-infectious neuroinflammatory conditions leading to cerebral oedema.

### 7.6.4 **Tier Three** (Summarised in Table 7.7)

#### 7.6.4.1 Pentobarbital Coma

It is the most aggressive level of management of raised ICP and is associated with the greatest risk of adverse events. Most of the recommendations here are derived by consensus, as literature is sparse. When most of the pharmacological agents and

**Table 7.7** Management of intracranial hypertension: tier three

| *The following interventions should be considered if ICP remains >22 mmHg despite all Tier Two goals being met:* |
|---|
| • Ensure that medical therapy with hypertonic saline is maximised (e.g., serum sodium 155–160 mEq/L) |
| • Consider revised ICP threshold of 25 mmHg with strict adherence to CPP >60 mmHg |
| • Initiate continuous EEG (if not already present) |
| • Decompressive surgical interventions include |
| – Placement of a ventricular drain |
| – Evacuation of extra-axial lesion (e.g., epidural hematoma) |
| – Resection of intracerebral lesion (e.g., lobar haemorrhage) |
| – Removal brain parenchyma (e.g., cerebellar mass) |
| – Uni- or bilateral decompressive craniectomies in patients without evacuable lesions (cerebral oedema after stroke, meningoencephalitis or non-infectious neuroinflammatory conditions) |
| Craniectomy solely for management of ICP does not improve long-term neurological outcome |
| Consider decompressive craniectomy/craniotomy in patients with a surgically evacuable lesion |
| • Barbiturate Coma |
| – If not a surgical candidate, and refractory to all above interventions, consider pentobarbital coma |
| Pentobarbital 10 mg/kg IV over 10 min, then 5 mg/kg/h × 3 h, then 1 mg/kg/h IV infusion |
| Titrate pentobarbital to the minimal dose required to achieve EEG burst suppression—3–5 bursts/min (= 1–2 bursts per screen) |
| – Discontinue all other sedative agents and paralytics after pentobarbital loading doses complete (4 h) |
| – Consider invasive hemodynamic monitoring (such as pulmonary artery catheter) due to the negative inotropic effects of pentobarbital |
| – Once ICP ≤ 22 mmHg for 48 h, wean pentobarbital dose over the next 48–72 h |
| • Discontinue or decrease tube feeds to trophic rate (10–20 mL/h) |
| • Moderate hypothermia (target core temperature 32–34 °C) |

surgical interventions fails to reduce ICP, then electrical activity of brain is suppressed using pharmacological agents, so that existing blood supply can meet the demand and further damage to brain can be prevented. Most commonly used agent for this purpose is pentobarbital which is given as a bolus 10 mg/kg over 30 min–2 h followed by 5 mg/kg/h × 3 h and then maintained @ infusion of 1–4 mg/kg/h titrated to the target ICP. The use of pentobarbital usually causes severe hypotension, and blood pressure may have to be supported by vasopressors. The pentobarbital is titrated by electroencephalogram (EEG) monitoring to achieve burst suppression or to achieve the target ICP. The pentobarbital infusion should be continued for 24–96 h till underlying disease processes raising ICP are treated and thereafter it is slowly tapered [37–39]. There are various side effects of pentobarbital, including respiratory depression, hemodynamic instability, immune system suppression, and paralytic ileus. Other agents can also be used for achieving burst suppression, including thiopentone and propofol.

#### 7.6.4.2 Hypothermia

Hypothermia acts sim as the pentobarbital coma, by reducing the cerebral metabolic activity. Hypothermia, in addition to suppression of electrical activity of the brain, also reduces basal component of cellular metabolism. There is a predictable decrease in ICP with moderate hypothermia (target core temperature 32–34 °C). Hypothermia may be induced with external cooling devices, cold fluid infusion through the intravenous route, and specially designed invasive cooling catheters [40–45]. There are various adverse effects of hypothermia such as shivering, electrolyte disturbances, cardiac arrhythmias, and sepsis. There may be rebound severe intracranial hypertension during rewarming so, rewarming should be done slowly.

#### 7.6.4.3 Hyperventilation

In patient with impending herniation not responsive to another modalities hyperventilation may be initiated to achieve mild to moderate hypocapnia ($PaCO_2$ 25–35 mmHg). Hyperventilation causes cerebrovascular constriction resulting in reduction in cerebral blood volume, in turn reducing ICP. It should be considered only for brief period during acute phase, as prolonging hyperventilation for more than 6–8 h initiates compensatory mechanisms, buffers the changes in pH caused by hyperventilation and reduces its efficacy. In addition, such hyperventilation can cause intense cerebral vasoconstriction that may aggravate ischaemic insults [25]. The cerebral ischaemia caused by hyperventilation, should be instituted in the presence of a monitor that can assess cerebral oxygenation such as jugular venous oximetry, near-infrared spectroscopy (NIRS) or brain tissue oxygen probe.

## 7.7 Newer Monitoring Modalities

Patients may benefit from the use of additional neuromonitoring, such as jugular venous oximetry, near-infrared spectroscopy, brain tissue oxygenation and cerebral microdialysis. The working principle these monitors is based on the measurement of balance in cerebral metabolic demand and supply. These complementary neuromonitoring techniques may benefit in selected patients, but the overall effect on outcome is not apparent.

There are various studies in the literatures showing that a significant parenchymal hypoxia (as detected by brain tissue oxygen sensors) can occur even when ICP and CPP are normal [46, 47]. Similarly, cerebral metabolic by-products as detected by cerebral microdialysis, including brain interstitial lactate, pyruvate, glucose, and glutamate, are the indicators of the balance of metabolic demand supply and may alter independent of ICP and CPP [48]. Currently, dynamic indices of cerebral autoregulation as detected by transcranial Doppler-derived CBF velocity such as mean index (Mx) and autoregulatory index (ARIx) express the real-time correlation between MAP or CPP and ICP. Autoregulation failure is strongly associated with poor prognosis [49, 50].

## 7.8 Summary

The absolute values of ICP and MAP may not be consistently the same for all individuals. These values may vary from individual to individual. These values are affected by the complex interplay of physiological disturbances in metabolic supply and demand at the tissue level. Hence, the goals of MAP and ICP should be customised for each patient. For example, an awake patient in whom ICP is >20 mmHg or a CPP below 50 mmHg, and there is no symptom, may not require any intervention.

*Checklist for management of patients with raised intracranial pressure:*

- *Tier Zero*
  - Take care of airway, breathing, circulation
  - Raise headend of the bed >30°
  - Ensure adequate sedation
  - Correct Hypoxia, Hypotension, Hypercarbia, Hypo/hyperglycaemia, hyponatraemia and hyperthermia
  - Treat vasogenic oedema with steroids
  - Maintain CPP 60–70 mmHg
- *Tier One*
  - Mannitol 0.5–1 g/kg IV bolus or 3% saline 10–20 cc/
  - CSF drainage
  - Transient hyperventilation
  - Appropriate sedation
- *Tier Two*
  - Repeat hypertonic saline bolus (23.4%)
  - Consider sedative bolus and infusion
  - Get EEG to rule out non-convulsive seizures
  - Consider decompressive craniotomy
- *Tier Three*
  - Pentobarbital bolus and infusion with EEG guided titration
  - Induce hypothermia
  - Hyperventilation to be used under the guidance of cerebral oxygen monitor
  - MAP augmentation to improve CPP

## Multiple Choice Questions

1. Which of the following statements is *not* true regarding raised intracranial pressure?
   (a). Normal values of ICP range from 10 to 15 mmHg in adults
   (b). Normal values of ICP range from 7 to 8 mmHg in full term infants
   (c). The values higher than 20–25 mmHg need to be treated
   (d). The values more than 40 mmHg can be immediate life-threatening

2. The following statements are true regarding signs and symptoms of raised intracranial pressure, *except*.
   (a). Cushing's triad includes: hypertension, bradycardia and irregular respiration
   (b). Subfalcine herniation may lead to contralateral leg weakness
   (c). Central transtentorial herniation may lead to Diabetes insipidus in late stages
   (d). Uncal herniation presents as decorticate and decerebrate posture and Cheyne-Stokes respiration
3. Which of the following is *not* a radiological finding of raised intracranial pressure
   (a). Loss of sulci-gyri and grey-white matter distinction
   (b). Effacement of lateral ventricles
   (c). Opening of perimesencephalic cisterns
   (d). Midline shift
4. Which of the following is true regarding intracranial pressure monitoring?
   (a). Subarachnoid bolt should be zeroed at the level of external auditory meatus
   (b). Intraparenchymal catheter is considered as gold standard technique
   (c). Intraparenchymal can be re-zeroed after insertion
   (d). Intraventricular catheter must be re-zeroed each time the level of the patient's head is altered
5. All of the following can cause secondary brain damage, except.
   (a). Hypothermia
   (b). Hypoxia
   (c). Severe Hypocapnia
   (d). Hypovolemia
6. Which of the following statement is true regarding initial management of raised intracranial pressure
   (a). Adequate cerebral perfusion pressure should be maintained at first place
   (b). Positive end-expiratory pressure must be avoided as it increases intracranial pressure
   (c). Airway, breathing and circulation should be managed initially in all the cases prior to raised intracranial pressure
   (d). Glasgow Coma Scale of more than 8 is an indication of securing the airway
7. All of the following can impede the cerebrospinal fluid drainage, *except*.
   (a). Abdominal compartment syndrome
   (b). Tight cervical collar
   (c). 30° head elevation
   (d). Hemothorax
8. Which of the fluids should not be used in initial resuscitation of patients with raised intracranial pressure
   (a). Plasma-lyte-A
   (b). 25% Dextrose
   (c). Normal Saline
   (d). 7.5% saline

9. Which of the following treatment modality in *not* included in tier-1?
   (a). Mannitol
   (b). Hypertonic saline
   (c). Hyperventilation
   (d). Hypothermia
10. Following are true about hypothermia, *except.*
   (a). It reduces cerebral metabolism beyond the isoelectrical activity
   (b). There may be rebound severe intracranial hypertension during rewarming
   (c). Moderate to severe hypothermia is beneficial in reducing intracranial pressure
   (d). There is a risk of severe dyselectrolytemia during rewarming phase

Answers: 1. (b), 2. (d), 3. (c), 4. (d), 5. (a), 6. (c), 7. (c), 8. (b), 9. (d), 10. (c)

## References

1. Welch K. The intracranial pressure in infants. J Neurosurg. 1980;52:693–9.
2. Castillo LR, Gopinath S, Robertson CS. Management of intracranial hypertension. Neurol Clin. 2008;26:521–41.
3. Treggiari MM, Schutz N, Yanez ND, Romand J-A. Role of intracranial pressure values and patterns in predicting outcome of traumatic brain injury: a systematic review. Neurocrit Care. 2007;6:104–12.
4. Ropper AH. Hyperosmolar therapy for raised intracranial pressure. N Engl J Med. 2012;367:746–52.
5. Mayer SA, Chong JY. Critical care management of increased intracranial pressure. J Intensive Care Med. 2002;17:55–67.
6. Nakagawa K, Smith WS. Evaluation and management of increased intracranial pressure. Continuum. 2011;17(5):1077–93.
7. Rangel-Castilla L, Gasco J, Nauta HJ, et al. Cerebral pressure autoregulation in traumatic brain injury. Neurosurg Focus. 2008;25:E7.
8. Figali AA, Zwane E, Fieggen AG, et al. Pressure autoregulation, intracranial pressure, and brain tissue oxygenation in children with severe traumatic brain injury. J Neurosurg Pediatr. 2009;4:420–8.
9. Eisenberg HM, Gary HE Jr, Aldrich EF, et al. Initial CT findings in 753 patients with severe head injury. A report from the NIH Traumatic Coma Data Bank. J Neurosurg. 1990;73:688–98.
10. Morgenstern L, Hemphill JC 3rd, Anderson C, et al. Guidelines for the management of spontaneous intracerebral hemorrhage: a guideline for healthcare professionals from the American Heart Association/American Stroke Association. Stroke. 2010;41:2108–29.
11. Connolly EJ, Rabinstein AA, Carhuapoma JR, et al. Guidelines for the management of aneurysmal subarachnoid hemorrhage: a guideline for healthcare professionals from the American Heart Association/American Stroke Association. Stroke. 2012;43:1711–37.
12. Bratton SL, Chestnut RM, Ghajar J, et al. Guidelines for the management of severe traumatic brain injury. J Neurotrauma. 2007;24(Suppl 1):S21–5.
13. Bhagat H, Mahajan S. Supratentorial Lesions. In: Prabhakar H, Mahajan C, Kapoor I, editors. Essentials of neuroanesthesia. 1st ed. New York: CRC Press; 2018. p. 541–53.
14. Caricato A, Conti G, Della CF, et al. Effects of PEEP on the intracranial system of patients with head injury and subarachnoid hemorrhage: the role of respiratory system compliance. J Trauma. 2005;58:571–6.

15. Joseph DK, Dutton RP, Aarabi B, et al. Decompressive laparotomy to treat intractable intracranial hypertension after traumatic brain injury. J Trauma. 2004;57:687–93.
16. Galicich JH, French LA, Melby JC. Use of dexamethasone in treatment of cerebral edema associated with brain tumors. J Lancet. 1961;81:46–53.
17. Quartey GR, Johnston JA, Rozdilsky B. Decadron in the treatment of cerebral abscess: an experimental study. J Neurosurg. 1976;45:301–10.
18. Qureshi A, Wilson D, Traystman R. Treatment of elevated intracranial pressure in experimental intracerebral hemorrhage: comparison between mannitol and hypertonic saline. Neurosurgery. 1999;44(5):1055–63.
19. Francony G, Fauvage B, Falcon D, et al. Equimolar doses of mannitol and hypertonic saline in the treatment of increased intracranial pressure. Crit Care Med. 2008;36(3):795–800.
20. Battison C, Andrews PJ, Graham C, et al. Randomized, controlled trial on the effect of a 20% mannitol solution and a 7.5% saline/6% dextran solution on increased intracranial pressure after brain injury. Crit Car Med. 2005;33:196–202.
21. Ichai C, Armando G, Orban JC, et al. Sodium lactate versus mannitol in the treatment of intracranial hypertensive episodes in severe traumatic brain-injured patients. Intensive Care Med. 2009;35:471–9.
22. Koenig MA, Bryan M, Lewin JL 3rd, Mirski MA, Geocadin RG, Stevens RD. Reversal of transtentorial herniation with hypertonic saline. Neurology. 2008;70:1023–9.
23. Kerr EM, Marion D, Sereika MS, et al. The effect of cerebrospinal fluid drainage on cerebral perfusion in traumatic brain injured adults. J Neurosurg Anesthesiol. 2000;12:324–33.
24. Coles JP, Minhas PS, Fryer TD, et al. Effect of hyperventilation on cerebral blood flow in traumatic head injury: clinical relevance and monitoring correlates. Crit Care Med. 2002;30:1950–9.
25. Muizelaar JP, Marmarou A, Ward JD, et al. Adverse effects of prolonged hyperventilation in patients with severe head injury: a randomized clinical trial. J Neurosurg. 1991;75:731–9.
26. Eberle BM, Schnuriger B, Inaba K, Gruen JP, Demetriades D, Belzberg H. Decompressive craniectomy: surgical control of traumatic intracranial hypertension may improve outcome. Injury. 2010;41:894–8.
27. Johnson RD, Maartens NF, Teddy PJ. Decompressive craniectomy for malignant middle cerebral artery infarction: evidence and controversies. J Clin Neurosci. 2011;18:1018–22.
28. Kelly DF, Goodale DB, Williams J, et al. Propofol in the treatment of moderate and severe head injury: a randomized, prospective double-blinded pilot trial. J Neurosurg. 1999;90:1042–52.
29. Pfefferkorn T, Eppinger U, Linn J, et al. Long-term outcome after suboccipital decompressive craniectomy for malignant cerebellar infarction. Stroke. 2009;40:3045–50.
30. Raco A, Caroli E, Isidori A, Salvati M. Management of acute cerebellar infarction: one institution's experience. Neurosurgery. 2003;53:1061–5.
31. Jiang JY, Xu W, Li WP, et al. Efficacy of standard trauma craniectomy for refractory intracranial hypertension with severe traumatic brain injury: a multicenter, prospective, randomized controlled study. J Neurotrauma. 2005;22:623–8.
32. Olivecrona M, Rodling-Wahlstrom M, Naredi S, et al. Effective ICP reduction by decompressive craniectomy in patients with severe traumatic brain injury treated by an ICP-targeted therapy. J Neurotrauma. 2007;24:927–35.
33. Taylor A, Butt W, Rosenfeld J, et al. A randomized trial of very early decompressive craniectomy in children with traumatic brain injury and sustained intracranial hypertension. Childs Nerv Syst. 2001;17:154–62.
34. Cooper DJ, Rosenfeld JV, Murray L, et al. Decompressive craniectomy in diffuse traumatic brain injury. N Engl J Med. 2011;364:1493–502.
35. Hofmeijer J, Kappelle LJ, Algra A, et al. Surgical decompression for space-occupying cerebral infarction (the Hemicraniectomy After Middle Cerebral Artery infarction with Life-threatening Edema Trial [HAMLET]): a multicentre, open, randomised trial. Lancet Neurol. 2009;8:326–33.

36. Vahedi K, Hofmeijer J, Juettler E, et al. Early decompressive surgery in malignant infarction of the middle cerebral artery: a pooled analysis of three randomised controlled trials. Lancet Neurol. 2007;6:215–22.
37. Brain Trauma Foundation. The use of barbiturates in the control of intracranial hypertension. J Neurotrauma. 1996;13:711–4.
38. Eisenberg HM, Frankowski RF, Contant CF, et al. High-dose barbiturate control of elevated intracranial in patients with severe head injury. J Neurosurg. 1988;69:15–23.
39. Perez-Barcena J, Llompart-Pou JA, Homar J, et al. Pentobarbital versus thiopental in the treatment of refractory intracranial hypertension in patients with traumatic brain injury: a randomized controlled trial. Crit Care. 2008;12:R112.
40. Jiang J, Yu M, Zhu C. Effect of long-term mild hypothermia therapy in patients with severe traumatic brain injury: 1-year follow-up review of 87 cases. J Neurosurg. 2000;93:546–9.
41. Liu WG, Qiu WS, Zhang Y, et al. Effects of selective brain cooling in patients with severe traumatic brain injury: a preliminary study. J Int Med Res. 2006;34:58–64.
42. Marion DW, Obrist WD, Carlier PM, et al. The use of moderate therapeutic hypothermia for patients with severe head injuries: a preliminary report. J Neurosurg. 1993;79:354–62.
43. Marion DW, Penrod LE, Kelsey SF, et al. Treatment of traumatic brain injury with moderate hypothermia. N Engl J Med. 1997;336:540–6.
44. Qiu W, Zhang Y, Sheng H, et al. Effects of therapeutic mild hypothermia on patients with severe traumatic brain injury after craniotomy. J Crit Care. 2007;22:229–35.
45. Shiozaki T, Sugimoto H, Taneda M, et al. Effect of mild hypothermia on uncontrollable intracranial hypertension after severe head injury. J Neurosurg. 1993;79:363–8.
46. Chang JJ, Youn TS, Benson D, et al. Physiologic and functional outcome correlates of brain tissue hypoxia in traumatic brain injury. Crit Care Med. 2009;37:283–90.
47. Longhi L, Pagan F, Valeriani V, et al. Monitoring brain tissue oxygen tension in brain-injured patients reveals hypoxic episodes in normal-appearing and in peri-focal tissue. Intensive Care Med. 2007;33:2136–42.
48. Chen HI, Stiefel MF, Oddo M, et al. Detection of cerebral compromise with multimodality monitoring in patients with subarachnoid hemorrhage. Neurosurgery. 2011;69:53–63.
49. Schmidt B, Czosnyka M, Raabe A, et al. Adaptive noninvasive assessment of intracranial pressure and cerebral autoregulation. Stroke. 2003;34:84–9.
50. Brady K, Joshi B, Zweifel C, et al. Real-time continuous monitoring of cerebral blood flow autoregulation using near-infrared spectroscopy in patients undergoing cardiopulmonary bypass. Stroke. 2010;41:1951–6.

# 8 Traumatic Brain Injury

Keshav Goyal and Rahul Yadav

## Key Points

- Knowledge and understanding of basic cerebral anatomy and physiology is required for successful management of TBI
- Prevention of secondary brain injury is possible by prevention of hypoxia and hypotension and early hemodynamic stability. Adequate resuscitation is important
- Focused neurological examinations shall be repeated in these patients to evaluate the deterioration or improvement. Frequent reassessment is required
- Resuscitate with isotonic crystalloids. Avoid hypotonic and glucose containing fluids. Treat shock aggressively
- Consider early need for transfer, admission, and consulting a neurosurgeon

## Case Scenario

A 25-year-old male was driving in SUV on Yamuna Expressway without seat-belt. He collided against a concrete divider at a speed of 90 km/h. There was no airbag in car and windshield was shattered. His initial GCS was 12 but on arrival to casualty after 1-h transfer, GCS score was 7.

K. Goyal (✉)
All India Institute of Medical Sciences, New Delhi, India

R. Yadav
INHS Asvini, Mumbai, India


P. U. Bidkar, P. Vanamoorthy (eds.), *Acute Neuro Care*,
https://doi.org/10.1007/978-981-15-4071-4_8

## 8.1 Introduction

TBI is the leading cause of death and disability worldwide. In the USA, approximately 1.7 million people sustain it each year. Of these, 275,000 are hospitalized, and 52,000 die. The total volume of TBI in India is unknown, but estimates suggest that there are more than a million trauma-related deaths in India per year, of which 50% are TBI related [1]. 50% of deaths due to TBI occur during the first few hours and 90% of the prehospital trauma-related deaths are due to TBI. Distribution of TBI patients coming for medical attention is 75% mild, 15% moderate, and 10% having severe brain injury. Road traffic accidents (RTA) and falls are the commonest causes. After the primary injury, secondary brain injury ensues which decides the long-term outcome. Secondary brain injury occurs at a microscopic cellular level (hypoxia) and macroscopic level (intracranial hematoma). Many patients after TBI, even mild, are left with neuropsychological and cognitive impairments, which render them socially and economically dependent. Protocolized care to prevent secondary brain injury will have a significant effect on public health by reducing morbidity and mortality. The first few hours after TBI are very critical in deciding the outcome.

## 8.2 Intracranial Anatomy and Physiology

**Skull:** Due to its rich blood supply, skull laceration can lead to major blood loss, even at times hemorrhagic shock leading to death.

**Cranium:** Base of the cranium is irregular. Acceleration and deceleration of the brain inside the cranium can thus lead to brain parenchymal injury. (Coup and Counter- coup injury).

**Meninges:** Three layers cover the brain: dura mater, arachnoid mater, and pia mater. Dura is the outermost and toughest of the three attaching firmly to the internal surface of the skull. Dura splits at certain points to house the large venous sinuses. Massive hemorrhage can occur if these venous sinuses are injured. The middle meningeal artery lies between the dura mater and the inner surface of cranium (epidural space). Skull fracture can injure this artery and lead to epidural hematoma. Rapidly expanding epidural hematoma can be lethal if not drained urgently. Epidural hematoma can also occur due to injury to dural sinuses and skull fractures but these are slowly expanding. There is a potential space between the dura and arachnoid mater called subdural space. The bridging veins traveling from the surface of the brain to the venous sinuses lie here and injury to these veins during head injury leads to the formation of subdural hematoma. Pia mater firmly attaches to the brain surface and the potential space between pia and arachnoid forms subarachnoid space where CSF is present and provides a cushion to the brain.

**Brain:** It comprises of cerebrum, brain stem, and cerebellum. The Cerebrum is divided into two hemispheres—right and left, separated by falx cerebri. Brainstem consists of the midbrain, pons, and medulla. Midbrain and upper pons contain reticular activating system responsible for alertness and arousal. Vital centers are present in the medulla that continues to form the spinal cord.

Cerebellum is responsible mainly for coordination and balance. Tentorium cerebelli separates supratentorial compartment from infratentorial compartment. Midbrain passes through the opening called tentorial notch or hiatus. Medial part of temporal lobe (uncus) generally herniates through the tentorial notch leading to ipsilateral pupillary dilatation with contralateral hemiparesis (Classic sign of uncal herniation).

**Ventricular System:** Ventricles and cisterns are CSF filled spaces and they communicate with each other. Edema and mass effect can cause effacement (of cisterns), compression, and shifting of these ventricles (midline shift) which is evident on CT scan of the brain.

**Intracranial Compartment and Physiology:** Two physiological concepts are prerequisite while managing the patients of TBI.

**Monroe–Kellie Doctrine:** The intracranial volume is composed of the brain, the CSF, and the blood in the blood vessels, which fill the cranial cavity. Thus, any increase in one of the components is at the expense of the other two. This concept (the *Monro-Kellie Doctrine*) is of great importance in the pathophysiology of head trauma. Following injury, the brain will swell. Because of the fixed space within a rigid skull, as the brain tissue swells, it occupies more volume inside the skull. Initially, with the brain swelling, blood and CSF volumes inside the skull decrease and compensate for the rise in pressure. As brain swelling continues, however, compensation fails, and intracranial pressure (ICP) begins to rise. As the ICP increases, the amount of blood that can enter the skull and perfuse the brain decreases, leading to further brain injury. As the ICP continues to rise, the only significant opening through which the pressure can be released is the foramen magnum at the base of the skull. A significant rise in ICP can cause the brain to herniate through the foramen magnum with catastrophic effects (Figs. 8.1 and 8.2).

**Cerebral Autoregulation (CAR):** The brain normally adjusts its blood flow in response to metabolic needs. The autoregulation of blood flow is adjusted based on the level of carbon dioxide ($CO_2$) in the blood. The normal level of $CO_2$ is 35–45 mmHg. An increase in the level of $CO_2$ (hypoventilation) promotes vasodilatation of vessels supplying the brain, whereas lowering the level of $CO_2$ (hyperventilation) causes vasoconstriction and decreases blood flow to the brain. ICP is considered dangerous when it rises above 15 mmHg; cerebral herniation may occur at pressures above 25 mmHg. The net pressure gradient causing blood flow through

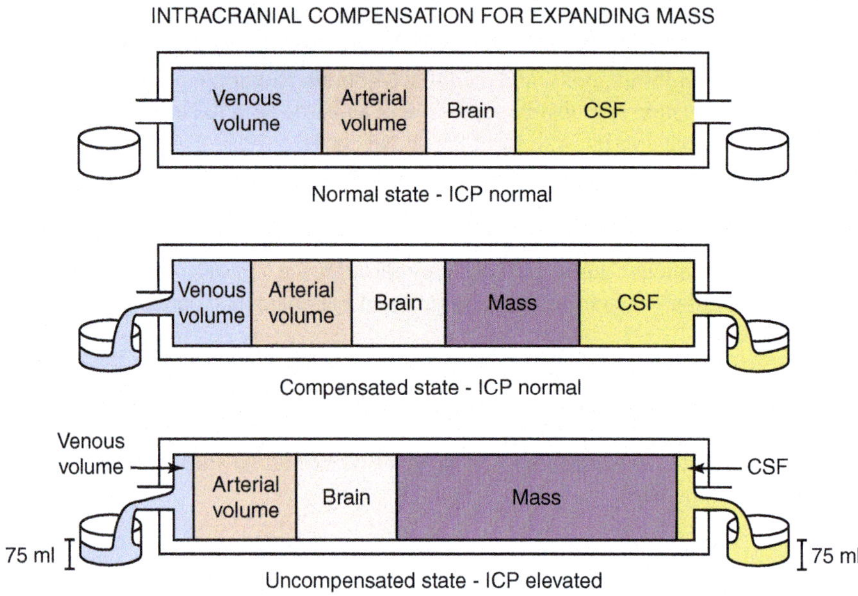


**Fig. 8.1** The Monro–Kellie doctrine regarding intracranial compensation for expanding mass

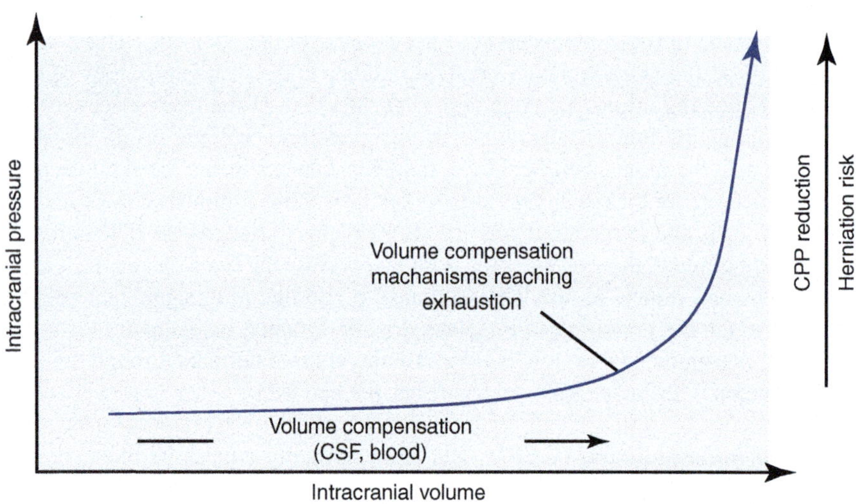


**Fig. 8.2** Relationship between intracranial pressure and volume, also known as brain compliance

the brain is termed the *cerebral perfusion pressure (CPP)*. Its value is obtained by subtracting the intracranial (intracerebral) pressure from the *mean arterial blood pressure (MAP)*.

$$\text{CPP} = \text{MAP} - \text{ICP}$$

When the ICP increases, the systemic blood pressure increases to try to preserve blood flow to the brain. The body senses the rise in systemic blood pressure, and this triggers a drop in the pulse rate as the body tries to lower the systemic blood pressure. With severe injury or ischemia, the pressure within the skull continues to rise until a critical point at which the ICP approaches the MAP, and there is no cerebral perfusion. All vital signs deteriorate, and the patient dies. Because CPP depends on both the arterial pressure and the ICP, hypotension also will have a devastating effect if the ICP is high.

Raised ICP may be clinically suspected by signs like dilated, non-reactive, or asymmetric pupils, progressive decline in neurological condition (fall in GCS >2), extensor posturing or low motor response, Cushing's response (Triad of hypertension, tachycardia followed by bradycardia, and irregular respirations).

Treatment of high ICP ought to begin early even before monitoring. Secondary brain injury can occur due to hypoxia, hypotension, hypercapnia, and hypocapnia. Every effort is made to prevent secondary brain injury by maintaining normal oxygenation and ventilation to maintain normocapnia. Cerebral perfusion should be maintained by maintaining normal intravascular volume, normal MAP, and reducing ICP. Hematomas and mass lesions that increase ICP and mass effect shall be evacuated early.

## 8.3 Diagnosis/Classification

Diagnosis is ascertained by mechanism of injury (e.g., RTA at a speed >50 km/h, fall >20 feet), physical signs of trauma (skull fracture, facial fractures, and scalp laceration) in a patient with neurological signs and symptoms.

### 8.3.1 Classification

#### 8.3.1.1 Skull Fractures

- Depressed vs Non- depressed
- Open vs closed
- Stellate vs linear

#### 8.3.1.2 Head Injury

**Focal**

- Extradural Hematoma (EDH)
- Subdural Hematoma (SDH)
- Intracerebral Hematoma or contusion (ICH)

**Diffuse**

- Concussion
- Multiple dot contusions
- Hypoxic ischemic injury
- Axonal Injury

### 8.3.2 Classification According to GCS

- Mild (GCS 13–15)
- Moderate (GCS 9–12)
- Severe (GCS ≤ 8)

### 8.3.3 Morphology

Head injury includes skull fractures and intracranial lesions like contusions, hematomas (EDH, SDH, and ICH), diffuse injuries (edema, hyperemia). Skull fractures may be in cranial vault or skull base. They may be linear or stellate and open or closed. Basilar skull fracture may lead to clinical signs like periorbital ecchymosis (raccoon eyes, panda eyes), retro auricular ecchymosis (battle's sign); CSF leak from the nose (rhinorrhea) or ear (otorrhea) and cranial nerve palsies especially seventh and eighth nerve (facial paralysis and hearing loss). CT with special bone window settings is required for fracture identification. As significant force is required for the skull to fracture, the possibility of intracranial hematomas is increased multifold. Suspicion is required especially in awake patients. These fractures may at times traverse the carotid canals and may damage carotid arteries. Open or compound fractures may lead to meningitis due to direct communication with the environment.

### 8.3.4 Focal Brain Injury

**Epidural Hematoma:** Relatively uncommon; and observed in 0.5% of brain-injured and 9% of comatose TBI patients. Typically, CT shows biconvex, lentiform shaped hematoma, usually due to middle meningeal artery laceration, may rarely be due to fracture or sinus bleed as well, above the dura and limited by suture line. Lucid interval (interval between the time of injury and neurological deterioration) is a classic feature (Fig. 8.3a).

**Subdural Hematoma:** More common; observed in 30% of patients with severe TBI. The same occurs due to the shearing of bridging veins traversing from the surface of the cortex to venous sinuses in the potential space between dura and arachnoid. CT shows hematoma generally concavo-convex shaped and along the contour of the brain. Brain damage is significant due to the presence of concomitant parenchymal injury (Fig. 8.3b).

**Contusions:** Common; observed in 20–30% of severe brain injury patients, generally involving frontal and temporal lobes, evolve over a period in size, and may coalesce to form intracerebral hematoma (ICH) with significant edema and mass effect. The need to undertake close monitoring and evaluation cannot be empha-

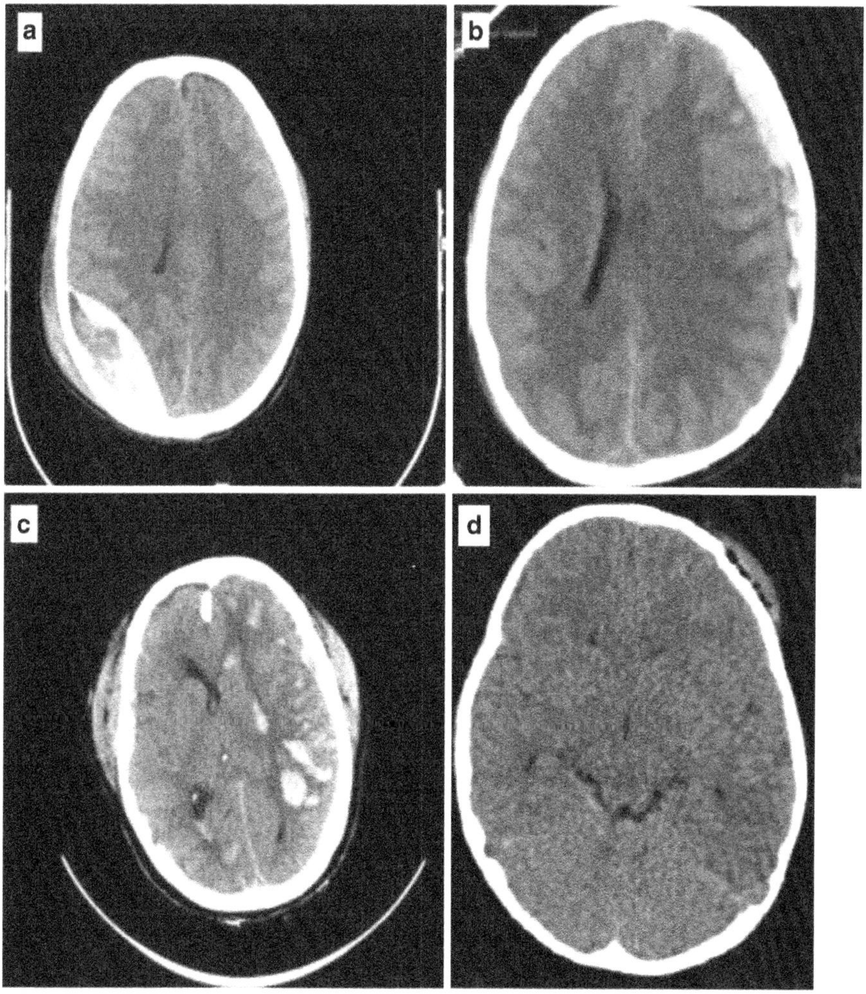


**Fig. 8.3** CT Scans of Intracranial Hematomas (**a**). Epidural hematoma (**b**). Subdural hematoma (**c**). Right intraparenchymal hemorrhage (**d**). Diffuse brain injury

sised more. CT is usually repeated within 24 h to see the progression of contusion (Fig. 8.3c).

**Diffuse Brain injuries:** Vary from mild concussion to severe ischemic hypoxic injuries. Initially CT appears normal without any mass lesion but the brain is diffusely swollen with loss of grey white matter distinction (Fig. 8.3d). Sometimes it may look like multiple punctate hemorrhages or contusions throughout the cerebral cortex.

*Glasgow Coma Scale (GCS)* is a common language among the health care workers that depicts the severity of head injury, prognosis, and improvement and/or worsening in a patient. The GCS should be seen following resuscitation but before the administration of any sedative or paralytic agents. When the mechanism of injury is not clear or history is lacking, non-traumatic causes (airway obstruction, tension pneumothorax, hypoglycemia, opiate overdose, and other poisonings) of decreased level of consciousness (LOC) must be considered. (Refer approach to comatose patient). During the assessment of GCS score in the presence of asymmetry (right/left, upper/lower), the best motor response is used to calculate the score. However, actual response on either side of the body, face, arm, and legs should be seen and noted.

Focused neurological examination consists of GCS, pupillary examination (size, reaction, symmetry), and lateralizing signs. This shall be repeated frequently during monitoring of these patients to elicit worsening (herniation) or improvement of their neurological status. Eye trauma may mimic or mask the signs of herniation. Pupil asymmetry is defined as >1 mm difference in diameter. A fixed pupil is defined as <1 mm response to bright light (Tables 8.1 and 8.2).

### 8.3.5 Early/Prehospital Care

50% of deaths due to TBI occur during the first few hours and 90% of the prehospital deaths in trauma are due to TBI. Basic measures include airway with cervical spine stabilization, maintenance of adequate oxygenation and ventilation. Providing adequate oxygenation and maintaining optimal blood pressure able to perfuse the brain is most important to prevent secondary brain injury. After stabilization by ABCDE, identification of mass lesion that requires surgical evacuation by computed tomography (CT) is critical. However, obtaining a CT should not delay the transfer of the patient to the appropriate neurosurgical facility. There is conflict regarding the adequate balance between early transfer to appropriate trauma center and best resuscitation at the site of injury. Ontario prehospital advanced life support (OPALS) study concluded that the addition of advanced life support in comparison to basic life support in the prehospital setting did not improve the outcome. Pediatric studies have even reported a worsened outcome after trying to perform advanced procedures and endotracheal intubation in the prehospital setting. In a large cohort trial, rapid sequence intubation (RSI) in TBI patients in the prehospital setting after using muscle relaxants was associated with higher mortality and decreased chances of favorable neurological outcome. The researchers observed that RSI doubled the scene time (13–26 min) and had more episodes of prolonged hypoxia and hypercapnia. Due to these concerns with advanced procedures like endotracheal intubation in the prehospital setting, supraglottic devices (LMA), or bag-mask ventilation is preferred. RSI and intubation using muscle relaxants ought to be used in the field only by a trained healthcare providers. Hypotension during initial hours worsens the outcome in these patients so isotonic normal saline is the preferred fluid for initial resuscitation.

**Table 8.1** Glasgow coma scale

| Behavior | Response | Score |
|---|---|---|
| Eye opening response | Spontaneously | 4 |
| | To speech | 3 |
| | To pain | 2 |
| | No response | 1 |
| Best verbal response | Oriented to time, place, and person | 5 |
| | Confused | 4 |
| | Inappropriate words | 3 |
| | Incomprehensible sounds | 2 |
| | No response | 1 |
| Best motor response | Obey commands | 6 |
| | Moves to localized pain | 5 |
| | Flexion withdrawal from pain | 4 |
| | Abnormal flexion (decorticate) | 3 |
| | Abnormal extension (decerebrate) | 2 |
| | No response | 1 |
| Total score | Best response | 15 |
| | Comatose client | 8 or less |
| | Totally unresponsive | 3 |

**Table 8.2** Pediatric Glasgow coma scale

| | Adult/child | Infant | Score |
|---|---|---|---|
| Eye opening | Same | Same | |
| Best verbal response | Oriented, appropriate | Coos and babbles | 5 |
| | Confused | Irritable cries | 4 |
| | Inappropriate words | Cries to pain | 3 |
| | Incomprehensible sounds | Moans to pain | 2 |
| | No response | No response | 1 |
| Best motor response | Obeys commands | Moves spontaneously | 6 |
| | Localizes to pain | Withdraws to touch | 5 |
| | Withdraws to pain | Withdraws to pain | 4 |
| | Flexion to pain | Flexion to pain | 3 |
| | Extension to pain | Extension to pain | 2 |
| | No response | No response | 1 |

**Airway:** Open, unobstructed, clear airway is required to maintain oxygen saturation greater than 90%. In the patient who is breathing spontaneously, the airway is monitored while maintaining spinal stabilization. Almost 10% of patients with severe head injury have associated cervical spine injury. Therefore, spinal stabilization is mandatory until the spine is cleared of any injury. Supplemental oxygen is delivered to all patients. All patients with severe TBI (GCS ≤8) should be intubated as they are unable to protect their airway. Bag mask ventilation or supraglottic airway devices are options in the prehospital setting until a definitive airway is established.

**Breathing:** Normal ventilation is the priority. Any injury hampering ventilation (pneumothorax, hemothorax, rib fracture) shall be ruled out. Normal ventilation (end-tidal $CO_2$ ($EtCO_2$) 35–40 mmHg) should be maintained and hyperventilation ($EtCO_2$ < 35 mmHg) avoided, unless there are signs of herniation. If there are clinical signs of herniation (e.g., unilaterally dilated pupil), then mild hyperventilation ($EtCO_2$ 28–35 mmHg) can be used as a temporary measure to reduce ICP (until signs of herniation resolve or until further assessment by emergency room personnel).

**Circulation:** Blood pressure is maintained (SBP > 90 mmHg in adults and age-specific in children). Avoidance of hypotension is particularly important in the first 6 hrs post-injury [2]. Hypotension is treated urgently with 1–2 L of isotonic crystalloid in adults and 20 mL/kg bolus in children. Hypotonic fluids (5% dextrose) should be avoided as the same may exacerbate cerebral edema. Any systemic injury, immediate and life-threatening, causing hypotension should be looked for and treated.

**CPP:** The goal is approximately 50–70 mmHg. A CPP of 45–60 mmHg may be the target in children. If serum lactate is not elevated, the administration of a vasopressor may be indicated to maintain cerebral perfusion. For anemic, actively bleeding patients, and children a red blood cell (RBCs) transfusion earlier may be prudent. Generally isolated TBI patients are not hypotensive but if a shock is there, mostly it is hemorrhagic shock which is associated with tachycardia. If a patient of head injury has hypotension with bradycardia not responding to fluid resuscitation, spinal cord injury should be suspected. Inotropes ought be started early.

**Additional Intervention:** Diagnose hypoglycemia, and, if hypoglycemic, give D50 (50 mL IV push in adults and 5 mL/kg of D10 in children). Frequent neurological examination should be repeated during the resuscitation. GCS after resuscitation is more valuable to define the severity of head injury.

## 8.4 Neurological Examination: Disability (D)

Focused Neurological Examination: After hemodynamic stability, a focused neurological examination is performed. It consists of GCS score, pupillary reaction, and focal neurological signs. Confounding factors like alcohol, intoxication, and other injuries may be enquired but should not be considered to be the cause of impaired consciousness until head injury is ruled out. Motor response is elicited by pinching trapezius muscle or applying supraorbital ridge pressure. Best motor response is considered in case of variable response on either side or discrepancy in upper and lower extremity response. Doll's eye response shall be withheld until cervical spine injury is ruled out. Neurological examination shall be performed preferably before intubation and before sedation and paralysis. Short-acting sedatives and paralytics are used to allow frequent neurological examinations.

**CT Scan/Neuroimaging:** Patient must be hemodynamically stable before transfer for CT. Immediate surgical intervention for life-threatening systemic hemorrhage may mean that neuroimaging (e.g., CT) is not performed initially. Emergency neurosurgical procedures, such as ventriculostomy (EVD), may be reasonable in some as a life-saving measure.

Non-contrast CT remains the neuroimaging modality of choice because of its faster acquisition and giving all practical information. The primary purpose of the initial CT is to identify any hemorrhagic mass lesions that warrant surgery. Significant findings on CT include scalp swelling, subgaleal hematoma at the region of impact, skull fractures (better seen in bone windows), intracranial hematomas, contusions, midline shift (mass effect), and obliteration of basal cisterns. As a general guide, an extra-axial hematoma (epi- or subdural) >1 cm in thickness, an intraparenchymal hematoma >3 cm in diameter, and a > 5 mm midline shift associated with a hematoma maybe considered for surgery [3].

Acute blood is generally hyperdense, but, in some patients, it may be iso- or hypodense more so if the patient is coagulopathic or anemic. Contusions can be hyperdense, hypodense, or have a "salt and pepper" appearance. Caution is required in patients on anticoagulation and antiplatelet therapy, hematoma and contusion can form and enlarge rapidly. Rapid normalization of coagulation abnormalities is warranted. Intracranial air suggests an open skull fracture, craniofacial trauma, or injury to an air sinus. Vault and facial fractures may be associated, so the bone window is preferable to delineate these. Associated cervical spine injuries occur in up to 10% of head-injured patients, hence radiologic imaging of TBI should include C-spine, preferably after the primary survey. Unless the C-spine is cleared for any injury or instability, the immobilization should be maintained by a rigid collar or manual in-line mobilization.

Surgical decision-making is often guided by the amount of mass effect and midline shift. Therefore, it should be determined whether the perimesencephalic cisterns are open, compromised, or closed, and the degree of midline shift at the level of the third ventricle is quantified [4].

## 8.5 Management (Fig. 8.4)

**Initial Casualty Management:** Preventing secondary brain injury by maintaining the airway, preventing hypoxia, hypocarbia, hypotension remains the priority. Definitive airway shall be established in casualty. Adequate resuscitation is completed in the casualty if not done in the field. Maintenance of cerebral perfusion and preventing/treating brain herniation is required. There exists a difference between $EtCO_2$ and $PaCO_2$, capnography mostly underestimating actual $PaCO_2$. This is due to increase in ventilator dead space, which is common in sick patients and those with low cardiac output.

**Management of Mild Head Injury (GCS 13–15):** Patient of head injury with history of transient loss of consciousness, disorientation, and amnesia (anterograde or

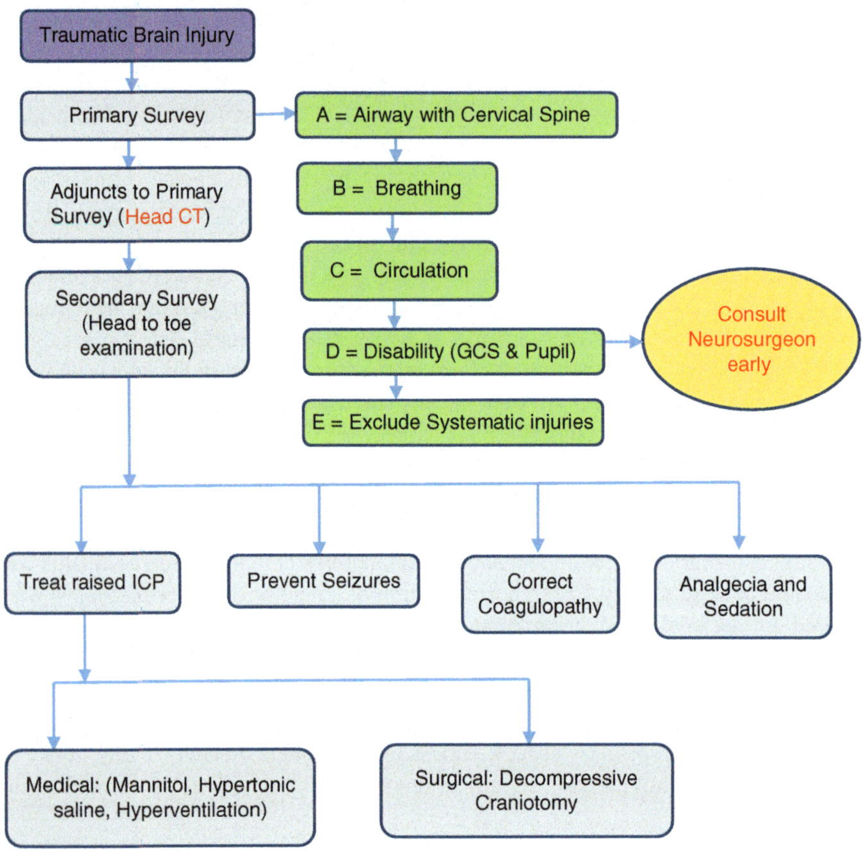


**Fig. 8.4** Management of TBI

retrograde) who otherwise is conscious and talking is considered a mild head injury. Mental status alterations shall never be attributed to confounding factors like alcohol or intoxication unless head injury is excluded. Mostly such patients recover completely but 3% of these may deteriorate. Serial neurological examination and documentation of GCS is important. CT scan is done in high and moderate risk of brain injury. CT scan acquisition shall not delay the transfer of a patient to a neurosurgical facility. Patient of mild head injury should be admitted to hospital and neurosurgeon consulted if the patient has abnormal CT or/and remains symptomatic. If such patients are asymptomatic without any neurologic abnormality and alert, they are observed and re-examined, and can be safely discharged to home along with a companion, in the absence of any neurological deficit. Instructions are directed to both the patient and companion to return to hospital in case of any deterioration in mental status, focal neurologic deficit and/or increasing headache (Table 8.3).

**Management of Moderate Head Injury (GCS 9–12):** 15% of patients of head injury arriving in casualty have moderate head injury. They are drowsy, confused, and can have focal neurologic deficits. After hemodynamic stability, serial

**Table 8.3** Indications of CT scan in mild head injury patients (26)

| High risk | Moderate risk |
|---|---|
| 1. GCS score less than 15 even at 2 h after injury | 1. Loss of consciousness (>5 min) |
| 2. Suspected open or depressed skull fracture | 2. Retrograde amnesia (>30 minu) |
| 3. Age more than 65 years | 3. Dangerous mechanism of injury (RTA at a speed >50 km/h, fall from a height > 20 feet, occupant ejected from vehicle, penetrating head injury) |
| 4. Vomiting (> 2 episodes) | 4. Moderate to severe headache |
| 5. Sign of basilar skull fracture | 5. Focal neurologic deficit |

neurological examination is must as approximately 10–20% of these patients can deteriorate. CT scan and neurosurgical consultation are required in all cases provided patients are hemodynamically stable. These patients require ICU admission where close monitoring and frequent neurological examinations are done. Repeat CT scan is done in the next 24 h if the patient deteriorates or the initial CT scan was abnormal. Moderate head injury patients can deteriorate rapidly to coma, with declining mental status leading to inability to protect their airway and hypoventilation. Urgent intubation may be required and further treatment similar to severe head injury is begun.

**Management of Severe Head Injury (GCS 3–8):** Approximately 10% of all head injury patients coming to casualty have severe head injuries. These patients remain comatose (GCS < 9) even after cardiopulmonary resuscitation and hemodynamic stabilization. Prompt diagnosis and management is very important. Primary survey (ABCDE), resuscitation and cardiopulmonary stabilization are achieved rapidly because the presence of hypotension doubles the risk of mortality, and the addition of hypoxia further worsens it. Early endotracheal intubation shall be performed in all patients with GCS < 9. Hyperventilation to be avoided during early hours after injury and should be used cautiously only when there is neurological deterioration and the presence of signs of herniation. Isolated head injury generally is not associated with hypotension unless there is associated spinal cord injury or in terminal stages when there is ensuing medullary failure. Neurological examination (GCS, pupillary examination) is considered after hemodynamic stabilization. If the patient remains hypotensive, then focused neurological examination should be performed and documented with hypotension. The cause of hypotension is searched for and treated before the neurosurgical evaluation in such cases.

If such patients are stable hemodynamically, then they should be admitted to ICU capable of neurosurgical care. Head to toe examination and AMPLE history is elicited.

Therapeutic agents to decrease ICP are administered. Serial focused neurological examinations are repeated frequently and any deterioration and improvement noted. Non-contrast CT scan is done in all these patients when hemodynamically stable. CT scan should be repeated whenever there is any neurological deterioration and routinely after 24 h of a previous scan to see the progress of hematoma and contusion.

**ICP Monitoring:** ICP monitoring is indicated in severe head injury (GCS < 9) with abnormal head CT or normal CT with the presence of any two of these clinical features: 1. Age > 65 years, 2. Hypotension SBP < 90 mmHg, 3. Decerebrate posturing.

### 8.5.1 Medical Treatment

**Intravenous Fluids:** Normovolemia is maintained by isotonic crystalloids or blood and blood products, as required. Hypovolemia is harmful. Hypotonic fluids are avoided as they worsen cerebral edema. Glucose containing fluids may result in hyperglycemia and have been implicated in causing cerebral ischemia. Isotonic fluids like normal saline and ringer lactate are preferred during resuscitation.

**Diuretics like Mannitol or Hypertonic Saline:** Mannitol 20% 0.5–1 g/kg can be given as a rapid bolus (within 5 min) intravenously provided the patient is hemodynamically stable. If hypotension along with signs of raised ICP is there, then instead of mannitol, hypertonic saline 3% NS (2–5 mL/kg) IV over 10 min can be administered. Mannitol should not be administered to a patient with hypotension as it will worsen hypovolemia by osmotic diuresis.

**Transient Hyperventilation:** Hyperventilation acts by reducing $PaCO_2$ and causing cerebral vasoconstriction. If there are signs of herniation, then as a temporizing measure hyperventilation with a target $PaCO_2$ of 28–35 mmHg may be used for a short period while awaiting definitive treatment. Aggressive and prolonged hyperventilation can lead to cerebral ischemia.

**Barbiturates:** Raised ICP refractory to usual measures may respond to barbiturates. They act by reducing cerebral metabolism and promoting cerebral vasoconstriction; thus culminating in reduction of ICP. They should not be used when the patient is already hypotensive, as the haemodynamic instability may be worsened.

**Coagulopathy:** There is high incidence (40–50% in severe TBI) of coagulopathy in TBI patients that can exacerbate secondary brain injury by increasing hematoma and preventing hemostasis. Recognition and correction of coagulopathy is important in the initial management of TBI. The mechanism involved is tissue factor release. Various factors associated are increased age, hypotension, low GCS (≤8), intraparenchymal lesions, penetrating injury, patients on anticoagulants and antiplatelets, and base deficit at presentation [5–7]. Routine coagulation parameters like prothrombin time (PT), INR, partial thromboplastin time (aPTT), platelet counts, and fibrinogen levels shall be monitored. Thromboelastography (TEG) can be performed at the bedside to give the dynamic status of coagulation. Fresh frozen plasma (FFP), platelet concentrates, Vitamin K is used routinely. Prothrombin Complex Concentrate (PCC) have been shown to more actively reverse warfarin-induced coagulopathy than FFP and vitamin K. It can be used even in patients on newer oral anti-coagulants (thrombin inhibitors and factor Xa Inhibitors). The benefit of platelet transfusion in patients on antiplatelet drugs is inconclusive. Desmopressin (0.3 mcg/kg IV) can be administered to patients in renal failure to temporarily improve uremic platelet function.

**Seizure Prophylaxis:** Posttraumatic seizures (PTS) must be prevented during the acute phase otherwise these can exacerbate the secondary brain injury. Prolonged seizures >30 min can at times lead to significant brain damage. Seizures can be classified as early (within 7 days of TBI) and late (>7 days after a head injury). Incidence of convulsive PTS is 5% in patients admitted to hospital with closed head injuries and 15% in those with severe TBI. The incidence of PTS may be even higher in children [7]. Non-convulsive seizures (NCSs) as monitored with continuous EEG (cEEG) are even higher, amounting to almost 30% in severe TBI patients. Several risk factors associated with an increased incidence of PTS are GCS <10, cortical contusion, subdural hematoma, epidural hematoma, intracerebral hematoma, depressed skull fracture, penetrating head injury, and seizure within 24 h of injury [8]. Phenytoin has proven efficacy in preventing early PTS in TBI patients [9]. Phenytoin (or fosphenytoin) is therefore recommended as seizure prophylaxis in all patients admitted to the hospital with moderate or severe TBI and an abnormal head CT scan. The seizure prophylaxis is stopped after 7 days if no seizures occur. Late prophylactic therapy (i.e., after 7 days) in patients without evidence of a previous seizure is not effective and may even cause harm to the patient. Anticonvulsants may inhibit brain recovery and early anticonvulsant therapy does not change long-term traumatic seizure outcome, so these drugs should be used only when necessary. Further concern for intermittent seizures may necessitate continuous EEG monitoring. Therefore, prophylactic use of antiepileptic medications is not recommended to prevent late PTS [10]. Levetiracetam is another AED that is commonly used and is supported by a growing volume of data. Muscle relaxants do not control seizures, they only mask clinical presentation but underlying brain damage is still going on. Muscle relaxants should not be used to treat seizures.

**Sedation:** Patients with severe TBI often require intubation for airway protection. Analgesia and sedation are required to ensure pain is relieved and that patients are not agitated. Short-acting agents with minimal hemodynamic effects may be chosen. This will allow frequent neurological examination as and when required. No single medication is superior in patients with severe TBI over others. Short-acting opioids and midazolam can be used. Dexmedetomidine infusion is also a promising agent which allows sedation, analgesia and patient remains arousable for examination as needed.

**Consultation:** Early neurosurgical consultation is required once the patient is stabilized hemodynamically. Patients with severe TBI should be transferred to a trauma center with neurosurgical capabilities.

**Surgery:** In general, extra-axial (extradural or subdural) hemorrhage or mass > 1 cm in thickness, midline shift >5 mm, ICH >3 cm in diameter, penetrating injury, depressed skull fracture, or refractory intracranial hypertension (ICH) are all indications for surgery. In general, acute extra-axial (i.e., extradural and subdural, hematomas >1 cm thick or associated with >5 mm of midline shift) hematomas should be considered for emergent surgery [11–15]. Similarly, intracerebral hematomas >50 mL in volume or > 3 cm in diameter particularly with mass effect should be considered for surgical evaluation with a neurosurgeon. Hematoma location is also important for decision-making. In the posterior fossa, minimal enlargement of a small lesion has the potential to result in brainstem compression. Midline cerebellar lesions may result in obstructive hydrocephalus. Depressed skull fractures that are displaced greater than the thickness of the skull table, and particularly those that are open or compound, typically require surgical repair. Any depressed fracture immediately over a major venous sinus requires surgical consideration. Blood loss from scalp wounds can be extensive, especially in children. Direct pressure bandage helps. Fractures of air sinuses, penetrating trauma, or craniofacial injuries all require special consideration. Decompressive craniectomy (DC), either a unilateral hemicraniectomy or bilateral frontal craniectomy, can be used to treat refractory intracranial hypertension. There is strong evidence that DC in select patients effectively controls ICP, though the effect on patient outcome is still being elucidated [16, 17] (Table 8.4).

**Pediatric Concerns:** TBI is the leading cause of injury-related pediatric deaths [18]. Interestingly, children have a remarkable ability to recover from seemingly devastating injuries so aggressive treatment should be done. The goals of initial management include rapid identification of intracranial injuries requiring surgical intervention and prevention of secondary brain insults that worsen outcome. For the most part, the approach and emergent care of a child with TBI are similar to adult management. Due to variations in verbal and motor skills, a pediatric Glasgow Coma Scale (GCS) was developed to assess disability and should be used in the setting of TBI. The standard GCS has been validated for use in children 3 years of age and older and the pediatric GCS should be used for infants through 2 years of age [19–22]. Predictors of poor outcome in children with severe TBI include hypoten-

**Table 8.4** Brain trauma foundation recommendations

| Positive (treat with) | Negative (do not use) | Neutral (risks and benefits are similar) |
|---|---|---|
| Nutrition | Steroids (level 1) | Seizure prophylaxis to treat early PTS |
| Early tracheostomy | Seizure prophylaxis to treat late posttraumatic seizures (PTS) | |
| Performing a large rather than a small decompressive craniectomy | Povidone -iodine use | |
| | Performing a bifrontal decompressive craniectomy instead of conservative treatment in diffuse injury | |

sion, hypothermia, and non-accidental trauma [23]. Spinal cord injury is less frequent in children compared to adults, but spinal precautions should be maintained at all times. Importantly, young children are at risk of spinal cord injury without radiographic abnormality (SCIWORA).

**Checklist**

| | |
|---|---|
| 1. | Airway with cervical spine immobilization ($SpO_2 > 90\%$) (A) |
| 2. | Breathing (B) |
| 3. | Systolic BP > 90 mmHg (C) |
| 4. | Focused neurological examination—Frequent re-evaluation (D) |
| 5. | Exclude systemic injuries (E) |
| 6. | Consult neurosurgeon |
| 7. | Head CT |
| 8. | Treat herniation |

## Multiple Choice Questions

1. Indications for craniotomy for acute epidural hematoma (EDH) include all of the following *except*:
   (a). Pupillary anisocoria
   (b). Midline shift greater than 5 mm
   (c). Hematoma volume greater than 30 $cm^3$
   (d). Lack of a lucid interval
2. The principal effect of mannitol in the treatment of elevated intracranial pressure (ICP) is:
   (a). Osmotic fluid removal from the brain
   (b). Decrease in cerebral blood flow
   (c). Free radical sequestration
   (d). Decrease in the cerebral metabolic rate
3. Which of these statements regarding basilar skull fractures is *not* true?
   (a). Basilar skull fractures occur in 7–16% of all patients with skull fractures
   (b). These fractures are often indicated by the presence of pneumocephalus on head CT in the absence of open cranial vault fractures
   (c). Prophylactic antibiotics have been demonstrated to reduce the risk of meningitis
   (d). These skull fractures are frequently accompanied by periorbital ecchymoses (raccoon's eyes) or postauricular ecchymoses (Battle's sign)
4. Which of the following statements regarding posttraumatic cerebrospinal fluid (CSF) fistulae is true?
   (a). CSF otorrhea is more likely to resolve spontaneously than CSF rhinorrhea
   (b). Posttraumatic CSF fistulae occur in 50% of all patients with basilar skull fractures
   (c). Less than one third resolve spontaneously
   (d). Meningitis occurs in less than 3%

5. Hypertonic saline has been demonstrated to:
   (a). Increase cerebral blood flow more than mannitol on an equimolar basis
   (b). Decrease intracranial pressure (ICP) more than mannitol on an equimolar basis
   (c). Have a shorter duration of action than mannitol
   (d). Have a greater risk of nephrotoxicity than mannitol
6. Risk factors for increase in the size of traumatic cerebral contusions/hemorrhages include:
   (a). Age older than 60 years
   (b). Elevation of partial thromboplastin time (PTT)
   (c). Deterioration of Glasgow Coma Scale (GCS) after resuscitation
   (d). All of the above
7. Which of these statements regarding prophylactic hypothermia in traumatic brain injury (TBI) is true?
   (a). Prophylactic hypothermia has been clearly demonstrated to benefit outcome from acute TBI in children.
   (b). Prophylactic hypothermia has a complication rate similar to other brain injury treatments in normothermic patients.
   (c). Prophylactic hypothermia decreases mortality, but does not improve outcome in adults with acute TBI.
   (d). Prophylactic hypothermia does not improve mortality or outcome in the treatment of adults and children with TBI.
8. Prophylactic anticonvulsants in the setting of traumatic brain injury (TBI) have been demonstrated to:
   (a). Decrease the incidence of early posttraumatic seizures
   (b). Decrease the incidence of both early and late posttraumatic seizures
   (c). Not alter the incidence of posttraumatic seizures but reduce the severity of posttraumatic seizures
   (d). Decrease the incidence of late posttraumatic seizures
9. Which of the following statements is true regarding the role of decompressive hemicraniectomy in the treatment of the patient with traumatic brain injury (TBI)?
   (a). Randomized prospective trials have shown that decompressive hemicraniectomy decreases mortality and improves outcomes
   (b). Decompressive hemicraniectomy may be effective in treating refractory intracranial pressure (ICP)
   (c). Decompressive hemicraniectomy has no role in the treatment of increased ICP in the patient with TBI and should only be used to treat the malignant middle cerebral artery (MCA) syndrome
   (d). Decompressive hemicraniectomy should never be performed in patients younger than 18 years
10. Indications for intracranial pressure (ICP) monitoring include all of the following *except*:
   (a). Severe alcohol withdrawal in the traumatic brain injury (TBI) patient
   (b). Glasgow Coma Scale (GCS) score 3–8 with an abnormal CT scan

(c). Normal head CT scan with any two of these features: age older than 40 years, unilateral or bilateral motor posturing, and systolic blood pressure (SBP) <90
(d). Patients with abnormal head CT scans with GCS greater than 8 who are undergoing prolonged general anesthesia or pharmacologic muscle relaxants and will not have a neurologic examination that may be assessed

11. Treatments designed to decrease intracranial pressure (ICP) should begin when:
    (a). ICP increases 10 mmHg from the pressure when the ICP monitor was placed
    (b). There is a presence of any midline shift on the head CT
    (c). ICP reaches a threshold of between 15 and 20 mmHg
    (d). ICP reaches a threshold of between 20 and 25 mmHg
12. Which of the following statements regarding barbiturate-induced coma is true?
    (a). Has been demonstrated to be beneficial in improving patient outcomes from severe traumatic injury when used in a prophylactic fashion
    (b). Is less effective than mannitol in lowering increased intracranial pressure (ICP)
    (c). Rarely induces systemic hypotension when infused at target rates
    (d). Causes an unacceptable increase in core body temperature

Answers: 1. (a), 2. (a), 3. (c), 4. (a), 5. (b), 6. (d), 7. (d), 8. (a), 9. (b), 10. (a), 11. (d), 12. (b)

## References


1. Maas AI. Traumatic brain injury in India: a big problem in need of data. Neurol India. 2017;65:257–8.
2. Garvin R, Venkatasubramanian C, Brown AL, Miller CM. Emergency neurological life support: traumatic brain injury. Neurocrit Care. 2015;23:S143–54.
3. Faul M, Xu L, Wald MM, Coronado VG. Traumatic brain injury in the United States: emergency department visits, hospitalizations, and deaths. Centers for Disease Control and Prevention, National Center for Injury Prevention and Control; 2010.
4. Katsnelson M, Mackenzie L, Frangos S, et al. Are initial radiographic and clinical scales associated with subsequent intracranial pressure and brain oxygen levels after severe traumatic brain injury? Neurosurgery. 2012;70:1095–105.
5. Stein SC, Smith DH. Coagulopathy in traumatic brain injury. Neurocrit Care. 2004;1:479–88.
6. Talving P, Benfield R, Hadjizacharia P, Inaba K, Chan LS, Demetriades D. Coagulopathy in severe traumatic brain injury: a prospective study. J Trauma. 2009;66:55–61.
7. Cap AP, Spinella PC. Severity of head injury is associated with increased risk of coagulopathy in combat casualties. J Trauma. 2011;71:S78–81.
8. Temkin NR, Dikmen SS, Wilensky AJ, Keihm J, Chabal S, Winn HR. A randomized, double-blind study of phenytoin for the prevention of post-traumatic seizures. N Engl J Med. 1990;323:497–502.
9. O'Neil BR, Handler MH, Tong S, Chapman KE. Incidence of seizures on continuous EEG monitoring following traumatic brain injury in children. J Neurosurg Pediatr. 2015; 8:1–10.
10. Bratton SL, Chestnut RM, Ghajar J, et al. Guidelines for the management of severe traumatic brain injury XIII. Antiseizure prophylaxis. J Neurotrauma. 2007;24(Suppl 1):S83–6.

11. Bullock MR, Chesnut R, Ghajar J, et al. Surgical management of depressed cranial fractures. Neurosurgery. 2006;58:S56–60.
12. Bullock MR, Chesnut R, Ghajar J, et al. Surgical management of posterior fossa mass lesions. Neurosurgery. 2006;58:S47–55.
13. Bullock MR, Chesnut R, Ghajar J, et al. Surgical management of traumatic parenchymal lesions. Neurosurgery. 2006;58:S25–46.
14. Bullock MR, Chesnut R, Ghajar J, et al. Surgical management of acute subdural hematomas. Neurosurgery. 2006;58:S16–24.
15. Bullock MR, Chesnut R, Ghajar J, et al. Surgical management of acute epidural hematomas. Neurosurgery. 2006;58:S7–15.
16. Cooper DJ, Rosenfeld JV, Murray L, et al. Decompressive craniectomy in diffuse traumatic brain injury. N Engl J Med. 2011;364:1493–502.
17. Sahuquillo J, Arikan F. Decompressive craniectomy for the treatment of refractory high intracranial pressure in traumatic brain injury. Cochrane Database Syst Rev. 2006:CD003983.
18. Langlois JA, Rutland-Brown W, Thomas KE. Traumatic brain injury in the United States: emergency department visits, hospitalizations, and deaths. Centers for Disease Control and Prevention, National Center for Injury and Prevention Control, Atlanta 2006 (Statistical data).
19. Morray JP, Tyler DC, Jones TK, et al. Coma scale for use in brain injured children. Crit Care Med. 1984;12:1018–20.
20. Kapapa T, Konig K, Pfister U, et al. Head trauma in children, part 1: admission, diagnosis, and findings. J Child Neurol. 2010;25:146–56.
21. Simpson D, Reilly P. Pediatric coma scale. Lancet. 1982;2:450.
22. James HE. Neurologic evaluation and support in the child with an acute brain insult. Pediatr Ann. 1986;15:16–22.
23. Vavilala MS, Bowen A, Lam AM, et al. Blood pressure and outcome after severe pediatric traumatic brain injury. J Trauma. 2003;55(6):1039–44.

# 9 Traumatic Spine Injury

Niraj Kumar and Ashish Bindra

**Key Points**

- Suspect spinal cord injury (SCI) in a trauma victim especially in polytrauma settings.
- Airway management in a trauma victim should be accompanied by cervical spine protection.
- Spinal immobilization should start with suspicion of trauma and should continue till spinal injury is ruled out.
- Excessive movement of the spine should be avoided during transport and shifting to prevent further neurological injury.
- Assessment of life-threatening injuries and achieving hemodynamic stability remains priority during primary survey.
- Exclude cervical spine injury either clinically or radiologically as quickly and effectively as possible in a neurologically intact person.
- In a conscious patient without any distracting injuries absence of pain and tenderness along the spine rules out the presence of spinal injury.
- In a patient with an altered level of consciousness imaging should be done as early as possible to rule out injury to the cervical spine.
- CT is the primary screening modality in SCI.
- Use of steroids in management of acute spinal cord injury is not recommended.
- In absence of facilities required for managing such patient arrangement should be made to transfer the patient to a higher center.

N. Kumar · A. Bindra (✉)
All India institute of medical sciences, New Delhi, India


P. U. Bidkar, P. Vanamoorthy (eds.), *Acute Neuro Care*,
https://doi.org/10.1007/978-981-15-4071-4_9

**Case Scenario**

A 26-year-old male suffered a motor vehicle accident. He is conscious, oriented, and able to follow commands. His vitals are Blood Pressure—84/60 mmHg, Heart Rate—55/m, Respiratory Rate—30/m. He has labored breathing and inability to move all four limbs.

## 9.1 Introduction

The incidence of Spinal cord injury (SCI) varies from 9.2 to 56.1 per million [1]. It is a huge social and economic burden across the globe. Management of SCI is an equally challenging condition for a clinician as well as the patient and his family. The majority of the victims are healthy male between 15 and 45 years of age [2]. Initial management of patients with spinal cord injury determines the outcome and overall quality of life a patient is going to have. The cervical spine being most mobile is the commonest site of SCI and accounts for more than 50% of total cases. It is followed by an injury to the thoracic, thoracolumbar, and lumbar spine. Cervical spine injury is associated with much higher mortality and morbidity compared to other sites [3]. In children upper cervical injury is commoner than lower cervical injury. Otherwise bony spinal injuries are less common in children who may suffer from SCI without evidence of radiological abnormality (SCIWORA). In such children the diagnosis of the injury is clinical and may be delayed due to lack of any findings on imaging. SCIWORA can be seen in 6–19% and 9–14% of spinal injuries in children and adults, respectively [4, 5].

The most common mechanism of SCI is fall especially in the elderly followed by road traffic accidents. Assault is another common mechanism of injury to the spinal cord in the developing world. Other causes include degenerative disease, tumors, infections, vascular lesions, and congenital deformities [6]. This chapter deals with the initial management of this neurological emergency (Fig. 9.1).

**Primary Injury:** It is caused at the time of initial impact. It can be direct damage to the cord by penetrating foreign objects or because of the impingement of the bony fragment. Usually compression, traction, or hemorrhage is responsible for the primary injury. A combination of mechanisms like axial loading, extension, flexion, lateral rotation, or distraction results in cervical spine injury.

**Secondary Injury:** The secondary injury starts immediately after the primary insult. Understanding pathophysiology of secondary injury is important as it is preventable, limits damage, and can improve prognosis. It occurs mainly as aftereffect to vascular and biochemical effects on primary injury. The initial injury causes immediate hemorrhage and rapid cell death but following it multiple secondary injury cascades are initiated which result in continued damage and cell death caus-

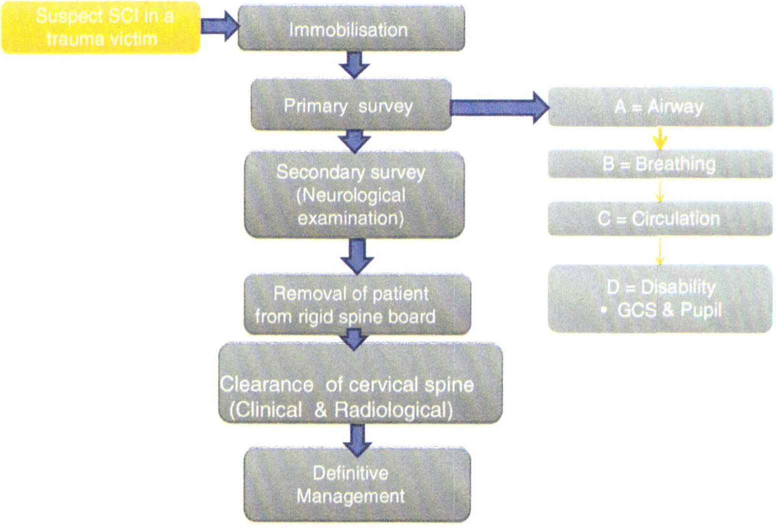


**Fig. 9.1** Algorithm for step wise approach to a patient with spinal cord injury

ing dysfunction and greater tissue loss [7]. The main aim of the management of SCI is prevention of this secondary injury.

## 9.2 When to Suspect a Spinal Column Injury

Spinal cord injury (SCI) should be suspected in a trauma victim especially in polytrauma settings. The mechanism of injury is an important indicator of the type of injury to be suspected. History of motor vehicle accident, fall from a height or assault points toward SCI along with the trauma to other organs. It should always be considered in an unconscious/intoxicated patient. Complaints of pain and tenderness along the spine and the presence of neurological deficits indicate SCI. SCI can be ruled out in a conscious patient without any tenderness or pain along the spine.

## 9.3 Immobilization

The initial goal of treatment of SCI is to protect and immobilize the cervical spine to prevent further injury due to unwarranted movement. Immobilization should be initiated at the scene of trauma or the first encounter with the patient and should continue until an unstable cervical injury is excluded by clinical criteria or radiography. A combination of the backboard, rigid cervical collar, head

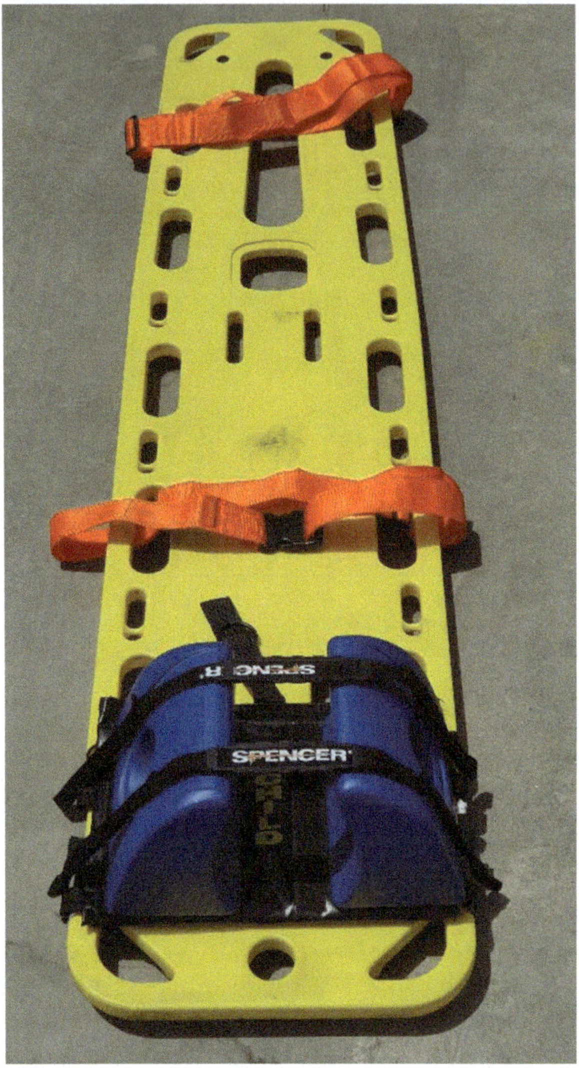


**Fig. 9.2** Long spine board for patient immobilization and transport

immobilization tape, and straps should ideally be used (Fig. 9.2). In absence of ideal conditions, head immobilization can be done on-site by giving lateral head support with bolstering devices like towel rolls, foam head blocks, or any other available material. Sometimes pain control and sedation may be required to achieve spinal immobilization in agitated patients. Immobilization is particularly important during patient transport and patient evaluation. Inappropriate mobility and excessive manipulation lead to neurological deterioration by the time patients reach treatment facilities. Apart from inadequate immobilization, factors like ischemia and increasing spinal edema are the main contributors to increasing neurological damage.

## 9.4 Management of a Patient with SCI

**Primary Survey:** It is the initial assessment and management of a trauma patient. It is conducted to detect and treat acute or imminent life threats and prevent complications from such injuries. A systematic approach using ABCDE is used [8].

### 9.4.1 A = Airway Management with Cervical Spine Stabilization

In trauma airway management is always accompanied by cervical spine stabilization. This is because various airway techniques and maneuvers used may hamper spinal stabilization and add to secondary neurologic injury of the spinal cord. Besides this spinal injury may itself pose a threat to airway patency. Patients with possible or known high cervical spine injury may require airway management on an urgent basis due to anticipated loss of protective airway reflexes and impending ventilatory failure. Every clinician should be aware of the complicated scenarios of the airway management and the possibility of diaphragmatic and phrenic nerve paralysis depending upon the level of spinal injury [9]. Airway obstruction may occur in these patients due to associated retropharyngeal hemorrhage or edema. Patients with complete cervical SCI above C5 are more likely to develop respiratory failure, hence its better do elective intubation and ventilation.

The main goal of airway management is the least spine movement during airway maneuvering. Jaw thrust maneuver should be preferred to head tilt and chin lift for airway opening and bag-mask ventilation. In a patient requiring emergent intubation; rapid sequence intubation (RSI) is the preferred method in conjunction with orotracheal intubation [10]. Manual in-line spinal stabilization (MILS) is recommended to prevent exacerbation of a cervical spinal cord injury during intubation. There are many techniques and devices available for intubation and clinician must be familiar with the pros and cons of each technique and select the best available option for intubating a patient with suspected cervical SCI.

Awake flexible fiberoptic intubation (FI) is the technique of choice for elective intubations in a cooperative patient. Awake FI is supposed to be the safest and most valuable method of airway management in a patient with a known or suspected cervical spine injury [11]. Video fluoroscopy-guided studies demonstrate the least cervical spine movement during fiberoptic-guided intubation [12]. However, presence of secretions and blood in airway and emergency settings may decrease the utility of FI. Use of video laryngoscope is becoming increasingly popular among emergency physicians and has added enormously to the armamentarium of difficult airway cart.

### 9.4.2 B = Breathing and Ventilation

The degree of respiratory impairment in SCI is dependent upon the extent and level of the neurological injury. High cervical injury results in paralysis or weakness of the diaphragm muscle leading to respiratory failure and usually requires intubation

**Table 9.1** Effect of level of spinal cord injury on respiratory system

| | | Clinical Implications |
|---|---|---|
| Above C3 | Loss of phrenic nerve leading to diaphragmatic paralysis | Requires early intubation if the lesion is complete and mechanical ventilation for prolonged period, inability to cough |
| C3-5 | Partial denervation of diaphragm | Prolonged ventilation may be required in up to 80% cases within 2 days of admission, inability to cough |
| Above T8 | Weakness of inspiratory intercostal and abdominal muscles | Inability to effectively clear secretions, may require short-/long-term ventilation, normal to weak cough |
| Below T8 | Weakness of abdominal and expiratory intercostal muscles | Normal to weak cough, may require ventilatory support if accompanied by other respiratory co-morbidities |

and elective ventilation. In addition paralysis or weakness of chest and abdominal muscle causes a decrease in maximum expiratory force resulting in reduced ability to cough out secretions. Retention of secretion eventually leads to the development of atelectasis and respiratory failure (Table 9.1).

Patients with SCI are better ventilated in supine position. Titration of tidal volumes is required to weigh the benefits of high tidal volume ventilation in prevention of atelectasis vis-a-vis risk of barotrauma and mechanical overinflation [13].

### 9.4.3 C = Circulation

High thoracic cord injuries can result in unstable hemodynamics due to loss of autoregulation [14]. Shock is a hemodynamic phenomenon distinguished by hypotension along with bradycardia secondary to loss of sympathetic innervations and unopposed parasympathetic activity. Because of reduced sympathetic activity, there is vasodilation and pooling of blood resulting in hypotension. Simultaneously because of unopposed parasympathetic activity bradycardia is a usual finding in such patients. Neurogenic shock should not be confused with spinal shock, the latter refers to a transient loss of spinal cord function (flaccidity, loss of reflexes) and can occur after spinal column injury. It is recommended to keep mean blood pressure (MAP) between 85 and 90 mmHg for the first 7 days after injury to maintain spinal cord perfusion [15, 16].

Fluid resuscitation should be started early however, patients may not respond to volume resuscitation. Fluid overload can result in pulmonary edema due to the impairment of pulmonary capillary integrity due to the initial catecholamine surge. Because of sympathetic paralysis, these patients usually require vasopressor to maintain MAP >85 mmHg [15]. Dopamine and noradrenaline are preferred agents having both alpha and beta adrenergic activity. Since phenylephrine is a pure alpha agonist, it can worsen bradycardia and is not a preferred agent except in lower thoracic lesions where hypotension is expected to be due to vasodilation. In a trauma patient coexistent hemorrhagic shock due to other injuries is also common and is characterized by hypotension and tachycardia. It has to be differentiated from neurogenic shock where bradycardia is a prominent finding. Coexisting neurogenic and hemorrhagic shock can be tricky to diagnose. Severe bradycardia is common due to unopposed vagal tone. It is usually treated with atropine or glycopyrrolate bolus and rarely pacing is required.

Bladder catheterization should be done in unstable patients. This will help in measurement of urinary output as well as avoid parasympathetic stimulation due to bladder distention and consequent bradycardia.

### 9.4.4 D = Disability

A quick neurological examination is an integral part of the primary survey. A patient with a head injury may have a co-existent spinal injury and vice versa. A basic neurologic examination in emergency settings should consist of an evaluation of initial Glasgow Coma Scale (GCS), pupillary response, and size and lateralizing signs. The inability to move any limb should be noted during disability evaluation.

### 9.4.5 E = Environment

The primary survey is completed with complete exposure of the patient along with the prevention of hypothermia. Hypothermia in trauma patients is detrimental. The classical triad of hypothermia, hemorrhage, and coagulation disorders is lethal for trauma patients.

## 9.5 Secondary Survey

After the completion of the primary survey and stabilization of vitals, the secondary survey is done for the head-to-toe examination of trauma victims with the aim to detect other significant but not immediately life-threatening injuries. Relevant history should also be obtained at this time. The secondary survey starts only after the completion of the primary survey.

The patient should be log rolled for completely visualizing the back if not done during the primary survey. Entire spine and para-vertebral musculature should be examined for the presence of areas of tenderness and/or deformity. A step-off spine denotes subluxation or vertebral fracture while the widening of inter-spinous space denotes a posterior ligament rupture.

### 9.5.1 Neurological Examination

During neurologic examination, particular attention should be given to sensory and motor examination at each spinal level. A serial neurologic examination is done to know the level of injury and its progression. Immobilization of the spine should

**Table 9.2** ASIA impairment scale [17]

| Asia grade | Scale | Description |
|---|---|---|
| A | Complete | No motor or sensory function in the lowest sacral segment |
| B | Sensory incomplete | Sensory but not motor function is preserved below neurological level |
| C | Motor incomplete | Less than 1/2 of the key muscles below the neurological spinal level have grade 3 or better strength |
| D | Motor incomplete | At least 1/2 of the key muscles below the neurological levels have grade 3 or better strength |
| E | Normal | Sensory and motor functions are normal |

**Table 9.3** Commonly referred dermatomes

| Root | Dermatome |
|---|---|
| C 5 | Deltoid |
| C 6 | Thumb |
| C 7 | Middle finger |
| C 8 | Little finger |
| T 4 | Nipple |
| T 8 | Xiphisternum |
| T 10 | Umbilicus |
| T 12 | Symphysis pubis |
| L 4 | Medial aspect of the calf |
| L 5 | Web space between the first and second toes |
| S 1 | The lateral border of the foot |

**Table 9.4** Commonly referred myotomes

| Roots | Muscle |
|---|---|
| C 4 | Deltoid |
| C 5 | Biceps |
| C 6 | Wrist extensors |
| C 7 | Triceps |
| T 1 | Finger abduction |
| L 2 | Hip flexors |
| L 3 | Knee flexors |
| L 4 | Ankle dorsiflexion |
| S 1 | Plantar flexion |

always be maintained while assessment. If there is a deformity, the highest level of dysfunction should be localized (Tables 9.2, 9.3, and 9.4).

### 9.5.2 Sensory and Motor Level

The sensory level may be defined as the caudal-most segment of the spinal cord having a normal sensory function; similarly, motor level refers to the lowest key muscle having at least grade 3/5 strength.

### 9.5.3 Complete Injuries and Incomplete Injuries

- Complete injuries mean there is no sensory or motor function below a particular spinal level.
- An incomplete injury implies some degree of sensory and motor function remaining below a particular spinal level. Incomplete injury has a better prognosis and functional recovery as compared to complete injury.

**American Spinal Injury Association (ASIA) Scale:** It is an assessment protocol which consists of sensory and motor examination to quantify the severity of the spinal cord injury. (Table 9.2).

## 9.6 Spine Board: Removal As Soon As Possible

In the emergency department (ED) itself patients should be taken off from the spine board, preferably within two hours to prevent potential complications. The backboard is mainly for transport [18, 19]. Pressure ulcers or sores can develop within hours especially at buttocks and heels. Elderly, obese, and hypotensive patients are more prone to develop pressure ulcers [18]. Log-rolling (turn side-to-side) movement is suggested every two hourly for the prevention of pressure sores in immobilized patients.

## 9.7 Clearance of Cervical Spine

It is important to rule out cervical spine injury as quickly as possible to decide for how long immobilization of spine to be continued and also plan definitive management. Previously it was a usual practice to obtain a full set of cervical spine X-ray films in any trauma patient with the suspicion of cervical spine injury. Reports from the National Emergency X-Radiography Utilization Study (NEXUS) modified the requirement of radiography in cervical injury patients [20]. According to the NEXUS criteria if a patient is fulfilling a set of five of the following clinical criteria, cervical spine injury can be excluded. In such circumstances, the cervical collar can be removed and radiography is not necessary.

### 9.7.1 NEXUS Low-Risk Criteria

1. Normal level of alertness.
2. No signs of intoxication.
3. Absence of midline tenderness.
4. Absence of focal neurological deficit.
5. No painful distracting injuries.

In the NEXUS study, these five criteria had a sensitivity 99%; specificity 12.9% for ruling out the cervical spinal injury [20]. In obtund and confused patients, evaluation is difficult and should be assumed to have an SCI and further radiography is suggested. According to some researchers, there might be an increase in X-ray utilization if we follow NEXUS low-risk criteria because of its low specificity (12.9%). Canadian C-spine rules (CCR) has a higher specificity (42.5%) compared to NEXUS criteria [21]. In CCR ability to turn his or her neck 45° to the right and left was used as a final step to clear the cervical spine.

### 9.7.2 Imaging

Plain X-ray or Computed tomography (CT) scan forms the basis of standard trauma protocols and can identify most fractures and ligamentous injuries [15]. Plain X-rays can be used as the first imaging method for the assessment of alignment or fracture in patients with SCI at places where CT is not available. In general, cervical X-rays in trauma patients include at least anteroposterior (AP), lateral, and open-mouth odontoid views. A lateral view of the cervical spine is very useful for assessment and can recognize fractures in about 60–80% of the cases [22, 23]. This percentage increases if AP and odontoid views are also taken along with lateral views. For an adequate view, all cervical vertebrae along with first thoracic (T1) need to be depicted [24]. The lower cervical spines may be unclear in some healthy or overweight patients; in such cases, pulling patient's hands toward their feet in a straight line may allow better visualization. If this maneuver is unsuccessful, a swimmer's view should be obtained for proper imaging of lower cervical and upper border of T1 vertebra.

CT is a widely used modality for the assessment of the suspected instability of the cervical spine in trauma patients. CT scan is replacing plain X-ray; the latter may be used as a primary screening if CT is not available [25]. Eastern Association for the Surgery of Trauma (EAST) guidelines also advocate CT as the primary method of screening for cervical spine injury in trauma patients [26]. CT is considered far better as compared to plain X-ray for the detection of cervical spine trauma in various studies [27]. In terms of time and cost it is advantageous to obtain a CT spine when head CT is also required to rule out head injury. CT is very sensitive for defining bone fractures in the spine. The main disadvantage of CT is increased radiation as compared to normal X-rays [28]. MRI is required for a detailed examination of ongoing compression of the spinal cord (hematoma, disc herniation, etc.) and surrounding soft tissue including ligaments. Although MRI provides a more detailed image of ligaments and soft tissues, hematoma, etc., it is of lesser value in fracture detection [23, 29]. MRI is seldom done in emergency settings due to the longer time required for the patient to be inside MRI gantry which can be risky for the patients with cardio-respiratory instability [30].

## 9.8 Definitive Management and Disposition

Definitive management of patients with SCI depends upon fracture stability and associated injuries (Fig. 9.3). For unstable injuries hospital admission and consultation of a spine surgeon is required. Immediate transfer to the higher center must be planned if the initial center doesn't have appropriate facilities to manage a case with SCI. Early admission to an intensive care unit should be considered in an unstable spine with polytrauma having cardiorespiratory insufficiency. Patients with minor undisplaced spinal fracture without neurologic deficit; analgesics and follow-up care may be considered [31, 32]. A closed reduction may be considered as a treatment option for some cases with cervical spine fracture with subluxation. This technique provides longitudinal traction using skull tongs or a halo fixator [33]. A halo fixator can restrict the mobility of cervical spinal to the extent of about 96% [34]. The management of such cases should be left on the discretion of the spine specialist.

Persistent compression of the spinal cord is a form of reversible secondary injury that should be treated by surgery as early as possible [35]. The main indications for spine surgery include unstable vertebral fracture or dislocation causing significant cord compression with neurologic deficits [36]. The primary goal for surgical intervention in SCI patients is to establish spinal stability and alleviate the pressure of the neural compartment.

**Venous Thromboprophylaxis:** Patients with spinal cord injury are likely to be bedridden for a prolonged period of time resulting in a high risk of deep vein thrombosis. The reported incidence is up to 40% during the first 3 months following injury

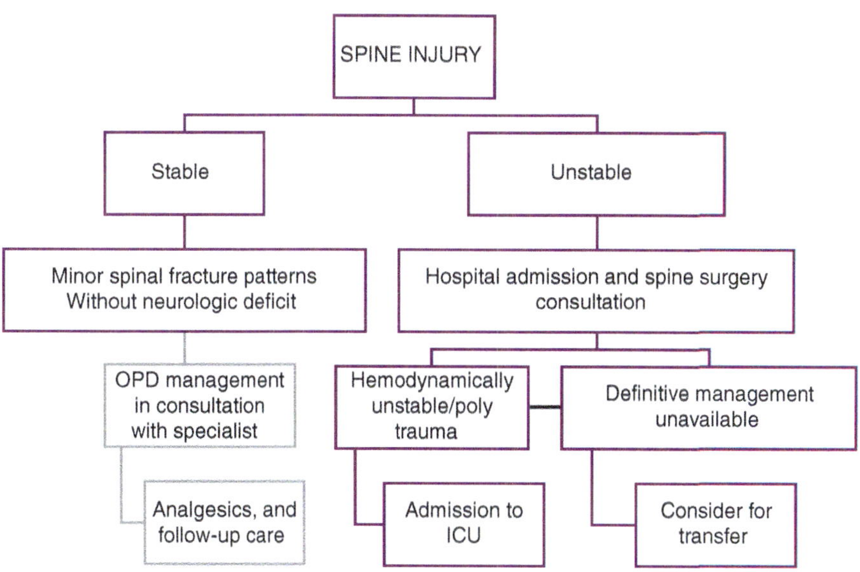


**Fig. 9.3** Definitive management of a patient with spinal cord injury

due to venous stasis and hypercoagulability. Current evidence supports the use of mechanical thromboprophylaxis in patients at risk of bleeding. Pharmacological prophylaxis with low molecular weight heparin is started after assuring adequate hemostasis preferably within 72 h after injury [37].

**Role of Steroids:** The current evidence does not support the use of steroids for the management of acute spinal cord injury owing to the harmful side effects associated with its use [38].

**Role of Therapeutic Hypothermia:** Currently there is no evidence to support the role of hypothermia in the management of acute spinal cord injury.

## 9.9 Summary

- Suspect SCI in any trauma victim especially in the setting of multiple injuries.
- Spinal immobilization should be started preferably at the point of accident and it should be continued until cervical spine injury is excluded or treated.
- Resuscitation and stabilization of vitals take priority over radiological investigations for which the patient has to be shifted.
- Spine board must be removed as quickly as possible to avoid the formation of pressure sores.
- CT is the screening modality in SCI patients. Plain X-rays can be used if CT is not available.
- Patient with SCI requires early consultation with the spine surgeon, in the absence of latter referral to higher center should be considered.
- Routine use of steroids in acute SCI is not recommended.

## Multiple Choice Questions

1. A 24-year-old construction worker is admitted to a trauma center following a history of fall from 20 feet. He has bradycardia, low blood pressure, labored breathing, and inability to move all four limbs. Which of the following injuries do you suspect in this patient?
   (a). Tension pneumothorax
   (b). Ruptured spleen
   (c). Fracture of cervical spine
   (d). All of the above
2. Which of the following region is the most common site for spinal column injury?
   (a). Cervical
   (b). Thoracic
   (c). Thoraco-lumbar
   (d). Lumbo-sacral

3. Which of the following is the sensory dermatome for thumb?
   (a). C5
   (b). C6
   (c). C7
   (d). C8
4. Which of the following statement is correct about the pathophysiology for the development of neurogenic shock in cervical spine injury?
   (a). Loss of sympathetic activity and preservation of parasympathetic activity
   (b). Loss of both sympathetic activity and parasympathetic activity
   (c). Preservation of sympathetic activity and loss of parasympathetic activity
   (d). Preservation of both sympathetic activity and parasympathetic activity
5. Which of the following is a characteristic feature of neurogenic shock?
   (a). Hypertension and tachycardia
   (b). Hypertension and bradycardia
   (c). Hypotension and tachycardia
   (d). Hypotension and bradycardia
6. Which of the following statements is correct about central cord syndrome?
   (a). There is a greater loss of motor strength of lower as compared to upper extremities
   (b). There is an equal loss of motor strength of both upper and lower extremities
   (c). There is an equal preservation of motor strength of both upper and lower extremities
   (d). There is a greater loss of motor strength of upper as compared to lower extremities
7. Which of the following statements is correct about an adequate cervical spine X-ray film in case of suspected cervical spine injury?
   (a). The upper three cervical vertebrae must be visualized
   (b). All seven cervical spine must be visualized
   (c). All seven cervical and first thoracic vertebra must be visualized
   (d). All seven cervical and upper three thoracic vertebrae must be visualized
8. How many individuals are required for logrolling a patient with an unstable spine?
   (a). 1
   (b). 2
   (c). 3
   (d). 4
9. Which of the following is the imaging modality of choice for screening an unconscious patient with suspected spinal cord injury?
   (a). Contrast-enhanced computed tomography
   (b). Noncontrast computed tomography
   (c). Magnetic resonance imaging
   (d). Focused assessment sonography in trauma

10. Which of the following should not be done for the management of patients with spinal cord injury?
    (a). Open mouth view X-ray in patients with suspected odontoid fracture
    (b). Using vasopressors to maintain a MAP 85–90 mmHg
    (c). Loading dose of methylprednisolone at the time of admission in patients with proven spinal cord injury
    (d). Immobilization on a long spine board

Answers: 1. (d), 2. (a), 3. (b), 4. (a), 5. (d), 6. (d), 7. (c), 8. (d), 9. (b), 10. (c)

## References

1. Mathur N, Jain S, Kumar N, Srivastava A, Purohit N, Patni A. Spinal cord injury: scenario in an Indian state. Spinal Cord. 2015;53(5):349–52.
2. Lowery DW, Wald MM, Browne BJ, Tigges S, Hoffman JR, Mower WR, et al. Epidemiology of cervical spine injury victims. Ann Emerg Med. 2001;38(1):12–6.
3. DeVivo MJ, Krause JS, Lammertse DP. Recent trends in mortality and causes of death among persons with spinal cord injury. Arch Phys Med Rehabil. 1999;80(11):1411–9.
4. Szwedowski D, Walecki J. Spinal cord injury without radiographic abnormality (SCIWORA) – clinical and radiological aspects. Pol J Radiol. 2014;79:461–4.
5. Pang D, Pollack IF. Spinal cord injury without radiographic abnormality in children--the SCIWORA syndrome. J Trauma. 1989;29(5):654–64.
6. Sekhon LH, Fehlings MG. Epidemiology, demographics, and pathophysiology of acute spinal cord injury. Spine. 2001;26(24 Suppl):S2–12.
7. Oyinbo CA. Secondary injury mechanisms in traumatic spinal cord injury: a nugget of this multiply cascade. Acta Neurobiol Exp (Wars). 2011;71(2):281–99.
8. ATLS Subcommittee, American College of Surgeons' Committee on Trauma, International ATLS Working Group. Advanced trauma life support (ATLS®): the ninth edition. J Trauma Acute Care Surg. 2013;74(5):1363–6.
9. Crosby ET. Airway management in adults after cervical spine trauma. Anesthesiology. 2006;104(6):1293–318.
10. Ollerton JE, Parr MJA, Harrison K, Hanrahan B, Sugrue M. Potential cervical spine injury and difficult airway management for emergency intubation of trauma adults in the emergency department--a systematic review. Emerg Med J. 2006;23(1):3–11.
11. Benumof JL. Management of the difficult adult airway. With special emphasis on awake tracheal intubation. Anesthesiology. 1991;75(6):1087–110.
12. Brimacombe J, Keller C, Künzel KH, Gaber O, Boehler M, Pühringer F. Cervical spine motion during airway management: a cinefluoroscopic study of the posteriorly destabilized third cervical vertebrae in human cadavers. Anesth Analg. 2000;91(5):1274–8.
13. Consortium for Spinal Cord Medicine. Early acute management in adults with spinal cord injury. J Spinal Cord Med. 2008;31(4):403–79.
14. Lehmann KG, Lane JG, Piepmeier JM, Batsford WP. Cardiovascular abnormalities accompanying acute spinal cord injury in humans: incidence, time course and severity. J Am Coll Cardiol. 1987;10(1):46–52.
15. Walters BC, Hadley MN, Hurlbert RJ, Aarabi B, Dhall SS, Gelb DE, et al. Guidelines for the management of acute cervical spine and spinal cord injuries: 2013 update. Neurosurgery. 2013;60(CN_suppl_1):82–91.
16. Yue JK, Winkler EA, Rick JW, Deng H, Partow CP, Upadhyayula PS, et al. Update on critical care for acute spinal cord injury in the setting of polytrauma. Neurosurg Focus. 2017;43(5):E19.

17. Roberts TT, Leonard GR, Cepela DJ. Classifications in brief: American spinal injury association (ASIA) impairment scale. Clin Orthop. 2017;475(5):1499–504.
18. Gefen A. How much time does it take to get a pressure ulcer? Integrated evidence from human, animal, and in vitro studies. Ostomy Wound Manage. 2008;54(10):26–8, 30–5
19. Oteir AO, Smith K, Stoelwinder JU, Middleton J, Jennings PA. Should suspected cervical spinal cord injury be immobilised?: a systematic review. Injury. 2015;46(4):528–35.
20. Hoffman JR, Mower WR, Wolfson AB, Todd KH, Zucker MI. Validity of a set of clinical criteria to rule out injury to the cervical spine in patients with blunt trauma. National Emergency X-Radiography Utilization Study Group. N Engl J Med. 2000;343(2):94–9.
21. Stiell IG, Clement CM, McKnight RD, Brison R, Schull MJ, Rowe BH, et al. The Canadian C-spine rule versus the NEXUS low-risk criteria in patients with trauma. N Engl J Med. 2003;349(26):2510–8.
22. West OC, Anbari MM, Pilgram TK, Wilson AJ. Acute cervical spine trauma: diagnostic performance of single-view versus three-view radiographic screening. Radiology. 1997;204(3):819–23.
23. Crim JR, Moore K, Brodke D. Clearance of the cervical spine in multitrauma patients: the role of advanced imaging. Semin Ultrasound CT MR. 2001;22(4):283–305.
24. Petri R, Gimbel R. Evaluation of the patient with spinal trauma and back pain: an evidence based approach. Emerg Med Clin North Am. 1999;17(1):25–39, vii–viii.
25. Daffner RH, Sciulli RL, Rodriguez A, Protetch J. Imaging for evaluation of suspected cervical spine trauma: a 2-year analysis. Injury. 2006;37(7):652–8.
26. Como JJ, Diaz JJ, Dunham CM, Chiu WC, Duane TM, Capella JM, et al. Practice management guidelines for identification of cervical spine injuries following trauma: update from the eastern association for the surgery of trauma practice management guidelines committee. J Trauma. 2009;67(3):651–9.
27. Holmes JF, Akkinepalli R. Computed tomography versus plain radiography to screen for cervical spine injury: a meta-analysis. J Trauma. 2005;58(5):902–5.
28. Adelgais KM, Grossman DC, Langer SG, Mann FA. Use of helical computed tomography for imaging the pediatric cervical spine. Acad Emerg Med Off J Soc Acad Emerg Med. 2004;11(3):228–36.
29. Holmes JF, Mirvis SE, Panacek EA, Hoffman JR, Mower WR, Velmahos GC, et al. Variability in computed tomography and magnetic resonance imaging in patients with cervical spine injuries. J Trauma. 2002;53(3):524–9; discussion 530.
30. Bozzo A, Marcoux J, Radhakrishna M, Pelletier J, Goulet B. The role of magnetic resonance imaging in the Management of Acute Spinal Cord Injury. J Neurotrauma. 2011;28(8):1401–11.
31. Bradley LH, Paullus WC, Howe J, Litofsky NS. Isolated transverse process fractures: spine service management not needed. J Trauma. 2008;65(4):832–6; discussion 836.
32. Homnick A, Lavery R, Nicastro O, Livingston DH, Hauser CJ. Isolated thoracolumbar transverse process fractures: call physical therapy, not spine. J Trauma. 2007;63(6):1292–5.
33. Bono CM. The halo fixator. J Am Acad Orthop Surg. 2007;15(12):728–37.
34. Botte MJ, Byrne TP, Abrams RA, Garfin SR. Halo skeletal fixation: techniques of application and prevention of complications. J Am Acad Orthop Surg. 1996;4(1):44–53.
35. Fehlings MG, Tetreault LA, Wilson JR, Kwon BK, Burns AS, Martin AR, et al. A clinical practice guideline for the Management of Acute Spinal Cord Injury: introduction, rationale, and scope. Glob Spine J. 2017;7(3 Suppl):84S–94S.
36. Huang Y-H, Yang T-M, Lin W-C, Ho J-T, Lee T-C, Chen W-F, et al. The prognosis of acute blunt cervical spinal cord injury. J Trauma. 2009;66(5):1441–5.
37. Dhall SS, Hadley MN, Aarabi B, Gelb DE, Hurlbert RJ, Rozzelle CJ, et al. Deep venous thrombosis and thromboembolism in patients with cervical spinal cord injuries. Neurosurgery. 2013;72(Suppl 2):244–54.
38. Bracken MB, Shepard MJ, Holford TR, Leo-Summers L, Aldrich EF, Fazl M, et al. Methylprednisolone or tirilazad mesylate administration after acute spinal cord injury: 1-year follow up: results of the third National Acute Spinal Cord Injury Randomized Controlled Trial. J Neurosurg. 1998;89(5):699–706.

# Acute Hemorrhagic Stroke

# 10

M. R. Rajani, Rajshree Deopujari, Shwetal Goraksha, and Joseph Monteiro

## Key Points

- ICH is a medical emergency—rapid diagnosis and emergent management of patients is important as early deterioration in the first few hours of onset is common
- Rapid neuroimaging is essential to differentiate between acute ischemic stroke and hemorrhagic stroke. Both CT and MRI are reasonable for initial evaluation within 6 hours of bleed; CT is faster, more easily accessible, and therefore more commonly used
- Once the diagnosis is confirmed, the main considerations are ABCs, control of elevated BP, correction of any coagulopathy, and assessing need for urgent surgical intervention
- Although emergency ICH protocol is mainly concerned with initial evaluation and treatment, the first few days following the event are critical for maintaining a secure airway, BP and ICP control, and identification of seizures to prevent secondary brain injury.

## Case Scenario

65-year-old right-handed, male, known case of hypertension since 10 years (irregular medication) is brought to EMS with chief complaints of:

- Headache since 1 day,
- Giddiness, inability to move left upper limb and lower limb since 6 am early morning

M. R. Rajani · R. Deopujari
Jaslok Hospital and research centre, Mumbai, India

S. Goraksha · J. Monteiro (✉)
P D Hinduja hospital and medical research centre, Mumbai, India


P. U. Bidkar, P. Vanamoorthy (eds.), *Acute Neuro Care*,
https://doi.org/10.1007/978-981-15-4071-4_10

- Drowsiness since 6 am
- two episodes of vomiting

Patient was apparently alright 1 day ago when he developed a holocranial headache not responding to simple pain-killer tablet. However, he ignored it and slept off. Next morning, he woke up early with a persistent headache, giddiness, and inability to move left upper and lower limb. He gradually became drowsy over the next 3 h, and also had two episodes of projectile vomiting on his way to EMS.

No history of chest pain/breathlessness/palpitation

No history suggestive of a seizure

Past history: Known case of hypertension (HTN) 10 years. (Compliance with medicines and follow-up poor)

Personal history: Social alcohol intake; no nicotine/illicit drug abuse

Family history: HTN in father

P—90 bpm, BP—220/110 mmHg, jugular venous pressure—Normal, no carotid bruit

No pallor/icterus/edema

CNS: E2-M4-V3, right gaze preference

Pupils: bilaterally equal and reactive to light, bilateral, papilledema on fundoscopy

Motor: Moves Right upper limb (UL) and lower limb (LL) vigorously, left UL 0/5, left LL 0/5

Plantars: Flexor on right/extensor on Left

No neck stiffness

Sensory and cerebellum could not be assessed

RS – AEBE, no adventitious sound

CVS: S1, S2 normal, no murmur

Patient was taken up for CT brain which showed right gangliocapsular bleed 25 × 14 mm with a midline shift of 12 mm

Patient was admitted to ICU with BP management and underwent craniectomy on the same evening. He was discharged on Day 10 with instruction for BP management, physiotherapy, and good nursing care with a Ryles tube in situ for feeding.

## 10.1 Introduction

Acute intracerebral hemorrhage (ICH) results from bleeding into the brain parenchyma either spontaneously or due to secondary causes. It accounts for 20–30% [1, 2] of all strokes in India and the rest of Asia. It is the most disabling form and has a high mortality rate (40–50%) [3, 4]. The risk of intracranial hypertension, early neurological deterioration, and poor long-term outcome stress the need for aggressive early management.

Guidelines are available for the management of ICH, though there are certain variations in the degree of evidence on treatment recommendations [5, 6]. The purpose of this protocol is to emphasize initial management with the goal of optimizing recovery.

## 10.2 Emergency Diagnosis and Assessment

ICH is a medical emergency. Rapid diagnosis and appropriate management of patients is very important as early deterioration in the first few hours of onset is common.

### 10.2.1 Risk Factors

Eighty-five percent of ICH is primary (spontaneous) due to arterial hypertension (60–70%) or amyloid angiopathy (30%) [1, 3]. Secondary ICH can be related to multiple causes—smoking, drug abuse (cocaine, amphetamines), oral anticoagulants, antiplatelets, coagulopathies, arteriovenous (AVM) or cavernous malformations, intracranial tumors, cerebral vasculitis, Moya-Moya syndrome, cerebral aneurysm rupture, and secondary transformation of an arterial or venous infarct [1]. Non- modifiable risk factors include male gender, older age, and African or Asian ethnicity.

### 10.2.2 Clinical Presentation

Acute hemorrhagic stroke usually presents as acute onset of focal neurological deficits, headache, and vomiting. It is difficult to differentiate between ischemic stroke and hemorrhagic stroke on the basis of clinical characteristics alone, thus neuroimaging is mandatory [7, 8].

Classic symptoms:

- Acute onset neurological deficit
- Vomiting
- Severe headache
- Altered or decreased consciousness
- Hypertension—systolic BP >220 mmHg
- Seizures
- Others—hemiparesis, cranial nerve palsies, sensory signs, and speech and gait abnormalities present depending on the location and extent of bleed.

### 10.2.3 Neuroimaging

Rapid neuroimaging is essential to differentiate acute ischemic stroke from hemorrhagic stroke.

Both CT and MRI are reasonable for initial evaluation within 6 h of bleed, but considering the time, cost, proximity to the emergency department (ED), patient tolerance, clinical status, and MRI availability, CT is commonly used as the primary modality.

CT is very sensitive for identifying acute hemorrhage and is considered as "gold standard." Gradient echo and T2 susceptibility-weighted MRI is as sensitive for the identification of prior hemorrhage [9].

Initial non-contrast CT will help to assess the size and location of hematoma, which influences outcome and treatment. Hypertensive bleeds are commonly seen in basal ganglia, thalamus, pons (brainstem), and cerebellum. AVM bleeds or cerebral amyloid angiopathy bleeds are usually lobar in location. Another strong predictor of patient outcome is the hematoma volume assessed by ABC/2 formula [7, 10].

(A = maximum length of the hematoma along the falx (cm), B = width perpendicular to A on the same head CT slice, and C = the number of slices, starting from the point at which the temporal lobe tips became visible, multiplied by the slice thickness.)

Hematoma expansion after the initial presentation of ICH is associated with worsening of clinical outcome [5, 7].

CT angiography (CTA) and contrast study may identify patients at risk of ICH expansion based on the presence of contrast within the hematoma called as "spot sign" [7, 11]. A larger number of contrast spots suggest a high risk of expansion [11, 12].

Thus the use of a "Stroke CT" which includes non-contrast CT as well as CTA may help identify patients at risk of hematoma expansion [5, 7].

CTA, CT venography, contrast CT, contrast-enhanced MRI, MRA, MRV, DSA catheter angiography can be used for evaluating underlying structural lesions including vascular malformations and tumors when there is clinical or radiological suspicion [5].

## 10.3 Medical Management

### 10.3.1 Initial Evaluation and Primary Intervention

The initial prehospital and ED resuscitation is same across the stroke subtypes till the diagnosis is made by neuroimaging.

### 10.3.2 Prehospital Management

The primary focus is to manage the ABCs and rapid transport to the closest facility prepared to care for patients with acute stroke [13].

### 10.3.3 ED Management

As with all emergency medical care, the initial assessment of ABC is critical. Once the diagnosis of ICH is confirmed with neuroimaging, disease-specific treatment can be started (Tables 10.1 and 10.2).

**Table 10.1** Intracerebral hemorrhage checklist for the first hour

| *Checklist* |
|---|
| – Complete blood count with platelets, PT, PTT, INR |
| – Head imaging results: hematoma size, location |
| – Glasgow Coma Scale (GCS) score |
| – Calculate ICH Score |
| – Interventions: |
| Coagulopathy reversal |
| Blood pressure lowering |
| Surgical hematoma evacuation (if indicated) |
| Airway/ventilation management |

Airway management gets priority. Supplemental oxygen should be given if $SpO_2$ is <95% [14].

Intubation should be done to protect airways:

- Decreased level of consciousness GCS(<8)
- Poor airway protection
- Impending ventilatory failure—$PaO_2$ <60 mmHg or $PaCO_2$ >50 mmHg
- Signs of raised intracranial pressure (ICP)

Rapid sequence induction is done with a goal of normoventilation.

An initial assessment of patients' condition and a quick focused neurological examination should be performed as part of the initial evaluation to assess the baseline severity of stroke.

The ICH score (Table 10.3) is the most widely used and externally validated clinical grading scale for patients with acute hemorrhagic stroke [15–19]. Each point increase in the ICH score is associated with an increased risk of mortality and poor functional outcome [7]. It is used as a communication tool among providers to chart the patients' condition rather than a prognostic tool.

### 10.3.4 Primary Intervention

Once the diagnosis of acute ICH is confirmed, the main considerations:

- Acute control of elevated blood pressure.
- Correction of any coagulopathy due to medications or underlying medical conditions.
- Assess the need for urgent surgical hematoma evacuation.

  Urgent treatment of time-sensitive issues like lowering blood pressure and reversal of coagulopathy should be initiated in ED itself, rather than waiting until transfer to an ICU, stroke unit, or another hospital. These decisions will guide further care such as transport from ED, repeat imaging, and need for ICP or EEG monitoring (Fig. 10.1).

**Table 10.2** Standardized ICH algorithm

| |
|---|
| *Prehospital care* |
| ABCs |
| Determine time of onset and circumstances |
| Perform prehospital stroke screen |
| Fingerstick for glucose |
| Brief medical history and medication list |
| Triage to stroke center |
| Perform prehospital notification of pending stroke patient |
| *ED care* |
| Emergent triage to high acuity area |
| Perform primary assessment—ABCs |
| Perform focused neurologic exam (GCS, NIHSS) |
| Obtain baseline screening labs (CBC and platelet count, electrolytes, PT/INR and PTT, glucose) |
| Obtain cerebrovascular imaging as soon as possible (non-con CT, stroke CT/CTA/CTP, or MRI) |
| Obtain a brief medical history and medication list |
| *After confirmation of ICH* |
| Reassess ABCs (consider intubation if comatose) |
| Initiate blood pressure intervention (target SBP <140 mmHg) |
| Quantify ICH volume (ABC/2 calculation) |
| Perform the ICH score (0–6) |
| Begin correction of anticoagulation as required |
| Correction of antiplatelet agents as required |
| Consult neurosurgery for potential hematoma evacuation or ICP monitor placement |
| Admit to NeuroICU/ stroke unit (may require transfer to another hospital) |
| *In-hospital setting* |
| Continue to reassess ABCs |
| Continue neurologic reassessment |
| ICP monitor and/or ventriculostomy for treatment of elevated ICP or hydrocephalus |
| Continue management of blood pressure |
| Place arterial blood pressure catheter as needed |
| Place central venous catheter as needed |
| Urine toxicology screen (if not already done) |
| Foley catheter (needed for most ICH patients early) |
| Feeding tube (goal to begin feeding within the first day) |
| DVT prophylaxis with sequential compression devices (consider heparin/LWMH within the first 3 days) recheck PT/INR and PTT (or specific labs for other oral anticoagulants) if patient was coagulopathic and receiving reversal agents |
| No anticonvulsant prophylaxis; treat clinical seizures; continuous EEG if level of consciousness impaired out of proportion to ICH or IVH |
| Consider the need for repeat head CT |
| Consider need for catheter cerebral angiography |

### 10.3.5 Blood Pressure

Hypertension is commonly associated with hemorrhagic strokes because of increased ICP, premorbid hypertension, pain, and stress [16]. It is a common risk factor in older people. The commonest sites of hypertensive bleed are basal ganglia (55%), thalamus (26%), cerebral hemisphere (11%), brainstem (8%), and cerebellum (7%) [1].

**Table 10.3** ICH score and 30-day mortality risk

| Feature | Finding | Points | ICH score | 30-day mortality (%) |
|---|---|---|---|---|
| Glasgow Coma Scale | 3–4 | 2 | 0 | 0 |
| | 5–12 | 1 | | |
| | 13–15 | 0 | | |
| Age | ≥80 years | 1 | 1 | 13 |
| | <80 years | 0 | | |
| Location | Infratentorial | 1 | 2 | 26 |
| | Supratentorial | 0 | | |
| ICH volume | ≥30 mL | 1 | 3 | 72 |
| | <30 mL | 0 | | |
| Intraventricular blood | Yes | 1 | 4 | 97 |
| | No | 0 | | |
| ICH score | | 0–6 | 5 | 100 |
| | | | 6 | 100 |

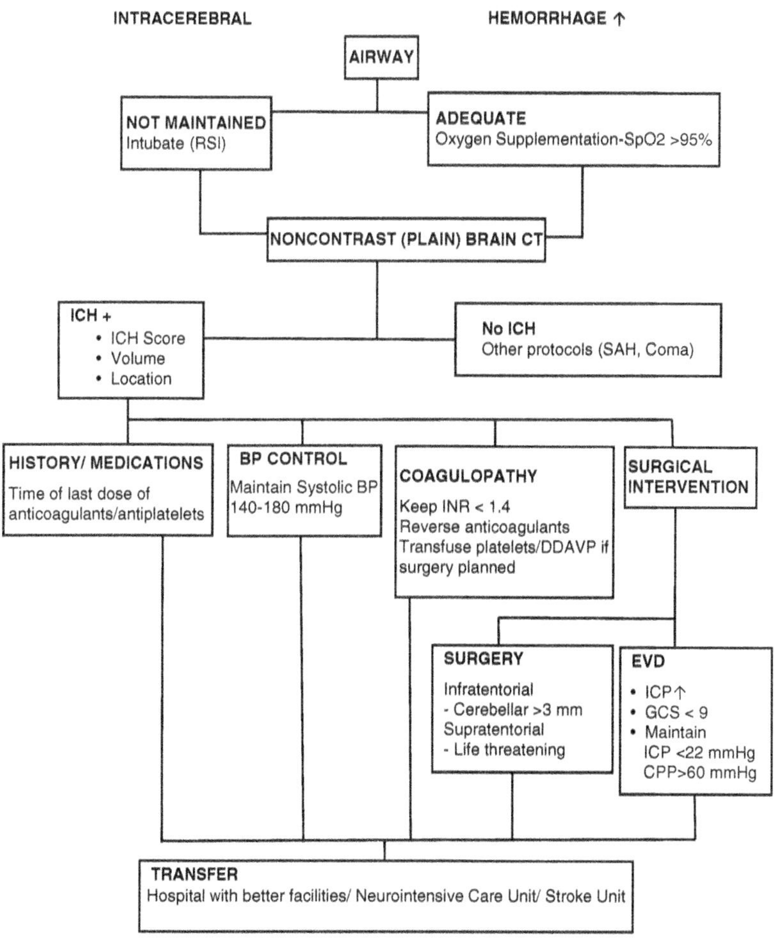


**Fig. 10.1** Management of Intracerebral hemmorrhage

Presence of hypertension influences both short-term and long-term outcomes in patients with ICH. High systolic blood pressure is associated with a higher risk of hematoma expansion either due to increased bleeding or due to elevated ICP from worsening edema [20, 21]. Cerebral and perihematomal edema are independent predictors of poor functional outcome [16, 22]. Intensive BP lowering in patients within the first 24 h after the onset of ICH has shown to reduce this edema, leading to better outcomes [23, 24].

There has been concern that acute lowering of BP could lead to ischemic brain injury in the perihematomal region, but this is not supported by recent studies [5, 25].

Blood pressure management has been remained controversial, but current studies favor rapid lowering of moderately elevated blood pressure, with the main concerns being reducing brain perfusion with lower BP, and hematoma expansion and increasing perihematomal edema among patients with increased BP [5–7].

Two trials "Intensive Blood Pressure Reduction In Acute Cerebral Hemorrhage" (INTERACT) and "Antihypertensive Treatment of Acute Cerebral Hemorrhage" (ATACH) suggested that acute lowering of SBP to <140 mmHg is safe [26–28], while INTERACT II showed better outcomes in intensive lowering of SBP to <140 mmHg, but showed no difference in hematoma expansion between two groups (standard threshold of <180 mm of Hg vs intensive threshold of <140 mmHg). ATACH 2 did not demonstrate a difference in outcome between treatment groups [21]. According to AHA stroke guidelines for ICH and European stroke guidelines, patients with SBP 150–220 mmHg, without contraindication to acute blood pressure treatment lowering of SBP to 140 mmHg is safe. But with new clinical trial results (ATACH 2), NCS recommends a target of SBP 140–180 mmHg with the specific threshold determined based on patient comorbidities and level of chronic hypertension [5–7].

Table 10.4 lists some commonly used drugs used to reduce BP in ICH. Basic principle of management of BP is that treatment should be started immediately, the drug should have a quick onset, should be easily titrated, and have minimal potential for overshoot. Beta-blockers and calcium channel blockers are commonly used. Labetalol, α and β antagonists, is given as an intravenous bolus of 5–20 mg.

**Table 10.4** Drugs to control BP

| Drug | Standard dose | Mechanism of action | Cautions |
|---|---|---|---|
| Labetalol | 10–20 mg bolus every 10 min, max 300 mg;0.5–2 mg/min infusion | Alpha and beta adrenergic receptor blocker | Bradycardia, bronchospasm, CHF, and hypotension |
| Enalaprilat | 0.625–1.2 mgq 6 hrly IV | ACE inhibitor | Precipitous fall in BP, variable response |
| Nicardipine | 5–15 mg/h infusion | L-type CCB | Severe AS, MI, hypotension |
| Esmolol | 0.5 mg/kg bolus,50–300 μg/kg/min | Beta-1 antagonist | Bradycardia, CHF, bronchospasm |

Nicardipine, calcium channel blocker, is given at 5 mg/h continuous infusion, titrated every 5–15 min, up to a maximum of 15 mg/h.

### 10.3.6 Coagulopathy

Antithrombotic medications are a risk factor (12–20%), for the occurrence of ICH, as well as for hematoma expansion [29, 30]. This incidence has increased with an aging population and the use of anticoagulant drugs for the treatment of IHD, stroke, systemic venous thromboembolism [29–31]. Vitamin K antagonists such as Warfarin is more commonly prescribed, but newer agents like dabigatran, rivaroxaban, and apixaban are increasingly being used. Coagulopathies can also occur due to underlying medical conditions like liver disease and hematological malignancies.

The second main primary intervention in ICH is to treat coagulopathy. Therefore as a part of the primary assessment, brief medical and drug history should be noted from the patient, relatives, or previous medical records especially for any antithrombotic drugs, and if possible the timing of the last dose should be noted. Urgent blood investigations including complete blood count, PT, INR, and APTT should be sent.

A general principle is that any ICH should be considered life-threatening due to the risk of hematoma expansion. Steps taken to treat coagulopathy should be based on history and lab investigations, more than size, location of hematoma, or clinical scores.

### 10.3.7 Reversal of Oral Anticoagulants

For patients with ICH taking vitamin K agonists such as Warfarin, rapid correction of INR (<1.4) is recommended [5, 7, 32]. Options include FFP, Vitamin K, PCC and $rFVII_a$ (recombinant factor $VII_a$), although PCC is now a recommended approach [5].

PCC are highly concentrated source of clotting factors containing 3 or 4 factors of coagulation cascade (II, VII, IX, and X) with nearly 25 times the concentration of coagulation factors than FFP (I, II, V, VII, IX, X, XI, XIII, and antithrombin) that can reverse the INR in minutes, faster than FFP, with fewer cardiopulmonary complications [7, 33]. A recent randomized controlled trial has shown the superiority of PCC over FFP for faster resolution of INR and smaller hematoma expansion [34].

FFP requires thawing after cross-matching by blood bank. It takes more time than PCC, and large volume infusions (10–15 mL/kg) putting the patient at risk of volume overload, pulmonary edema, and at risk of transfusion reaction. The recent guidelines (AHA) recommend weight-based dosing for PCC (or FFP only if PCC is not available) with dose adjusted based on INR [5].

Vitamin K injection can also help resynthesize depleted clotting factors but the peak action is 24 h if liver functions are normal, and longer in compromised patients. Current guidelines recommend the use of Vitamin K 10 mg slow IV in combination

**Table 10.5** Newer anticoagulants and their reversal agents

| Newer agents | Dose | Structure | Comment |
|---|---|---|---|
| Idarucizumab | 5 gm IV bolus | Humanized monoclonal antibody | Noncompetitive binding to dabigatran. Effective against dabigatran only |
| Andexanet alfa | 400 mg IV bolus at 30 mg/min bolus continuous infusion at 4 μg/min for 120 min | Modified recombinant derivative of human FXa, catalytically inactive | Competitive binding to direct FXa inhibitor |
| Aripazine/ciraparantag | 25–100 mg IV bolus, single dose | Small,512 Dalton water soluble molecule | Against oral factor Xa inhibitors and DTIs, as well as UFH & LMWH, argatroban, known as universal NOAC antidote. Biomarker of activity whole blood clotting time. |

*DTIs* Direct thrombin inhibitors, *UFH* unfractionated heparin, *LMWH* low molecular weight heparin, *NOACs* newer oral anticoagulants

with other more rapidly acting agents, but it has a longer duration of action than PCC or FFP [35].

rFVIIa has also shown to decrease hematoma growth in ICH patients without coagulopathy, but studies do not show an improved clinical outcome. It is therefore not recommended, but can be used in patients with liver failure related coagulopathy. Reversal of newer anticoagulants is more complicated. There are no randomized trials for reversal agents for newer oral anticoagulants (NOAC). Immediate drug discontinuation is needed. Activated charcoal (50 gm) can absorb NOACs, if administered within 2 h of exposure [36]. Additional administration of PCC, rFVIIa or aPCC, FEIBA (factor VIII inhibitor bypassing activity) can be considered [37].

Specific agents are available for the reversal of newer anticoagulants (Table 10.5). Hemodialysis can be tried in dabigatran (Direct thrombin inhibitor) overdose, but less for more protein bound agents like rivaroxaban, apixaban (Direct Xa inhibitor). Direct Xa inhibitors do not have specific reversal agents. The currently recommended approach is to use FEIBA or 4 factor PCC with the addition of charcoal if the last dose is within 2 h [7, 35].

Protamine sulfate can reverse unfractionated heparin at a dose equivalence of 1 mg for 100 U of UFH with the maximum dose of 50 mg. It is used if heparin was given within the last 2 h [5]. If the last dose of heparin was given >4 h before ICH onset, reversal is unnecessary. Protamine is also given to reverse LMWH given within the prior 8 h, however, the reversal may be incomplete.

### 10.3.8 Antiplatelets Induced ICH

Up to 30% of patients with symptomatic ICH give a history of antiplatelet intake. There are conflicting results about its use increasing the risk of hematoma expansion and increased risk of mortality [38]. A randomized controlled trial (PATCH study) has shown no improvements in outcome by giving platelet transfusion to patients with ICH on antiplatelet agents. On the contrary, they are associated with significantly increased risk of death and more adverse events. As per AHA guidelines [5], the usefulness of platelet transfusion in ICH patients with a history of antiplatelet use is uncertain and not recommended. However recent guidelines from NCS recommend platelet transfusion for patients on antiplatelet medication who are undergoing neurosurgical procedures [7, 35]. They also recommend a single dose of intravenous DDAVP 0.4µg/kg in these patients. Many studies have suggested that platelet dysfunction measured by platelet function assay may help in directing hemostatic interventions, reducing hematoma expansion, and improving clinical outcomes [39].

## 10.4 Surgical Treatment of ICH

The role of surgery for most patients with spontaneous ICH remains controversial. Theoretical benefits include prevention of brain herniation, decreasing ICP, decreasing the pathophysiological impact of the hematoma on surrounding tissue by decreasing mass effects or cellular toxicity of blood products.

### 10.4.1 Surgery in Supratentorial ICH

The role of surgery in the management of supratentorial ICH is a matter of debate. The STICH trial was undertaken to determine whether early surgery reduces mortality and improves neurological outcomes compared with conservative management for patients where there is uncertainty of preferred treatment. They found early surgical evacuation of supratentorial ICH was not harmful, but there was no difference in long-term mortality or functional outcome [40]. But subgroup analysis showed benefit in superficial (1 cm from the cortical surface) lobar hemorrhages with those with GCS score <8 showed poorer outcomes. STICH 2 trial compared the outcomes of early vs conservative treatment in conscious patients with superficial lobar hemorrhages (10–100 mL) with intraventricular extension within 48 h of symptom onset.

Minimally invasive techniques including endoscopic hematoma aspiration or instillation of thrombolytic agents as Urokinase or rTPA into the hematoma with aspiration of contents are also being studied but the effectiveness of these measures is uncertain [41].

According to AHA guidelines [5]:

- Early hematoma evacuation is not beneficial compared with hematoma evacuation when patient deteriorates.
- In deteriorating patients, surgical evacuation of hematoma might be a life saving measure.
- Decompressive craniectomy with or without hematoma evacuation might reduce mortality for patients with supratentorial ICH who are in coma, have large hema-

toma with significant midline shift, or have elevated ICP refractory to medical management.
- The effectiveness of minimally invasive clot evacuation with stereotactic or endoscopic aspiration with or without thrombolytic usage is uncertain.

### 10.4.2 Surgery in Infratentorial ICH

According to studies, emergency surgery is beneficial in patients with cerebellar hemorrhages who are deteriorating neurologically or who have brainstem compression and/or hydrocephalus from ventricular obstruction [5, 42, 43].

Initial treatment of the patients with ventricular drainage alone rather than surgical evacuation is not recommended [5, 6]. However, for brainstem hemorrhages, no clear guidelines exist for surgical management and are best treated conservatively. Correction of coagulopathy is very important in patients undergoing surgical hematoma evacuation.

## 10.5 Secondary Interventions

Although emergency ICH protocol is mainly concerned with initial evaluation and treatment, the first 24 h is critical for BP and ICP control, maintaining a secured airway, identification of seizures to prevent secondary brain injury.

### 10.5.1 Hospital Admission

Patients with ICH are usually medically and neurologically unstable especially within the first few days after onset. Admission to a dedicated neurological ICU or Stroke Unit is associated with lower mortality rates [5, 7]. All primary interventions such as control of airway and blood pressure, correction of coagulopathy, treatment of acute seizures should be done without any delay in the initial presenting hospital, before shifting the patient to another hospital for neurological ICU management, neuro intervention or neurosurgical procedures.

### 10.5.2 ICP Management

Elevated ICP is undoubtedly an important factor in ICH management. Intraventricular hemorrhage in ICH is associated with hydrocephalus and elevated ICP.

Current guidelines for ICP monitoring in ICH is similar to TBI.

- Patients with GCS < 8 that is presumed related to large hematoma with mass effect.
- Hydrocephalus
- Patients with significant IVH.
- Clinical evidence of transtentorial herniation.

An ICP <20 mmHg, MAP <130 mmHg, and CPP around 70 mmHg should be maintained depending on the status of cerebral autoregulation [39, 44].

Ventricular drainage can be considered in patients with decreased or loss of consciousness. Ventricular catheters can measure both ICP and drain CSF; therefore, they should be used in patients with hydrocephalus.

### 10.5.3 DVT Prophylaxis

These patients are at an increased risk for the development of DVT; current guidelines recommend use of intermittent pneumatic compression devices and elastic stockings after hospital admission, as well as initiation of LMWH or low dose unfractionated heparin within 1–4 days following onset (after documentation of cessation of bleeding) [5, 45].

### 10.5.4 Temperature Control

Fever in ICH could be due to infections or central causes. Duration of fever correlates with worse outcome and needs to be treated. Paracetamol in Acute Ischemic Stroke (PAIS) trial randomizing stroke patients to either paracetamol 6 g or placebo group showed improved outcomes in the paracetamol group [46].

### 10.5.5 Glucose Management

Avoiding both hypoglycemia and hyperglycemia is important, as this will influence the outcome [5, 47].

### 10.5.6 Seizures

ICH as compared to ischemic stroke can cause a higher proportion of seizures (10.6% vs. 8.6%). The majority of early seizures occur at or near the onset of ICH [48]. Cortical involvement is the most important factor. Incidence and impact of seizures on outcomes vary across different studies—30-day risk is about 8%. In a large single-center study, prophylactic anticonvulsants significantly reduced the seizure occurrence in lobar ICH [49]. However, most of the studies suggest that prophylactic anticonvulsants (esp. phenytoin) are associated with worse functional outcomes [50, 51]. Current guidelines do not recommend prophylactic anticonvulsants, although some practitioners still use a short prophylactic course (1 month) in patients with lobar ICH and those undergoing surgical hematoma evacuations [5, 7]. Acute management is with intravenous benzodiazepines such as lorazepam (0.05–0.1 mg/kg) followed by a loading dose of phenytoin (10–15 mg/kg), fosphenytoin (15–20 mg/kg), or sodium valproate (15–45 mg/kg). Levetiracetam is recommended especially in children, and is thought to be more effective for prophylaxis without suppression of cognitive abilities. (July 2011 neurocrit care) [52] Carbamazepine, lamotrigine, sodium valproate, and topiramate are also recommended first-line anticonvulsants for both focal and secondary generalized seizures. Clinical or EEG seizures in patients with a change in mental status should be treated with anticonvulsant drugs. Continuous EEG should be considered in patients with decreased level of consciousness that is disproportionate to the degree of brain injury [5, 7].

## 10.6 Pediatric Considerations

ICH occurs less frequently in children but can be as devastating and life-threatening. It could be traumatic or spontaneous. Vascular malformations are the most common cause, AVMs almost 50% with 5–10% mortality and 50% neurological morbidity risk. Cavernous malformations represent 20–25% of spontaneous ICH in children; the hemorrhage is usually smaller with better outcomes [53]. Other causes include bleeding diathesis, thrombocytopenias, intracranial tumors, Moya-Moya disease, cerebral venous thrombosis, and sickle cell disease. Thus during neuroimaging, CT contrast and CTA or MRA should be considered. The pediatric ICH score is slightly different from adults, taking into account the volume of hemorrhage as a percentage of total brain volume, and the presence of hydrocephalus and herniation [54]. Emergent management is similar to adults regarding ABCs. The treatment was based on the child's presentation, the precipitating cause, and the radiological findings. It is essential to avoid hypotension (calculated as <fifth percentile, i.e. <70 mmHg + Age in years> ×2) and hypertension (maintain SBP <140 mmHg). Drugs to control BP are nicardipine and esmolol. Nicardipine 0.5 mcg/kg/min, titrated by 0.5 mcg/kg/min every 15 min to a maximum of 5 mcg/kg/min. In older children (adult weight) 2.5 mg/h, titrated by 2.5 mg/h every 15 min up to a maximum of 15 mg/h. Surgical evacuation of ICH if there is impending herniation, and same-sitting or staged surgical resection of the offending lesion is done. Coagulopathy should also be evaluated and treated in children with ICH who present with coagulation abnormalities to prevent hematoma expansion and before surgical treatment.

### 10.6.1 Communication

When handing over, referring or accepting a patient with ICH, following points should be noted:

- Age
- Hematoma volume and location
- GCS
- ICH Score

- Hydrocephalus present ±
- Blood pressure
- Coagulation parameters and reversal treatment
- Plan for surgery

## Multiple Choice Questions

1. A patient presents to the emergency department with a severe headache and is suspected of having an intracerebral bleed. What is the next step in the investigation?
   (a) Brain MRI
   (b) CT of the brain with contrast
   (c) CT of the brain without contrast
   (d) Lumbar puncture
2. A 62-year-old lady with a history of atrial fibrillation on Warfarin, comes to ED with right-sided weakness. BP is 195/120 mmHg, irregular heart rate approximately 92 bpm and blood sugar of 325 mg/dL and INR >6. Emergent noncontrast CT brain revealed an intracerebral hemorrhage in the left internal capsule bordered by edema. All the following should be given to the patient except
   (a) Insulin
   (b) Fresh frozen plasma
   (c) IV labetalol
   (d) Phenytoin
   (e) IV Vitamin K
3. An elderly patient on warfarin with a cerebellar hemorrhage is in the intensive care unit. Appropriate reversal agents for his coagulopathy were previously administered and the patient's last INR was 1.2 this morning. His mental status suddenly declines. Which of the following is true regarding the management of this patient when managing spontaneous intracranial hemorrhage (ICH)?
   (a) Osmotic agents may be used to decrease the amount of intracranial hemorrhage (ICH)
   (b) Consider emergent decompressive surgery
   (c) The hyperosmolar agent hypertonic saline is superior to mannitol in the treatment of increased intracranial pressure
   (d) Immediately administer 2 units of fresh frozen plasma and the appropriate weight-based dose of prothrombin complex concentrate
4. The commonest site of intracranial hypertensive bleed is
   (a) Cerebellum
   (b) Basal ganglia
   (c) Brainstem
   (d) Hippocampus
   (e) Cerebral hemispheres

5. Which of the following is recommended to treat coagulopathy in spontaneous intracerebral hemorrhage?
   (a) Fresh frozen plasma
   (b) Vitamin K
   (c) Prothrombin complex concentrate
   (d) rVIIIa
6. Decompressive surgery in intracerebral bleed is indicated in
   (a) All supratentorial bleeds
   (b) Infratentorial—when cerebellar bleed >3 cm
   (c) GCS >9
   (d) ICP <22 mmHg
7. Excluding trauma, which statement is true about intracranial hemorrhage?
   (a) 55% of intracranial hemorrhage is intracerebral
   (b) Basal ganglia hemorrhage is most common
   (c) 60% is due to amyloid angiopathy
   (d) Often asymptomatic
8. An 85-year-old male was brought to the emergency department with a right-sided facial droop and weakness of the right arm which occurred suddenly while watching the athletic event on television. He has a history of hypertension, hyperlipidemia, chronic obstructive pulmonary disease, and benign prostatic hyperplasia. A workup revealed intracranial hemorrhage on the left. What percentage of strokes are hemorrhagic?
   (a) 1–5%
   (b) 20–30%
   (c) 50%
   (d) 80%
9. A 91-year-old female becomes acutely unresponsive in her assisted living care facility. She is taken to the hospital for a stroke workup and found to have a right frontal intraparenchymal hemorrhage with intraventricular extension. The estimated blood volume of the hemorrhage is 65 mL. She takes warfarin for non-valvular atrial fibrillation and has an INR of 2.1. She has hypertension, diabetes mellitus, asthma, gastroesophageal reflux disease, and stress incontinence. On initial exam, her eyes do not open to painful stimuli, she moans and withdrawals to noxious stimuli in the right arm and has extensor posturing in the left arm with extension of bilateral legs. What is her 30-day mortality based on the intracerebral hemorrhage score?
   (a) 26%
   (b) 72%
   (c) 97%
   (d) 100%
10. Current guidelines for ICP monitoring in ICH include all except:
    (a) Patients with GCS >8.
    (b) Hydrocephalus.
    (c) Patients with significant IVH.
    (d) Clinical evidence of transtentorial herniation.

Answers: 1. (c), 2. (d), 3. (b), 4. (b), 5. (c), 6. (b), 7. (b), 8. (b), 9. (c), 10. (a).

## References


1. Kumar S. Hypertension and hemorrhagic stroke. Hypertens J. 2017;3(2):89–93.
2. Kamalakannan S, et al. Stroke in India. Indian J Med Res. 2017;146:175–85. https://doi.org/10.4103/ijmr.IJMR-516-15.
3. Feigin VL, Lawes CM, Bennett DA, et al. Worldwide stroke incidence and early case fatality reported in 56 population- based studies: a systematic review. Lancet Neurol. 2009;8(4):355–69.
4. Broderick J. Intracerebral hemorrhage. In: Gorelick P, Alter M, editors. Handbook of neuro-epidemiology. New York: Marcel Dekkar Inc.; 1994. p. 141–67.
5. Morgenstern LB, Hemphill JC 3rd, Anderson C, Becker K, Broderick JP, Connolly ES Jr, Greenberg SM, Huang JN, RL MD, Messé SR, Mitchell PH, Selim M, Tamargo RJ. On behalf of the American heart guidelines for the management of spontaneous intracerebral hemorrhage: association stroke council and council on cardiovascular nursing. A guideline for healthcare professionals from the American Heart Association/American Stroke Association. Stroke. 2010;41:2108–29. https://doi.org/10.1161/STR.0b013e3181ec611b.
6. Steiner T, Al-Shahi Salman R, Beer R, et al. European stroke organisation (ESO) guidelines for the management of spontaneous intracerebral hemorrhage. Int J Stroke. 2014;9:840–55.
7. Hemphill JC III, Lam A. Emergency neurological life support: Intracerebral hemorrhage. Neurocrit Care. 27(1):89–101. https://doi.org/10.1007/s12028-017-0453-0.
8. Garrett JS, Zarghouni M, Layton KF, Graybeal D, Daoud YA. Validation of clinical prediction scores in patients with primary intracerebral hemorrhage. Neurocrit Care. 2013;19:329–35. https://doi.org/10.1007/s12028-013-9926-y.
9. Ji R, Shen H, Pan Y, Wang P, Liu G, Wang Y, Li H, Zhao X, Wang Y, China National Stroke Registry (CNSR) Investigators. A novel risk score to predict 1-year functional outcome after intracerebral hemorrhage and comparison with existing scores. Crit Care. 2013;17:R275. https://doi.org/10.1186/cc13130.
10. Kothari R, Brott T, Broderick J, Barsan W, Sauerbeck L, Zuccarello M. The ABCs of measuring intracerebral hemorrhage volume. Stroke. 1996;27:1304–5.
11. Goldstein JN, Fazen LE, Snider R, Schwab K, Greenberg SM, Smith EE, Lev MH, Rosand J. Contrast extravasation on CT angiography predicts hematoma expansion in intracerebral hemorrhage. Neurology. 2007;68:889–94. https://doi.org/10.1212/01.wnl.0000257087.22852.21.
12. Wada R, Aviv RI, Fox AJ, Sahlas DJ, Gladstone DJ, Tomlinson G, Symons SP. CT angiography "spot sign" predicts hematoma expansion in acute intracerebral hemorrhage. Stroke. 2007;38:1257–62. https://doi.org/10.1161/01.STR.0000259633.59404.f3.
13. Acker JE 3rd, Pancioli AM, Crocco TJ, Eckstein MK, Jauch EC, Larrabee H, Meltzer NM, Mergendahl WC, Munn JW, Prentiss SM, Sand C, Saver JL, Eigel B, Gilpin BR, Schoeberl M, Solis P, Bailey JR, Horton KB, Stranne SK. Implementation strategies for emergency medical services within stroke systems of care: a policy statement from the American Heart Association/American Stroke Association expert panel on emergency medical services systems and the stroke council. Stroke. 2007;38:3097–115. https://doi.org/10.1161/STROKEAHA.107.186094.
14. Prasad K, Kaul S, Padma MV, et al. Stroke management. Ann Indian Acad Neurol. 2011;14(Suppl 1):S82–96.
15. Hemphill JC 3rd, Farrant M, Neill TA Jr. Prospective validation of the ICH score for 12-month functional outcome. Neurology. 2009;73:1088–94. https://doi.org/10.1212/WNL.0b013e3181b8b332.
16. Rost NS, Smith EE, Chang Y, Snider RW, Chanderraj R, Schwab K, FitzMaurice E, Wendell L, Goldstein JN, Greenberg SM, Rosand J. Prediction of functional outcome in patients with primary intracerebral hemorrhage: the FUNC score. Stroke. 2008;39:2304–9. https://doi.org/10.1161/STROKEAHA.107.512202.

17. Clarke JL, Johnston SC, Farrant M, Bernstein R, Tong D, Hemphill JC 3rd. External validation of the ICH score. Neurocrit Care. 2004;1:53–60.
18. van Asch CJ, Velthuis BK, Greving JP, van Laar PJ, Rinkel GJ, Algra A, Klijn CJ. External validation of the secondary intracerebral hemorrhage score in the Netherlands. Stroke. 2013;44:2904–6. https://doi.org/10.1161/STROKEAHA.113.002386.
19. Bruce SS, Appelboom G, Piazza M, Hwang BY, Kellner C, Carpenter AM, Bagiella E, Mayer S, Connolly ES. A comparative evaluation of existing grading scales in intracerebral hemorrhage. Neurocrit care existing grading scales in intracerebral hemorrhage. Neurocrit Care. 2011;15:498–505. https://doi.org/10.1007/s12028-011-9518-7.
20. Rodriguez-Luna D, Piñeiro S, Rubiera M, Ribo M, Coscojuela P, Pagola J, Flores A, Muchada M, Ibarra B, Meler P, Sanjuan E, Hernandez Guillamon M, Alvarez-Sabin J, Montaner J, Molina CA. Impact of blood pressure changes and course on hematoma growth in acute intracerebral hemorrhage. Eur J Neurol. 2013;20:1277–83. https://doi.org/10.1111/ene.12180.
21. Anderson CS, Heeley E, Huang Y, et al. Rapid blood-pressure lowering in patients with acute intracerebral hemorrhage. N Engl J Med. 2013;368:2355–65.
22. Goldstein LB, Simel DL. Is this patient having a stroke? JAMA. 2005;293:2391–402. https://doi.org/10.1001/jama.293.19.2391.
23. Fiebach JB, Schellinger PD, Gass A, Kucinski T, Siebler M, Villringer A, Olkers P, Hirsch JG, Heiland S, Wilde P, Jansen O, Röther J, Hacke W, Sartor K, KompetenznetzwerkSchlaganfall B5. Stroke magnetic resonance imaging is accurate in hyperacute intracerebral hemorrhage: a multicenter study on the validity of stroke imaging. Stroke. 2004;35:502–6. https://doi.org/10.1161/01.STR.0000114203.75678.88.
24. Sahni R, Weinberger J. Management of intracerebral hemorrhage. Vasc Health Risk Manag. 2007;3(5):701–9.
25. Zazulia AR, Diringer MN, Videen TO, et al. Hypoperfusion without ischemia surrounding acute intracerebral hemorrhage. J Cereb Blood Flow Metab. 2001;21:804–1039.
26. Qureshi AI, Palesch YY, Barsan WG, et al. Intensive blood pressure lowering in patients with acute cerebral hemorrhage. N Engl J Med. 2016;375:1033–4338.
27. Antihypertensive Treatment of Acute Cerebral Hemorrhage Investigators. Antihypertensive treatment of acute cerebral hemorrhage. Crit Care Med. 2010;38:637–4840.
28. Anderson CS, Huang Y, Wang JG, et al. Intensive blood pressure reduction in acute cerebral haemorrhage trial (INTERACT): a randomised pilot trial. Lancet Neurol. 2008;7:391–9.
29. Huhtakangas J, Tetri S, Juvela S, Saloheimo P, Bode MK, Hillbom M. Effect of increased warfarin use on warfarin-related cerebral hemorrhage a longitudinal population-based study. Stroke. 2011;42:24312435. https://doi.org/10.1161/STROKEAHA.111.615260.
30. Rådberg JA, Olsson JE, Rådberg CT. Prognostic parameters in spontaneous intracerebral hematomas with special reference to anticoagulant treatment. Stroke. 1991;22:571–6. https://doi.org/10.1161/01.STR.22.5.571.
31. Flaherty ML, Kissela B, Woo D, Kleindorfer D, Alwell K, Sekar P, Moomaw CJ, Haverbusch M, Broderick JP. The increasing incidence of anticoagulant-associated intracerebral hemorrhage. Neurology. 2007;68:116–21. https://doi.org/10.1212/01.wnl.0000250340.05202.8b.
32. Holbrook A, Schulman S, Witt DM, Vandvik PO, Fish J, Kovacs MJ, Svensson PJ, Veenstra DL, Crowther M, Guyatt GH, American College of Chest Physicians. Evidence-based management of anticoagulant therapy: antithrombotic therapy and prevention of thrombosis, 9th ed: American College of Chest Physicians Evidence-Based Clinical Practice Guidelines. Chest. 2012;141(2 Suppl):e152S–84S. https://doi.org/10.1378/chest.11-2295.
33. Sarode R, Milling TJ Jr, Refaai MA, et al. Efficacy and safety of a4-factor prothrombin complex concentrate in patients on vitamin K antagonists presenting with major bleeding: a randomized plasma-controlled, phase IIIb study. Circulation. 2013;128:1234–43.
34. Steiner T, Poli S, Griebe M, et al. Fresh frozen plasma versus prothrombin complex concentrate in patients with intracranial haemorrhage related to vitamin K antagonists(INCH): a randomised trial. Lancet Neurol. 2016;15(6):566–73.

35. Frontera JA, Lewin JJ III, Rabinstein AA, et al. Guideline for reversal of antithrombotics in intracranial hemorrhage: a statement for healthcare professionals from the Neurocritical care society and Society of Critical Care Medicine. Neurocrit Car. 2016;24:6–46e.
36. Kaatz S, Kouides PA, Garcia DA, Spyropolous AC, Crowther M, Douketis JD, Chan AK, James A, Moll S, Ortel TL, Van Cott EM, Ansell J. Guidance on the emergent reversal of oral thrombin and factor Xa inhibitors. Am J Hematol. 2012;87(Suppl 1):S141–5. https://doi.org/10.1002/ajh.23202.
37. Enriquez A, Lip GY, Baranchuk A. Anticoagulation reversal in the era of the non-vitamin K oral anticoagulants. EP Eur. 2016;18(7):955–64.
38. Roquer J, Rodriguez Campello A, et al. Previous antiplatelet therapy is an independent predictor of 30- day mortality after spontaneous supratentorial intracerebral hemorrhage. J Neurol. 2005;252(4):412–6.
39. Bratton SL, Chestnut RM, Ghajar J, McConnell Hammond FF, Harris OA, Hartl R, Manley GT, Nemecek A, Newell DW, Rosenthal G, Schouten J, Shutter L, Timmons SD, Ullman JS, Videtta W, Wilberger JE, Wright DW. Guidelines for the management of severe traumatic brain injury, IX: cerebral perfusion thresholds [published correction appears in J Neurotrauma. 2008;25:276–278]. J Neurotrauma. 2007;24(suppl 1):S59–S64194.
40. Mendelow AD, Gregson BA, Fernandes HM, Murray GD, Teasdale GM, Hope DT, Karimi A, Shaw MD, Barer DH, STICH investigators. Early surgery versus initial conservative treatment in patients with spontaneous supratentorial intracerebral haematomas in the international surgical trial in Intracerebral Haemorrhage (STICH): a randomised trial. Lancet. 2005;365(9457):387–9.
41. Auer LM, Deinsberger W, Niederkorn K, et al. Endoscopic surgery versus medical treatment for spontaneous intracerebral hematoma: a randomized study. J Neurosurg. 1989;70:530–5.
42. Firsching R, Huber M, Frowein RA. Cerebellar haemorrhage: management and prognosis. Neurosurg Rev. 1991;14:191–4.
43. Kirollos RW, Tyagi AK, Ross SA, van Hille PT, Marks PV. Management of spontaneous cerebellar hematomas: a prospective treatment protocol. Neurosurgery. 2001;49:1378–86. discussion 86-7
44. Chambers IR, Banister K, Mendelow AD. Intracranial pressure within a developing intracerebral haemorrhage. Br J Neurosurg. 2001;15(2):140–1.
45. Nyquist P, Bautista C, Jichici D, et al. Prophylaxis of venous thrombosis in neurocritical care patients: an evidence-based guideline: a statement for healthcare professionals from the Neurocritical care society. Neurocrit Care. 2016;24:4725.
46. Den Hertog HM, van der Worp HB, et al. The Paracetamol (acetaminophen) in stroke (PAIS) trial: a multicentre,randomised, placebo-controlled, phase III trial. Lancet Neurol. 2009;8(5):434–40.
47. Vespa PM. Intensive glycemic control in traumatic brain injury: what is the ideal glucose range? Crit Care. 2008;12:175.
48. De Herdt V, Dumont F, Hénon H, Derambure P, Vonck K, Leys D, Cordonnier C. Early seizures in intracerebral hemorrhage: incidence associated factors, and outcome. Neurology. 2011;77:1794–800. https://doi.org/10.1212/WNL.0b013e31823648a6.
49. Passero S, Rocchi R, Rossi S, Ulivelli M, Vatti G. Seizures after spontaneous supratentorial intracerebral hemorrhage. Epilepsia. 2002;43:1175–80.
50. Naidech AM, Garg RK, Liebling S, Levasseur K, Macken MP, Schuele SU, Batjer HH. Anticonvulsant use and outcomes after intracerebral hemorrhage. Stroke. 2009;40:3810–5. https://doi.org/10.1161/STROKEAHA.109.559948.
51. Messé SR, Sansing LH, Cucchiara BL, Herman ST, Lyden PD, Kasner SE, CHANT investigators. Prophylactic antiepileptic drug use is associated with poor outcome following ICH. Neurocrit Care. 2009;11:38–44. https://doi.org/10.1007/s12028-009-9207-y.
52. Beghi E, D'Alessandro R, Beretta S, Consoli D, Crespi V, Delaj L, Gandolfo C, Greco G, La Neve A, Manfredi M, Mattana F, Musolino R, Provinciali L, Santangelo M, Specchio LM,

Zaccara G, Epistroke Group. Incidence and predictors of acute symptomatic seizures after stroke. Neurology. 2011;77:1785–93. https://doi.org/10.1212/WNL.0b013e3182364878.

53. Srinivasan VM, et al. Management of intracerebral hemorrhage in pediatric neurosurgery. Surg Neurol Int. 2016;7(Suppl 44):S1121–6.
54. Beslow LA, et al. Pediatric intracerebral hemorrhage score a simple grading scale for intracerebral hemorrhage in children. Stroke. 2014;45:66–70.

# 11 Aneurysmal Subarachnoid Hemorrhage

Charu Mahajan, Indu Kapoor, and Hemanshu Prabhakar

**Key Points**

- The most common presenting feature is onset of sudden severe headache which is categorically considered as the worst headache of life and reaches a peak within seconds
- Noncontrast CT scan is the investigation of choice for initial detection of subarachnoid blood
- Patients of SAH should be rapidly and safely transferred to high-volume centers having neurosurgical facility for further management
- A goal to maintain systolic blood pressure below 160 mmHg and mean arterial blood pressure less than 110 mmHg is considered reasonable in patients with unclipped aneurysms.
- Nimodipine is the only pharmacologic agent which has a definitive role in improving the outcome
- Poorer the SAH grade of the patient, more is the chance of development of extracranial complicatons like NSM, pulmonary edema, electrolyte imbalance

**Case-Scenario**

A 64-year-old female was brought to the emergency department of a tertiary care center by his son. She was apparently alright till 10 h back when she complained of sudden onset of severe headache followed by two episodes of vomiting and transient loss of consciousness. She was a known hypertensive for last 15 years,

C. Mahajan · I. Kapoor · H. Prabhakar (✉)
All India Institute of Medical Sciences, New Delhi, India


P. U. Bidkar, P. Vanamoorthy (eds.), *Acute Neuro Care*,
https://doi.org/10.1007/978-981-15-4071-4_11

on Tab amlodipine 10 mg BD. On examination, patient had a GCS score of E4V5M6 (drowsy), with pupils bilaterally equal in size and reacting to light. There was presence of neck rigidity with no other motor/sensory deficits. Heart rate—92/min, BP—178/102 mmHg, $SpO_2$—95% on face mask with oxygen flow @ 6 L/min. Chest and CVS examination findings were normal. Samples for lab testing were sent. Noncontrast CT head revealed blood in the right sylvian fissure. Cerebral DSA was carried out which confirmed the presence of right middle cerebral artery (M1) aneurysm 5.23 × 3.42 × 2.32 mm.

## 11.1 Introduction

Aneurysmal subarachnoid hemorrhage (aSAH) is an acute neurological emergency that often strikes without a warning. The time-critical care requires an early emergency response within minutes to hours. As our country lacks a well-established prehospital emergency medical services, many patients do not receive care as early as they should and present to the emergency department usually after hours or even days. Our chapter discusses the clinical features, early resuscitation and stabilization, means of prompt diagnosis, early management goals, definitive therapy, and management of early complications, both cranial and systemic.

"Brain attack," as the name implies, is an acute neurological intervention that requires immediate medical attention. aSAH is its non-traumatic hemorrhagic version which is associated with quite high mortality and morbidity even in this era. The aSAH patients who reported to a tertiary care center in India had mortality as high as 45.4% at 3 months follow-up [1]. This does not include those patients who die before reaching any medical institute. The initial complications and aneurysmal rebleed are major dreaded factors affecting early mortality and need to be attended to promptly. This makes it important that emergency care providers follow evidence-based protocol care during early window period of SAH, which may at its best help in early diagnosis and help provide optimum care to improve the outcome.

Unlike western nations, our country lacks a well-developed and uniform emergency medical services (EMS) access numbers which makes the quality of care heterogeneous. The fundamentals for providing optimum prehospital care like healthcare resources, widespread education, training, and strengthening of the EMS system is still a distant dream. However, the emergency department services have improved over the years with better vital signs monitoring, point-of-care clinical diagnostics, and early referral systems.

Emergency neurological care of SAH patients includes quick appropriate identification of clinical features, maintaining the airway, breathing and circulation, point-of-care tests, neurosurgeon consultation, and urgent interventions. Figure 11.1 depicts the early management of patients having SAH.

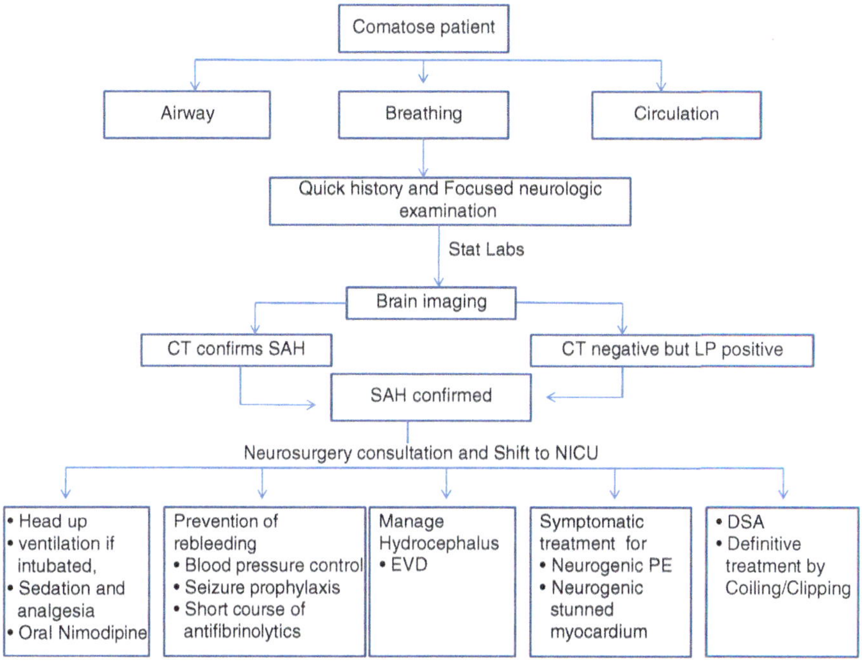


**Fig. 11.1** Algorithm for management of SAH patient. *CT* Computed tomography head, *LP* lumbar puncture, *EVD* External ventricular drainage, *DSA* Digital Subtraction angiography, *PE* Pulmonary edema, *NICU* Neurosurgical intensive care unit

## 11.2 Clinical Presentation

The mean age of presentation in India is around 50 years which is similar to world trends; and male: female ratio varies from 1:1 to 1:1.5 [1, 2]. The most common presenting feature is the onset of sudden severe headache which is categorically considered as the worst headache of life and reaches a peak within a few seconds. The other associated signs and symptoms may include nausea, vomiting, brief loss of consciousness, neck stiffness, third nerve palsy, retinal hemorrhage, or even focal neurological deficits. A typical history along with neck pain and stiffness are strongly suggestive of SAH [3]. Depending on the severity of bleed, patients may present in an altered mental state or even in a comatose state. Correct diagnosis at this stage is imperative as it is easy to miss patients with no/subtle focal neurological signs as having migraine. This group of patients may present later with a rebleed and fare a poorer outcome [4]. It is neither recommended to subject every patient with a headache to Computed tomography (CT) or lumbar puncture (LP). The four aspects of patient's history which helps to identify SAH includes (a) abrupt onset (b) worst in severity when compared to earlier headaches (c) quality of headache compared to prior headaches (d) associated findings like nausea/vomiting, syncope, seizures, diplopia [5]. Neurologically intact patients may be relieved by intake of analgesics for headache. On the other hand, comatose patients require urgent care. The provision of prehospital care in our Indian setup lacks, though if available it should concentrate on maintaining the airway, establishing intravenous access and rapid transfer to the nearest tertiary care center.

## 11.3 Differential Diagnosis

It is important to rule out conditions which mimic hemorrhagic stroke like pituitary apoplexy, intracerebral bleed, tumor bleed, hypertensive encephalopathy, cervical/cerebral artery dissection, cerebral venous sinus thrombosis, reversible cerebral vasoconstriction syndrome, meningitis, or migraine [6]. A good history and neurological examination helps to rule out these conditions and brain imaging aids in confirming the diagnosis.

## 11.4 Resuscitation and Stabilization

Once the patient reaches the hospital, the level of consciousness and arousability is assessed by stimuli of increasing intensity. Patients are categorized as A—alert and oriented, V—respond to verbal command, P—responding to pain, and U—unresponsive [7]. Alternatively, consciousness can also be assessed by a quick Glasgow coma scale (GCS) scoring. Table 11.1 enumerates the steps to be followed after hospital admission. If the patient is not responsive, the first step is resuscitation and stabilization. An intravenous access should be established as soon as the patient presents to the hospital. The primary and secondary survey should be followed. Maintaining A—Airway, B—Breathing, and C—Circulation is the first step in the management of comatose patient. A patent airway has to be ensured and the need for endotracheal intubation is assessed. The cervical spine should be immobilized in comatose patent until it is cleared by radiology later. Hypoxia and hypotension should be rapidly corrected to prevent any secondary brain injury. A rapid focused neurological examination in a comatose patient includes assessment of GCS, pupillary reaction, and other neurological deficits. Hypoglycemia should be ruled out at bedside by glucometer testing. Blood samples for complete blood count, coagulation profile, renal function tests, and serum electrolytes should be collected and sent. Lab testing should also include a toxicology screen to rule out poisoning. Chest X-ray and an Electrocardiography (ECG) are also obtained to see any abnormal findings and to serve as a baseline investigation for comparing changes that develop later. Brain imaging with a noncontrast computed tomography (NCCT) should be done as early as feasible.

In the first hour of presentation, the patient should be evaluated for the following

1. Noncontrast CT scan
2. Laboratory investigations
3. 12 lead ECG
4. Neurosurgical consultation
5. Address initial complications

**Table 11.1** Checklist for a suspected case of SAH admitted to hospital

| |
|---|
| • Secure IV line, send blood samples for testing |
| • ABC approach |
| • Assess GCS, pupillary size, and reaction |
| • Endotracheal intubation (GCS≤8, airway requires protection, not able to maintain oxygenation) |
| • Brain imaging |
| • Neurosurgeon consultation |
| • Shifting to an intensive care unit |
| • Communication of vitals, SAH scores, and medications given |
| • Mechanical ventilation with normocapnia, if poor grade SAH or features of raised ICP—hyperventilation may be instituted to $PaCO_2$ levels of 30–35 mmHg |
| • Head-up position, avoid Valsalva or stressful stimuli |
| • Sedation and analgesia for patients on ventilator |
| • Ryles tube insertion |
| • Maintain blood pressure, fluid resuscitation, treat dysrhythmias and shock |
| • Arterial line and central venous line depending on requirement |
| • Start Nimodipine 60 mg orally QID |
| • Treat hypertension |
| • Correct coagulopathy if present |
| • Treat seizures with midazolam and phenytoin |
| • Short course of antifibrinolytics (optional). |
| • Treat hydrocephalus by EVD |
| • DSA as soon as possible |
| • Definitive treatment by coiling/clipping |
| • Close neurological monitoring and TCD evaluation |
| • Induced hypertension if vasospasm present |
| • Angioplasty (pharmacological/balloon) if refractory |

## 11.5 Diagnosis of SAH and its Confirmation

Noncontrast CT scan is the investigation of choice for initial detection of subarachnoid blood which appears as a hyperdense shadow in basal cisterns, fissures, and even within the ventricles. A CT scan performed within 6 h of ictus by a third generation CT scanner is almost 100% sensitive and specific for the detection of subarachnoid blood [8]. However, sensitivity is time-dependent and it may fail to detect blood in older, smaller bleeds and when performed in anemic patients. If CT is negative but patients have a high suspicion of SAH, they should be subjected to LP only after ruling out midline shift, obstructive hydrocephalus, and cerebral edema [9]. The Cerebrospinal fluid collected via LP should be evaluated for RBC count in the final fourth tube (which should be equal to the RBC count present in first tube) and xanthochromia (yellowish discoloration). LP is also time-dependent and is almost 100% sensitive at 12 h postbleed. Magnetic resonance imaging (MRI) may be done in CT negative cases where time to ictus is already >72 h. Fluid attenuated inversion recovery sequence of MRI is an excellent alternative to CT scan but may not be easily available in our Indian context. Moreover, after a negative MRI, it is still recommended to do LP [10].

Once the diagnosis of SAH is confirmed, further aneurysm localization is carried out by performing a digital subtraction angiogram (DSA). The AHA/ASA guidelines recommend carrying out computed tomography angiography (CTA) or magnetic resonance angiography (MRA) in cases where DSA cannot be performed promptly [9]. The CTA and MRA can localize an aneurysm but cannot provide any information on whether it has bled or not. So, it may not help in differentiating a ruptured aneurysm from an unruptured aneurysm. However, in our Indian scenario, the availability of DSA or CTA/MRA is limited to specialized centers only, and patients of SAH should be rapidly and safely transferred to these centers for further management.

## 11.6 Grades of SAH

Grading the SAH patients is vital for effective communication among medical staff, assessing the prognosis of the patient, and evaluating the risk of intervention. Though several SAH scales have been proposed, the popular ones are Hunt and Hess grade and World Federation of Neurological Surgeons (WFNS) grade [11, 12]. The Hunt and Hess grade includes five scores and higher the grade, poor is the prognosis. Grade 1 is an asymptomatic patient or having mild headache with slight nuchal rigidity. Patients having moderate–severe headache, cranial nerve palsy (III, VI), and nuchal rigidity are grouped as grade 2. Grade 3 patients have mild, focal deficit, lethargy, or confusion. Grade 4 patients have stupor, hemiparesis (moderate–severe), and decerebrate rigidity. Grade 5 patients are moribund, in a deep coma with decerebrate rigidity. Presence of hypertension, chronic obstructive airway disease, severe atherosclerosis, diabetes mellitus, or if arteriography depicts vasospasm, the patient is allocated to a grade higher. Modified Hunt and Hess classification includes also grade 0 (unruptured aneurysm) and grade 1a (fixed neuro deficit in absence of acute meningeal reaction) [13]. WFNS is another 5-point grading that takes GCS and major focal deficit into account for computation of grade. Grade 1 includes patients having GCS 15 with no major focal deficit. Grade 2 and grade 3 include patients having GCS 13–15 without and with major focal deficits, respectively. Grade 4 includes all patients with or without major focal deficits with GCS 7–12. Grade 5 includes patients having GCS 3–6 with or without major focal deficits.

Many scales are radiology based, common ones being Fisher scale, modified Fisher scale, and Claassen CT rating scale [14–16]. Fisher scale quantifies the amount of subarachnoid blood on the CT scan image and helps to predict the risk of cerebral vasospasm. It includes four grades, grade 1: No blood visible, grade 2: diffuse, <1 mm thin layer, grade 3: Localized clot or >1 mm thick, grade 4: intracerebral or intraventricular blood with diffuse or no subarachnoid blood. The incidence of vasospasm is greatest in grade 3. Fisher scale was subsequently modified to give a five-grade scale in which the risk of vasospasm increased with each subsequent higher grade [15].

There are many other comprehensive scales also which take into account several factors to obtain risk stratification [17–19]. Though, they are accurate, but are elaborate and time-consuming resulting in their limited use.

## 11.7 Definitive Treatment

The patient is shifted to ICU for further management while definitive treatment is being planned. Patients should be taken up for definitive treatment as soon as feasible [9]. Many factors guide the decision for choosing the best modality of treatment, either surgical clipping or endovascular coiling. The main factors are the age of the patient, comorbidities, location of the aneurysm, size of the neck of the aneurysm, presence of hematoma, patient affordability, and technical expertise availability. For an aneurysm which is considered to be equally suitable for either treatment, endovascular coiling is the preferred treatment modality. Patients who have a middle cerebral artery aneurysm or a large intraparenchymal hematoma are preferably surgically operated. Endovascular coiling is preferred in elderly patients >70 years, WFNS IV/V grade patients, and basilar artery aneurysms [9]. Though wide-necked aneurysms are easier to clip, balloon remodeling and use of stents enable successful coiling but may be associated with a higher morbidity. Flow diverters are a new class of endovascular stents which are placed in parent vessel across the aneurysm [20]. The high mesh density prevents the flow of blood into the aneurysmal sac and causes subsequent complete occlusion of the aneurysm. However, it requires the administration of dual anti-platelet therapy.

## 11.8 ICU Management

An awake patient is shifted to a calm, quiet place in ICU with head end of bed elevated to 15–30°. Analgesics, anti-emetics are administered and intramuscular injections or other stressful stimuli are completely avoided. Intubated patients are provided analgo-sedation and mechanically ventilated to keep arterial carbondioxide levels of around 30–35 mmHg. Continuous monitoring of ECG, blood pressure, and oxygen saturation is carried out. A 12-lead ECG, a chest X-ray should be obtained and all investigations should be reviewed.

Oral nimodipine 60 mg every four hourly is administered to all patients for 21 days as it is the only drug proven to improve the outcome [21]. Poor grade patients may require Ryle's tube insertion before starting therapy. Definitive treatment either endovascular coiling or surgical clipping depends on aneurysm factors (size, site, morphology) surgeon's expertise, and patient factors (age, comorbidities, cost of procedure). Early treatment helps in eliminating the risk of rebleed as well as the institution of therapies for vasospasm.

Initial concerns which need to be attended to are:

1. Blood pressure
2. Risk of rebleeding

3. Seizures
4. Coagulopathy
5. Hydrocephalus
6. Decline in neurological status
7. Neurogenic pulmonary edema
8. Cardiogenic stunned myocardium

### 11.8.1 Blood Pressure Control

Hypotension decreases cerebral perfusion in acute brain injury and should be avoided and treated promptly. This may require fluid resuscitation and even vasopressors. Hypertension in the acute phase of hemorrhage may be a consequence of SAH itself due to sympathetic surge as a compensatory mechanism to maintain CPP.

In an unclipped aneurysm, blood pressure control is highly recommended to prevent rebleeding. A goal to maintain systolic blood pressure below 160 mmHg and mean arterial blood pressure less than 110 mmHg is considered reasonable [9, 22]. Other factors like patients age, comorbidities, and the past history of hypertension should also be considered before the setting of blood pressure goals. For this purpose, short-acting, easily titrable drugs like nicardipine and labetalol are preferred. However, these drugs may not be easily available, so a decision of selection of an antihypertensive agent should be based on local availability of the best possible drug. Cerebral vasodilators like nitroglycerine and sodium nitroprusside are avoided because of their cerebral vasodilatory action.

### 11.8.2 Prevention of Rebleed

The risk of rebleed is highest in the first 6 h and is associated with worse outcomes [23]. Strict blood pressure control and early aneurysm obliteration are two main strategies that prevent rebleeding from an aneurysm. The role of antifibrinolytics arises in situations where a definitive treatment cannot be carried out on time. So to prevent rebleed in that window period, a short course of antifibrinolytics for less than 3 days might help but it does not improve the outcome [24]. The associated side effects like thromboembolism and cerebral ischemia warrant a short course of these drugs.

### 11.8.3 Global Cerebral Edema

Cerebral edema secondary to inflammation or circulatory disturbances is often evident on CT. It is seen more commonly in patients who present with a history of loss of consciousness and higher Hunt and Hess grade. Its incidence is around 8% and is associated with poor outcome [25]. Measures to reduce cerebral edema may improve the outcome.

### 11.8.4 Coagulopathy

Patients with abnormal coagulation tests should be urgently treated based on the history and type of drugs used. Platelet count below 50,000 should be treated by platelet transfusion. Patients on warfarin need an injection of vitamin K along with prothrombin complex concentrates. Patients on aspirin and clopidogrel may be given platelet transfusion before clipping of aneurysm.

### 11.8.5 Acute Hydrocephalus

Several factors are associated with the development of hydrocephalus after subarachnoid hemorrhage. Few important predictive factors are intraventricular hemorrhage, admission level of consciousness, hypertension, and increasing age [26]. Acute hydrocephalus may occur due to the presence of blood clots in the ventricles, thereby preventing the free flow of CSF. The associated mass effect and inflammation also plays a role in its pathogenesis. It can be an important factor causing early brain injury [27]. Poor grade SAH patients are likely to have associated intracranial hypertension due to cerebral edema, hematoma, and development of acute hydrocephalus. The incidence of acute hydrocephalus is about 18% with approximately 30% recovering spontaneously [28]. Standard measures to lower intracranial pressure (ICP) are instituted in these patients. When progressively increasingly hydrocephalus is associated with altered level of consciousness, external ventricular drain (EVD), or a lumbar drain (if third and fourth ventricles are free of blood and there is no intracranial space-occupying hematoma) is inserted to allow drainage of CSF and lowering of ICP. The possible complications of EVD insertion are aneurysmal rebleeding, brain parenchyma hemorrhage, over drainage, and infection.

### 11.8.6 Seizures

Many factors predispose an aSAH patient to early seizures, few of which are thick intracerebral clot, Middle cerebral artery (MCA) aneurysm, and poor neurological grade. It may result in rebleeding which carries a poor prognosis. A short course of anti-epileptic drugs <7 days may be considered in the immediate posthemorrhagic period [9]. Long-term use of these drugs is associated with cognitive decline and no clear-cut advantage.

### 11.8.7 Cardiac Abnormalities

Cardiac abnormalities are common in patients having SAH and may be manifested as abnormal ECG depicting a variety of changes like sinus tachycardia, arrhythmias, ST depression or elevation, QT prolongation, and even wall motion abnormalities [29]. At times, in the absence of reliable past history, it may be difficult to differentiate it from preexisting cardiac disease. Raised Troponin levels are a common finding in SAH but usually the levels are lower than that found in myocardial infarction [30]. Neurogenic stunned myocardium (NSM) is a state seen in acute brain injury that is secondary to the sympathetic surge and catecholamine release resulting in ECG changes, raised cardiac enzymes levels, and left ventricular dysfunction. Basal segments and mid-ventricular part of left ventricle is commonly involved. The clinical picture resembles Takotsubo cardiomyopathy (TC) which commonly involves the apical portion of myocardium. The prevalence of TC in SAH varies from 1.2% to 26% [31, 32]. These patients are managed symptomatically by continuous hemodynamic monitoring and administration of vasopressors or inotropes as required. If complicated by cardiogenic shock and pulmonary edema, it requires intubation and mechanical ventilation.

### 11.8.8 Neurogenic Pulmonary Edema

Neurogenic pulmonary edema (PE) is thought to be due to the raised ICP which results in a sympathetic surge and release of catecholamines [33]. Patients present with dyspnea, tachypnea, tachycardia, and basal rales. Features of cardiogenic pulmonary edema will be cardiomegaly, Kerley B lines, and pleural effusion. At times, it may be difficult to separate the two entities especially in an old patient having preexisting compromised cardiac function and there may occur overlap of both conditions. This requires lowering of ICP, oxygen inhalation, or endotracheal intubation with mechanical ventilation.

### 11.8.9 Electrolyte Disorders

Electrolyte disorders like hyponatremia, hypernatremia, hypokalemia, and hypomagnesemia are common in these patients. Hypernatremia, hypokalemia, and hypomagnesemia are associated with poor outcome [34]. The initial lab values should be serially followed for any subsequent derangements. Syndrome of inappropriate antidiuretic hormone secretion (SIADH), cerebral salt wasting syndrome (CSW), or diabetes insipidus (DI) may develop resulting in fluid and electrolyte disturbances. This requires appropriate diagnosis and management.

### 11.8.10 Others

Fever is a common finding in these patients arising as a result of reaction to breakdown products of blood in subarachnoid hemorrhage. Control of fever with cold sponging and antipyretics is essential for the prevention of secondary brain damage. No clear-cut hemoglobin threshold for blood transfusion has been described in the literature. Though anemia is associated with poor outcomes, blood transfusion has not been proven to improve the outcome. However, when delayed cerebral ischemia is present, blood transfusion may have a beneficial role [35]. Another study measuring CBF and oxygen extraction fraction using O-PET demonstrated improved cerebral delivery especially to vulnerable regions in patients at risk for DCI [36].

### 11.8.11 Decline in Neurological Status

Early decline in neurological status may be due to hypotension, rebleeding, hydrocephalus, or seizures (epileptic or non-epileptiform). These factors should be considered and appropriate therapy instituted accordingly.

## 11.9 Summary

Aneurysmal SAH is a cerebrovascular emergency that needs to be taken care of in a high-volume center. Prompt recognition, early resuscitation, stabilization, and urgent referral to a neurosurgical specialty may help in the optimal management of this condition. Early goals concentrate on prevention of secondary brain injury, prevention of rebleeding, supportive treatment related to extracranialsystems and early definitive therapy. The early brain injury has an impact on the overall outcome and thus needs to be promptly managed.

## Multiple Choice Questions

1. A patient having moderate headache with nuchal stiffness belongs to which grade on Hunt and Hess scale?
   (a) I
   (b) II
   (c) III
   (d) IV
2. Which one is least likely to be present in a patient admitted with a history of aneurysmal SAH?
   (a) ECG abnormalities
   (b) Hyponatremia
   (c) Hypothermia
   (d) Hydrocephalus
3. The gold standard for the detection of ruptured cerebral aneurysms in acute SAH is
   (a) CT
   (b) MRA
   (c) CTA
   (d) DSA

4. Which of the following complications carries the highest mortality in acute SAH?
   (a) Rebleeding
   (b) Electrolyte abnormalities
   (c) ECG changes
   (d) Hyperthermia
5. The only proven pharmacological agent which improves outcome in patients having aneurysmal SAH is
   (a) Magnesium
   (b) Clazosentan
   (c) Nimodipine
   (d) Erythropoietin
6. Patient having aneurysmal bleed with large intraparenchymal hematoma is preferably taken up for
   (a) Surgical clipping
   (b) Coiling
   (c) Flow divertor placement
   (d) Conservative management
7. Which one is not true about antifibrinolytics administration in SAH?
   (a) Delay in definitive treatment is expected
   (b) Prevents vasospasm
   (c) Should be given for <72 h
   (d) May cause cerebral ischemia
8. Which one is true about seizures in SAH?
   (a) Prophylactic therapy should be given for 1 month.
   (b) Short course of anti-epileptic drugs <7 days may be considered.
   (c) Long-term use is associated with a good outcome.
   (d) Levetiracetam is proven to be better than phenytoin.
9. Which one is a feature of neurogenic stunned myocardium?
   (a) Troponin levels will be higher than that in MI
   (b) No past history of cardiac disease
   (c) Wall motion abnormalities correlating with coronary vascular distribution
   (d) Abnormal coronaries.
10. All are components of early brain injury except
   (a) Microthrombosis
   (b) Decreased glutamate
   (c) Cortical spreading depolarisation
   (d) High ET-1.

Answers: 1. (b), 2. (c), 3. (d), 4. (a), 5. (c), 6. (a), 7. (b), 8. (b), 9. (b), 10. (b).

## References


1. Sodhi HS, Savardekar AR, Mohindra S, Chhabra R, Gupta V, Gupta SK. The clinical profile, management, and overall outcome of aneurysmal subarachnoid hemorrhage at the neurosurgical unit of a tertiary care center in India. J Neurosci Rural Pract. 2014;5:118–26.
2. Aggarwal A, Dhandapani S, Praneeth K, et al. Comparative evaluation of H&H and WFNS grading scales with modified H&H (sans systemic disease): a study on 1000 patients with subarachnoid haemorrhage. Neurosurg Rev. 2018;41:241–7.
3. Carpenter CR, Hussain AM, Ward MJ, Zipfel GJ, Fowler S, Pines JM, Sivilotti ML. Spontaneous subarachnoid hemorrhage: a systematic review and meta-analysis describing the diagnostic accuracy of history, physical examination, imaging, and lumbar puncture with an exploration of test thresholds. Acad Emerg Med. 2016;23(9):963–1003.
4. Kowalski RG, Claassen J, Kreiter KT, et al. Initial misdiagnosis and outcome after subarachnoid hemorrhage. JAMA. 2004;291:866–9.
5. Edlow JA. Diagnosis of subarachnoid hemorrhage in the emergency department. Emerg Med Clin North Am. 2003;21:73–87.
6. Abraham MK, Chang WW. Subarachnoid hemorrhage. Emerg Med Clin North Am. 2016;34:901–16.
7. Romanelli D, Farrell MW. AVPU (alert, voice, pain, unresponsive). Treasure Island: Stat Pearls Publishing; 2019.
8. Blok KM, Rinkel GJ, Majoie CB, et al. CT within 6 hours of headache onset to rule out subarachnoid hemorrhage in nonacademic hospitals. Neurology. 2015;84(19):1927–32.
9. Connolly ES Jr, Rabinstein AA, Carhuapoma JR, et al. Guidelines for the management of aneurysmal subarachnoid hemorrhage: a guideline for healthcare professionals from the American Heart Association/American Stroke Association. Stroke. 2012;43(6):1711–37.
10. Edlow JA, Figaji A, Samuels O. Emergency neurological life support: subarachnoid hemorrhage. Neurocrit Care. 2015;23(Suppl 2):S103–9.
11. Hunt WE, Hess RM. Surgical risk as related to time of intervention in the repair of intracranial aneurysms. J Neurosurg. 1968;28(1):14–20.
12. Teasdale GM, Drake CG, Hunt W, et al. A universal subarachnoid haemorrhage scale: report of a committee of the world federation of neurosurgical societies. J Neurol Neurosurg Psychiatry. 1988;51(11):1457.
13. Hunt WE, Kosnik EJ. Timing and perioperative care in intracranial aneurysm surgery. Clin Neurosurg. 1974;21:79–89.
14. Fisher CM, Kistler JP, Davis JM. Relation of cerebral vasospasm to subarachnoid hemorrhage visualized by computerized tomographic scanning. Neurosurgery. 1980;6:1–9.
15. Frontera JA, Claassen J, Schmidt JM, Wartenberg KE, Temes R, Connolly ES Jr, et al. Prediction of symptomatic vasospasm after subarachnoid hemorrhage: the modified fisher scale. Neurosurgery. 2006;59:21–7.
16. Claassen J, Bernardini GL, Kreiter K, Bates J, Du YE, Copeland D, Connolly ES, Mayer SA. Effect of cisternal and ventricular blood on risk of delayed cerebral ischemia after subarachnoid hemorrhage: the Fisher scale revisited. Stroke. 2001;32:2012–20.
17. Ogilvy CS, Carter BS. A proposed comprehensive grading system to predict outcome for surgical management of intracranial aneurysms. Neurosurgery. 1998;42:959–68.
18. Naval NS, Kowalski RG, Chang TR, Caserta F, Carhuapoma JR, Tamargo RJ, The SAH. Score: a comprehensive communication tool. J Stroke Cerebrovasc Dis. 2014;23:902–9.
19. Ogilvy CS, Cheung AC, Mitha AP, Hoh BL, Carter BS. Outcomes for surgical and endovascular management of intracranial aneurysms using a comprehensive grading system. Neurosurgery. 2006;59:1037–42.
20. Lozupone E, Piano M, Valvassori L, Quilici L, Pero G, Visconti E, Boccardi E. Flow diverter devices in ruptured intracranial aneurysms: a single-center experience. J Neurosurg. 2018;128:1037–43.

21. Pickard JD, Murray GD, Illingworth R, Shaw MD, Teasdale GM, Foy PM, Humphrey PR, et al. Effect of oral nimodipine on cerebral infarction and outcome after subarachnoid haemorrhage: British aneurysm nimodipine trial. BMJ. 1989;298(6674):636–42.
22. Diringer MN, Bleck TP, Claude Hemphill J 3rd, et al. Critical care management of patients following aneurysmal subarachnoid hemorrhage: recommendations from the neurocritical care society's multidisciplinary consensus conference. Neurocrit Care. 2011;15(2):211–40.
23. Tanno Y, Homma M, Oinuma M, et al. Rebleeding from ruptured intracranial aneurysms in north eastern province of Japan: a cooperative study. J Neurosci. 2007;258:11–6.
24. Starke RM, Kim GH, Fernandez A, et al. Impact of a protocol for acute antifibrinolytic therapy on aneurysm rebleeding after subarachnoid hemorrhage. Stroke. 2008;39(9):2617–21.
25. Claassen J, Carhuapoma JR, Kreiter KT, Du EY, Connolly ES, Mayer SA. Global cerebral edema after subarachnoid hemorrhage: frequency, predictors, and impact on outcome. Stroke. 2002;33(5):1225–32.
26. Graff-Radford NR, Torner J, Adams HP, Kassell NF. Factors associated with hydrocephalus after subarachnoid hemorrhage: a report of the cooperative aneurysm study. Arch Neurol. 1989;46:744–52.
27. Chen S, Luo J, Reis C, Manaenko A, Zhang J. Hydrocephalus after subarachnoid hemorrhage: pathophysiology, diagnosis, and treatment. Biomed Res Int. 2017;2017:8584753.
28. Lu J, Ji N, Yang Z, Zhao X. Prognosis and treatment of acute hydrocephalus following aneurysmal subarachnoid haemorrhage. J Clin Neurosci. 2012;19:669–72.
29. Wartenberg KE, Mayer SA. Medical complications after subarachnoid hemorrhage. Neurosurg Clin North Am. 2010;21(2):325–38.
30. Naidech AM, Kreiter KT, Janjua N, et al. Cardiac troponin elevation, cardiovascular morbidity, and outcome after subarachnoid haemorrhage. Circulation. 2005;112:2851–6.
31. Lee VH, Connolly HM, Fulgham JR, Manno EM, et al. Tako-tsubo cardiomyopathy in aneurysmal subarachnoid hemorrhage: an underappreciated ventricular dysfunction. J Neurosurg. 2006;105:264–70.
32. Mayer SA, Li Mandri G, Sherman D, et al. Electrocardiographic markers of abnormal left ventricular wall motion in acute subarachnoid haemorrhage. J Neurosurg. 1995;83:889–96.
33. Chen S, Li Q, Wu H, et al. The harmful effects of subarachnoid hemorrhage on extracerebral organs. Biomed Res Int. 2014;2014:858496.
34. Alimohamadi M, Saghafinia M, Alikhani F, et al. Impact of electrolyte imbalances on the outcome of aneurysmal subarachnoid hemorrhage: a prospective study. Asian J Neurosurg. 2016;11:29–33.
35. Kumar MA, Levine J, Faerber J, Elliott JP, Winn HR, et al. The effects of red blood cell transfusion on functional outcome after aneurysmal subarachnoid hemorrhage. World Neurosurg. 2017;108:807–16.
36. Dhar R, Zazulia AR, Derdeyn CP, Diringer MN. RBC transfusion improves cerebral oxygen delivery in subarachnoid hemorrhage. Crit Care Med. 2017;45:653–9.

# Acute Ischemic Stroke

# 12

Ponniah Vanamoorthy and Prasanna Udupi Bidkar

**Key Points**

- AIS is a time sensitive neuro-emergency where revascularization therapy should be initiated without any delay.
- Transfer of AIS patients to a comprehensive stroke center where EVT facility is available improves the outcome.
- Systems of care including stroke rapid response team like code stroke help reduce the time to initiate therapy
- Emergent brain imaging is a key factor in deciding subsets of stroke and initiating therapy in AIS
- IVT should be administered without delay in all the eligible patients
- Tight Blood Pressure control of BP < 180/105 mmHg has to be achieved with cIV infusion of anti-hypertensives
- All patients eligible for revascularization should undergo CTA for detection of LVO
- Eligible candidates with LVO and presenting within 6 h of LKW are treated with EVT
- Eligible candidates with LVO and presenting 6–24 h of LKW undergo additional imaging like CT or MRI perfusion to identify salvageable area and treatment with EVT
- All the stroke patients to be cared preferably at subspecialized units where rehabilitation is available

P. Vanamoorthy (✉)
MGM Health Care, Chennai, India

P. U. Bidkar
Jawaharlal Institute of Postgraduate Medical Education and Research, Pondicherry, India



P. U. Bidkar, P. Vanamoorthy (eds.), *Acute Neuro Care*,
https://doi.org/10.1007/978-981-15-4071-4_12

## 12.1 Introduction

Stroke is the second leading cause of death worldwide next to ischemic heart disease [1]. There are over 13.7 million new strokes each year and ischemic stroke remains to be the most common type with 9.5 million new cases [2]. There are 67.5 million ischemic stroke survivors worldwide and 2.7 million deaths occur from ischemic stroke. Each year 51.9 million years of healthy life is lost due to ischemic stroke-related death and disabilities. Most strokes occur in the age group greater than 44 years, but stroke is also common in young (7% of new ischemic stroke and 10% of survivors are under the age of 44). Men and women are more or less equally affected (52% of new cases of stroke occur in men vs 48% in women) [3, 4]. The conventional risk factors for the development of stroke are hypertension, diabetes mellitus, hyperlipidemia, smoking, obesity, and a sedentary lifestyle [5]. Great progress has been made in the treatment of ischemic stroke with the evolution of intravenous thrombolysis (IVT) and endovascular treatment (EVT). For these treatments to be effective, they should be initiated early from the time of symptom onset. This is possible only by having systems of care and coordination between the specialties. In a typical large vessel occlusion about 1.9 million neurons, 14 million synapses, 12 km of myelinated fibers are lost each minute without revascularization [6]. This signifies "Time is brain" and time lost is brain lost. Delay in initiating emergent revascularization therapies will result in the worst outcomes.

## 12.2 Recognition of Stroke

Stroke can occur in the community or in the hospital. The first responders in the community is usually the family member, the paramedics, or a nursing home practitioner. Stroke is recognized by the following acronym BEFAST (Table 12.1) [7].

**B**alance—Acute or sudden onset of loss of balance or co-ordination
**E**ye signs—Blurred or unclear vision /double vision/ Gaze preference
**F**acial weakness—Facial asymmetry
**A**rm and/or Leg weakness
**S**peech difficulty/slurring of speech
**T**ime is Brain: Time to activate stroke system and stroke clock.

Stroke is a clinical diagnosis and rapid neuroimaging usually a Non-Contrast CT (NCCT) head is performed to rule out hemorrhage and to initiate time-sensitive interventions. Ischemic stroke is caused by an abrupt and sustained reduction in regional cerebral blood flow (CBF) leading to cell death. Within hours, patients often have a central zone of irreversibly damaged tissue destined to die known as the infarct core and a surrounding zone of damaged tissue that may recover with abrupt restoration of CBF known as the penumbra. Secondary stroke prevention targets a variety of mechanisms, including cardioembolism, artery to artery thromboembolism, occlusive arterial disease, and small vessel disease that caused AIS. However, the detailed mechanism of AIS is not necessarily relevant to the choice of acute treatment.

**Table 12.1** Identification of stroke

| | Acute onset of one the following | | |
|---|---|---|---|
| 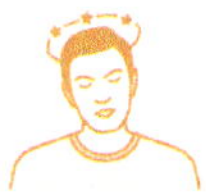 | **Imbalance Dizziness**<br>Is there a sudden loss of Balance or coordination? | B | ☐ |
| 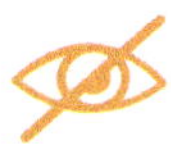 | **Blurred/unclear Vision**<br>Is there a double vision or unable to see out of one eye? | E | ☐ |
| 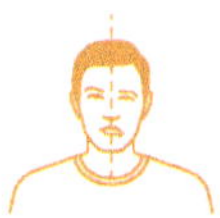 | **Facial Drooping**<br>Ask the patient to smile. Is one side of the face drooping? | F | ☐ |
| 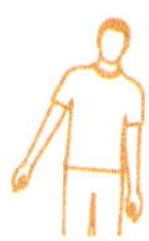 | **Arm/ Limb Weakness**<br>Have the Patient raise both arms in air. Does one arm drift downward? | A | ☐ |
| 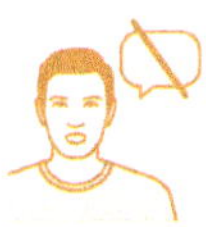 | **Speech difficulty/Slurring**<br>Slurring of words/ unable to speak/ can't repeat a simple sentence/ hard time being understood | S | ☐ |
|  | **Time to activate "STROKE Team"**<br>Start **"STROKE CLOCK"** | T | ☐ |

Once a stroke is recognized, the time of onset of symptoms or the time last known well (LKW) or last seen normal (LSN) has to be ascertained apart from checking blood pressure and capillary blood sugar (CBG). These are very crucial in deciding the eligibility of these patients for revascularization therapies. Wake-up strokes constitute a significant proportion of the stroke and LKW / LSN is used to describe as the time of onset is not known. LKW or LSN is the time usually when the patients were at their previous baseline or symptom-free state.

It is recommended to transfer the patients to the hospital with the facility and expertise for EVT. At present the guidelines recommend initiating IVT before transferring to such centers although this has been challenged by many authors favoring direct shifting to EVT facility without time delay. Time should not be wasted in detailed neurological assessments or detailed laboratory investigations. Most commonly time is wasted in doing ECG, chest X-ray, and other laboratory tests which are unwarranted at this stage.

**Table 12.2** Prehostpital check list

- ☐ Is the Patient Awake / Responding to call or Stimuli?
- ☐ Is the Breathing Spontaneous and smooth with RR < 20 breaths/ minute and SpO2 > 94%?
- ☐ Is Systolic Blood Pressure > 100 mmHg?
- ☐ Are Pupils Equal?
- ☐ CBG > 50 mgs/dl

## 12.3 Prehospital Care

Stroke centers with trained paramedics can easily recognize a stroke and they play a vital role in the stroke system of care in reducing the time delay to administer therapies. The key information that the paramedical team conveys to the stroke center is the time of onset of symptoms or the time last seen normal (LSN), blood pressure, and capillary blood sugar (CBG). A prehospital checklist (Table 12.2) would help decide the in-house stroke team to by-pass the emergency room. An awake patient with a normal breathing pattern and who is hemodynamically stable with stroke symptoms can be taken directly to CT. Various prehospital scales are being used to identify stroke and large vessel occlusion (LVO). Cincinnati prehospital stroke severity scale is evaluated to have high accuracy in identifying TIA and also stroke severity [8, 9]. Noorian et al. did a comparative analysis of 8 prehospital scales including Los Angeles motor scale (LAMS) and conclude that the LAMS performed in the field by paramedics shows good sensitivity and specificity in identifying LVO AIS patients among all cerebral ischemia patients [10].

Mobile stroke units have the facility to do CT and transfer the image for interpretation to the stroke team and IVT can be initiated in the ambulance. Currently there is only one mobile stroke unit in India and in the future many such would come if found to be cost-effective.

Though guidelines recommend initiating IVT before transferring to EVT facility, [11] many authors favor direct shifting to EVT facility without time delay.

## 12.4 Stroke Team and Code Stroke

Systems of care have been found to impart positive outcomes in time-sensitive emergencies including trauma, acute coronary syndrome, and stroke [12]. Depending on the expertise available in a hospital a stroke team is formed to provide round the clock stroke services. Such a team would typically compromise of a physician, nursing practitioner, clinical pharmacist, radiographer, technician, laboratory personal, attending staff, social worker, and a manager or counselors [13]. Once stroke code gets activated all team members get together and start evaluating the patient, check eligibility for IVT/EVT, and perform their specific roles.

Each member of the team has specific roles and responsibilities depending on the institution where they practice and upon an agreed protocol. In hospitals where endovascular treatment facilities are not available the emergency physician or a neurologist usually attends these patients and initiates IVT before shifting the patient to a facility and expertise for EVT. The target is to keep the door-to-needle time (DNT) to less than 60 min in all the patients and to 30 min in at least 50% of the eligible patients.

## 12.5 Emergency Room Assessment and Intervention

Patients can be shifted in ambulance stretcher (without a need to change to hospital trolley). Time should not be wasted in changing to hospital clothes. Before shifting to radiology, the key things to be optimized (if compromised) are the airway, breathing, and circulation (ABC). Oxygen supplementation should be given if $SPO_2 < 94\%$ through a face mask [15]. Most often AIS patients present with hypertension. When the cause for stroke is not known at this stage it is reasonable to reduce the SBP to target 185 mmHg as all the stroke patients except for when they present late (out of window period) require blood pressure control to be eligible for revascularization [16]. Two large bore IV cannulas are to be secured in both arms and a balanced crystalloid infusion initiated at 50 ml per hour in one line, while the other is dedicated for IVT. Simultaneously blood has to be collected for labs. Hypotension with systolic blood pressure (SBP < 90 mmHg) should be aggressively treated with vasopressors as it is associated with poor outcomes [17].

Time should not be delayed in detailed history or neurological examination. A serious neurological issue like Raised ICP and Herniation (CODE BRAIN) and Status Epilepticus should be quickly recognized and treated. The National Institute of Health Scale (NIHSS) (Table 12.3) is a recognized tool to document and communicate the neurological deficit in the setting of AIS [18]. NIHSS range from 0 to 42 points with a score of 0–5 points suggests a mild stroke, 6–15 a moderate stroke, and greater than 15 a severe stroke.

Apart from establishing the symptom of the onset of stroke a brief medical history including history of medications, particularly the use of anticoagulants is important in the decision making for treatment.

History and physical examination should be brief. A structured history and physical examination are not warranted at this stage. A simple way of obtaining this would be AMPL, which stands for Allergies, Medications, Past Illness, Last Meal, and Events in sequence.

The key information which has to be gathered are the time of symptom onset or LKW/LSN, history of Anticoagulation /Antiplatelets, bleeding tendencies, major surgeries, and serious cardiac symptoms. All patients are assumed to be full stomach for intervention and anesthesia.

**Table 12.3** National Institute of Health Stroke Scale

| Item | Title | Score | NIHSS |
|---|---|---|---|
| 1A | Loss of consciousness | 0 | Alert—keenly responsive |
| | | 1 | Drowsy—Arousable by minor stimulation |
| | | 2 | Stuporous—requires repeated stimulation |
| | | 3 | Comatose—responds only with reflex motor or autonomic effects or no response |
| 1B | LOC questions ask month and age | 0 | Answers both correctly |
| | | 1 | Answers one correctly |
| | | 2 | Both incorrect |
| 1C | LOC command ask to open and close eyes, grip | 0 | Obeys both correctly |
| | | 1 | Obeys one correctly |
| | | 2 | Both incorrectly |
| 2 | Best gaze | 0 | Normal |
| | | 1 | Partial gaze palsy—abnormal gaze in one or both eyes |
| | | 2 | Forced deviation or total gaze paresis |
| 3 | Visual fields | 0 | No visual loss or in coma |
| | | 1 | Partial hemianopia |
| | | 2 | Complete hemianopia |
| | | 3 | Bilateral hemianopia or cortical blindness |
| 4 | Facial palsy | 0 | Normal |
| | | 1 | Minor-flattened nasolabial fold or smiling asymmetry |
| | | 2 | Partial-total or near total paralysis of lower face |
| | | 3 | Complete–absent facial movement |
| 5A | Best motor RT arm | 0 | No drift-holds limb at 90° for full 10 s |
| | | 1 | Drifts down but does not hit bed |
| | | 2 | Some effort against gravity |
| | | 3 | No effort against gravity |
| | | 4 | No movement |
| 5B | Best motor LT arm | 0 | No drift-holds limb at 90° for full 10 s |
| | | 1 | Drifts down but does not hit bed |
| | | 2 | Some effort against gravity |
| | | 3 | No effort against gravity |
| | | 4 | No movement |
| 6A | Best motor RT leg | 0 | No drift-holds limb at 45° for full 5 s |
| | | 1 | Drifts down but does not hit bed |
| | | 2 | Some effort against gravity |
| | | 3 | No effort against gravity |
| | | 4 | No movement |
| 6B | Best motor LT leg | 0 | No drift-holds limb at 45° for full 5 s |
| | | 1 | Drifts down but does not hit bed |
| | | 2 | Some effort against gravity |
| | | 3 | No effort against gravity |
| | | 4 | No movement |
| 7 | Limb ataxia | 0 | Obeys or absent (coma) |
| | | 1 | Present in one limb |
| | | 2 | Present in 2 limbs |

**Table 12.3** (continued)

| Item | Title | Score | NIHSS |
|---|---|---|---|
| 8 | Sensory | 0 | Normal |
| | | 1 | Partial loss (pin prick is less sharp or dull on affected side) |
| | | 2 | Dense loss or in coma (unaware of touch on face, arm, or leg) |
| 9 | Best language | 0 | No aphasia |
| | | 1 | Mild to moderate (loss of fluency without significant limitation on ideas expression) |
| | | 2 | Severe(fragmentary expression need for listener inference or guessing) |
| | | 3 | Mute or in coma(no speech or auditory comprehension) |
| 10 | Dysarthria | 0 | Normal |
| | | 1 | Mild to moderate (slurs some words can be understood with some difficulty) |
| | | 2 | Unintelligible or worse(so slurred speech, out of proportion to dysarthria) |
| 11 | Inattention | 0 | No neglect or in coma |
| | | 1 | Partial neglect (visual, tactile, auditory, spatial, or personal inattention or extinction to b/l simultaneous stimulation in one of the sensory modalities) |
| | | 2 | Complete-profound inattention to one or more modalities (does not recognize own hand or orients to only one side of space) |
| Total Score | | | |

Detailed laboratory tests should not delay neuroimaging. CBG is essential and CBG <50 mgs% has to be corrected with dextrose solution. The platelet count and INR should be notified immediately once ready, especially when the patient is on oral anticoagulation. While securing two large-bore IV cannula in both the arms blood sample can be collected for complete blood count and INR or as per the hospital protocol pack of tests (Including renal function, liver function, and Trop I) can be sent. The laboratory personal should be notified to quickly inform the platelet count and INR especially when the patient is on oral anticoagulation. ECG, Chest X-Ray, ECHO is not warranted unless there is pressing serious coexisting cardiac symptoms.

If the prehospital checklist could be completed and stroke team informed, then emergency room (ER) can be bypassed [19] and patient shifted directly to radiology room, where members of stroke team evaluate and decide on eligibility for IVT and EVT. ER assessment and intervention can be done in the CT room when ER is bypassed. All resuscitative equipment should be made available at all times. An ER checklist (Table 12.4) with all the above information has to be duly filled any abnormality has to be informed in a loud voice to all members of the team.

**Table 12.4** ER checklist

- ☐ ABC Optimised?
- ☐ 2 IV Lines preferably 18 G,50 ml per hour Crystalloid in Line 1, Line 2 exclusive for IVT
- ☐ If BP > 185/110 mmHg Give Labetalol
- ☐ Clear Seizures
- ☐ Clear CODE BRAIN
- ☐ NIHSS
- ☐ AMPLE
- ☐ If CBG < 50 mgs% Give D50 50 mL bolus and recheck CBG
- ☐ LABS: Order Lab to report Platelets, INR, aPTT

## 12.6 Neuroimaging

Rapid imaging of the brain is the key to initiate IVT. Non-contrast CT (NCCT) is quick, possesses high sensitivity and specificity to detect ICH, and can be done in critically ill patients without any delay. Stroke is a clinical diagnosis and a normal NCCT does not rule out an acute ischemic stroke. Non-contrast CT can exclude alternate causes for neurological symptoms such as subdural hematoma, brain tumor, or other space-occupying lesions. An NCCT of the brain with no ICH or SAH usually is enough to decide eligibility for IVT in most cases (Fig. 12.1) [20].

A normal looking CT brain implies that infarct has not set in and revascularization in this instance should result in better outcomes. Some of the early signs in CT are hypo-attenuating brain tissue, obscuration of the lentiform nucleus, dense MCA sign (Implying large vessel occlusion of ICA/MCA) (Fig. 12.2a), insular ribbon sign, and loss of sulci effacement. Frank hypodensities especially involving large areas may be an established infarct and generally they are excluded from revascularization therapies (Fig. 12.2b).

NCCT allows differentiation between ischemic stroke and intracerebral hemorrhage and in the case of an ischemic stroke, allows quantification of the extent of early ischemic changes by applying the Alberta Stroke Program Early CT Score (ASPECTS), a 10-point score that subtracts a point for each region of parenchymal hypoattenuation within the anterior circulation [21, 22]. Scan quality, training, and experience affect the reliability of ASPECTS. Automated software (Fig. 12.3) is now available to calculate the ASPECT score [22]. Lower scores are predictive of a poor functional outcome with an increased risk of intraparenchymal hemorrhage associated with thrombolysis [23, 24].

IVT is usually initiated immediately after NCCT in the CT room. Once IVT is initiated for eligible patients after NCCT a CT angiogram (CTA) is performed for all the patients [25]. Patients with a large vessel occlusion (LVO) and eligible for EVT with LSN less than 6 h are transferred to neurointervention suite for EVT. Patients with LVO and LSN > 6 h and up to 24 h will undergo further imaging, either CT perfusion or MRI to check eligibility for EVT [26].

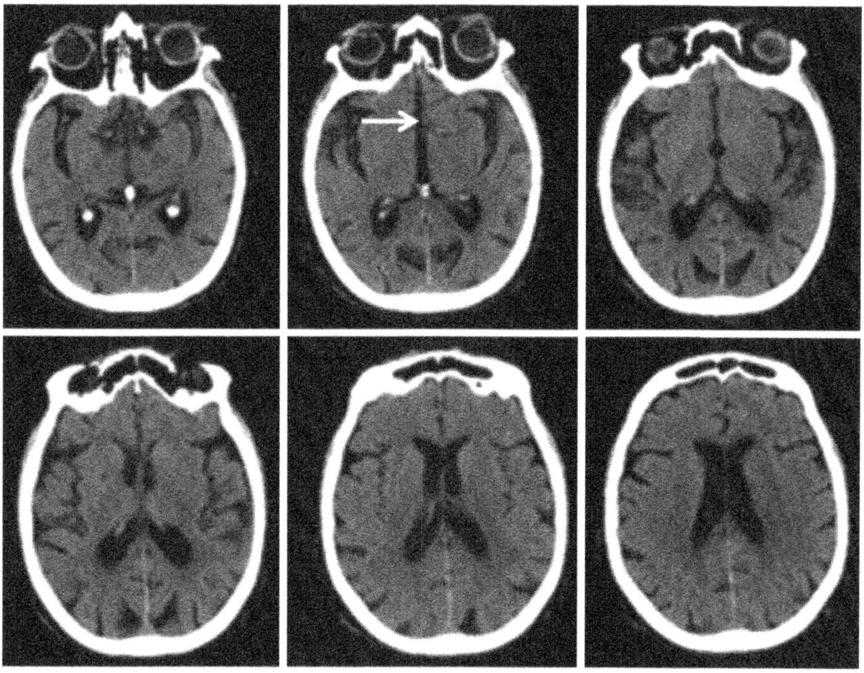

**Fig. 12.1** A 76-year-old male presented to the ER within 2 h of acute onset of facial weakness, right arm and leg weakness, and slurring of speech. NCCT of the brain performed show no ICH or no obvious hypodensity. Left MCA show Hyperdense MCA sign

CT angiography is used to identify proximal vessel occlusions as possible target lesions for endovascular treatment and should be a concurrent imaging study for patients with stroke (Fig. 12.4). Neurointerventionalists can plan an endovascular procedure with CT angiography information [27].

MRI DWI (Fig. 12.5) and FLAIR are more sensitive to detect ischemia/infarction, but they are time-consuming. DWI maps show early ischemic changes within minutes from stroke onset and a correlating apparent diffusion coefficient map visualizes the extent of cytotoxic edema caused by brain ischemia [28]. MRI is especially useful in detecting minor strokes and differentiating ischemic stroke from mimics in the setting of ischemic lesions of small volume, multiple embolic lesions, and in posterior circulation strokes where the skull base creates bony artifacts on NCCT. Logistics and critical nature of illness make CT the preferred modality although MRI has been used as a primary modality in some trials and centers to evaluate stroke.

Intensive efforts are underway to develop a practical and reliable way of assessing core and penumbra. With MRI, areas with diffusion–perfusion mismatch (i.e., DWI lesion within a larger area of PWI lesion) has been interpreted as penumbral tissue.

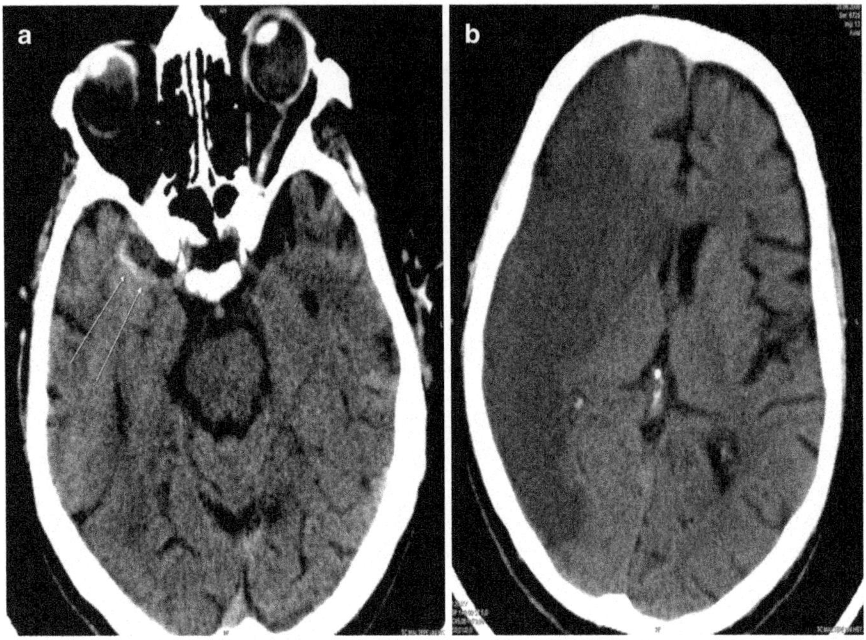

**Fig. 12.2** (**a**), NCCT show Right Hyperdense MCA sign. (**b**), 48 h later NCCT show Right Malignant MCA territory infarct

Time of light MR angiography enables a flow-dependent visualization of the brain arteries without the need for a contrast agent. Susceptibility weighted imaging allows for the detection of intracerebral hemorrhage with high sensitivity, and the detection of cerebral microbleeds not captured by NCCT, which might indicate underlying pathophysiology, such as cerebral amyloid angiopathy, and might be associated with an increased risk of intracranial hemorrhage after intravenous thrombolysis [29]. Specific MRI patterns of imaging acquisition and processing delays treatment initiation. The threshold for when sufficient information is available to make a correct therapeutic decision should be short. The chance of poor outcome with treatment increases while time passes with each additional test obtained [30].

To select eligible patients with LVO presenting in 6–24 h window period CT perfusion (CTP) (Fig. 12.6) is done to assess Mean Transit Time (MTT), CBF (cerebral Blood Flow), CBV (Cerebral Blood Volume), and other parameters to gain insight into the proportion and volume of tissue at risk of infarction. Quantitative perfusion thresholds are used to estimate Core (tissue that is already irreversibly damaged), Penumbra (tissue that is likely to infarct but salvageable with reperfusion and oligemia (tissue that is not threatened but might have reduced blood flow). A severe relative reduction of cerebral blood flow of <30% of the normal brain indicates irreversible injury in several trials, including late window treatment trials. Automated software now allows timely postprocessing of CT perfusion functional

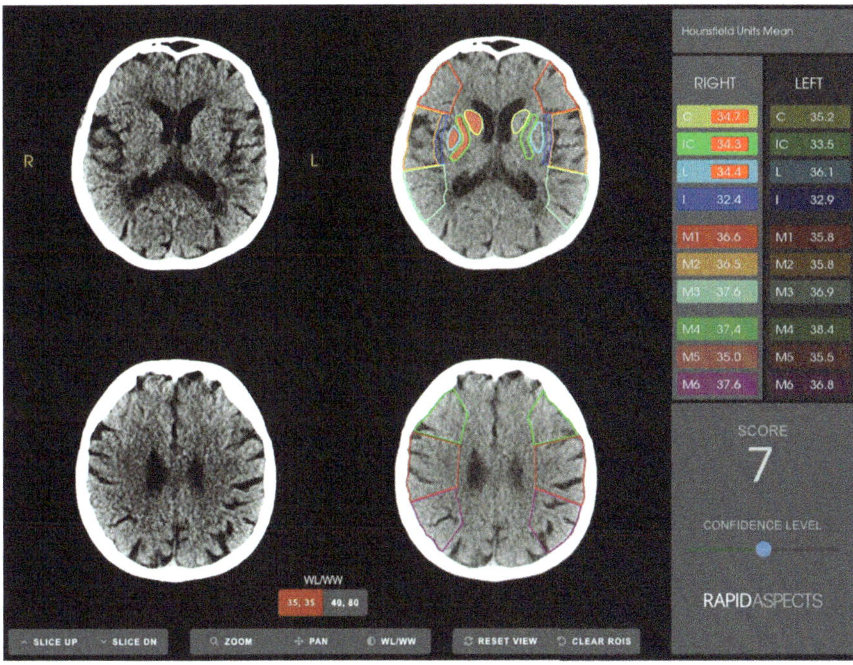


**Fig. 12.3** ASPECT scoring. Automated software output of ASPECT Score. *C* Caudate, *I* Insular ribbon, *IC* Internal Capsule, *L* Lentiform Nucleus, *M1* Anterior MCA Cortex, *M2* MCA Cortex Lateral to Insular Ribbon, *M3* Posterior MCA Cortex, *M4* Anterior MCA Superior territory, *M5* Lateral MCA Superior territory, *M6* Posterior MCA Superior territory

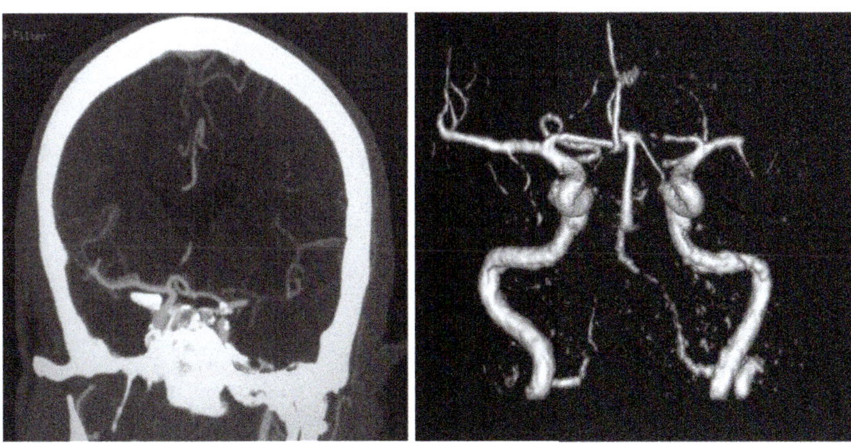

**Fig. 12.4** CT Angiogram show Large Vessel occlusion (LVO). Occlusion of Left MCA (M1)

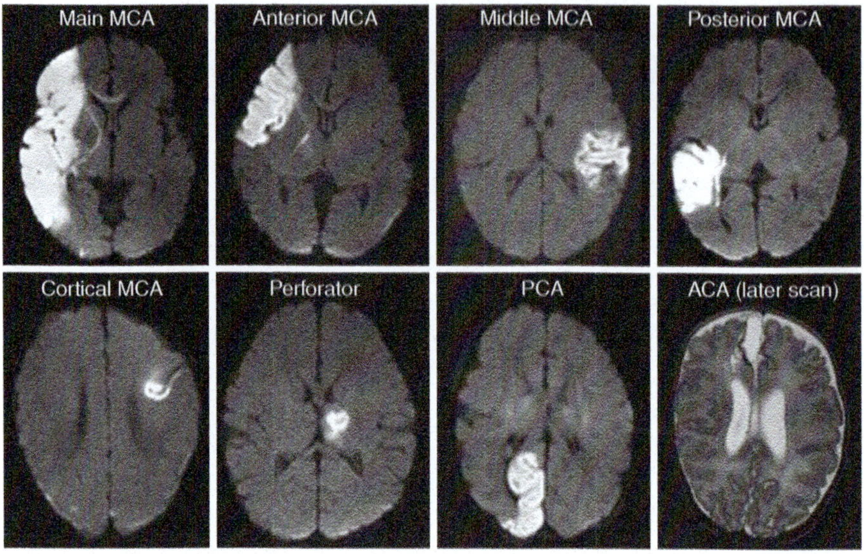


**Fig. 12.5** MRI DWI image showing diffusion restriction

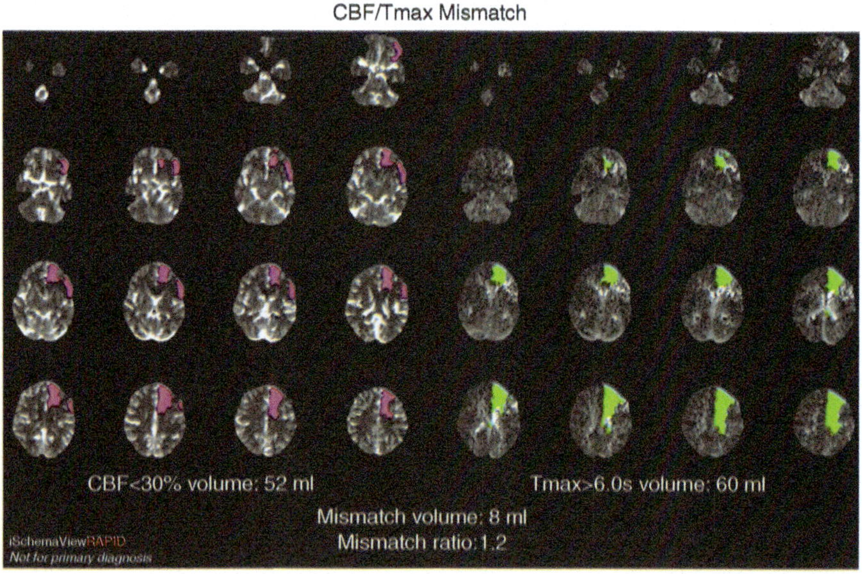


**Fig. 12.6** CT perfusion automated software output show core volume, mismatch ratio, and mismatch volume

**Table 12.5** Imaging–decision algorithm

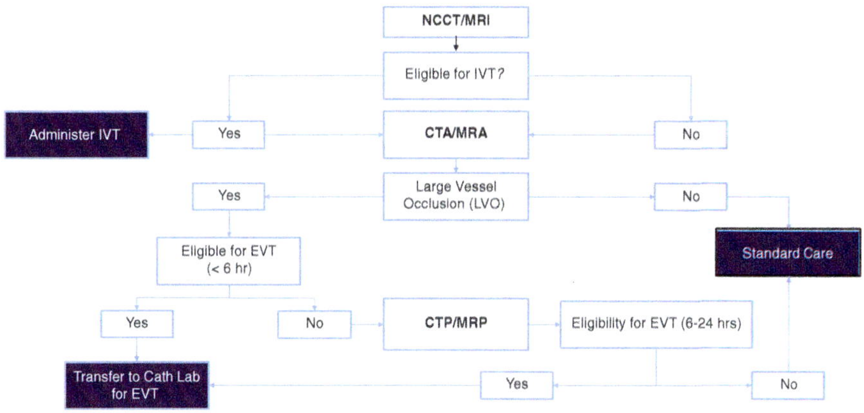


**Table 12.6** Imaging checklist

| NCCT Check List | CTA Checklist | | | CTP Check List | Other Findings |
|---|---|---|---|---|---|
| ☐ ICH/SAH : No /Yes | ☐ Level Of Occlusion | R | L | ☐ Core Volume: ▭ | ☐ Occlusion > 1 arterial Territory |
| ☐ Prominent Hypo density | MCA | M1 | | ☐ Mismatch Ratio > 1.8 | ☐ Tandem Occlusion |
| | | M2 | | ☐ Mismatch Volume >15 ml | ☐ EC Cervical Dissection |
| ☐ > 1/3rd MCA territory hypodensity | | M3 | | | ☐ Intracranial arterial Dissection |
| | ICA | | | | ☐ Aneurysm/AVM |
| ☐ Mass effect/MLS | ACA | | | | ☐ Intracranial Intraaxial Leision |
| | PCA | | | | |
| ☐ ASPECT Score: ▭ | VA | | | | ☐ Intracranial Extra-axial Leision |
| | ☐ BAO | | | | |

maps that are robust to common artifacts allowing rapid clinician interpretation (Fig. 12.6). However, care is required to avoid delaying treatment decisions because of the time taken to acquire, transfer, postprocess, and interpret CT perfusion data [30–33].

Neuroimaging is the cornerstone for revascularization therapies and an imaging–decision algorithm will help decide in patient eligibility (Table 12.5). A radiology checklist (Table 12.6) should be promptly filled up and the radiology eligibility check informed to all the team members.

## 12.7 Intravenous Thrombolysis (IVT)

The most effective treatment for acute ischemic stroke is timely reperfusion by either thrombolysis or thrombectomy. Reperfusion improves outcomes by reducing the volume of infarct. As time from initial stroke increases, the penumbra (viable but ischemic tissue) is quickly replaced by infarcted tissue (irreversibly lost brain tissue) [34]. Therefore, swift reperfusion preserves not only the penumbra tissue but also reduces the size of the final infarct core, thereby limiting the volume of damaged tissue and reducing disability from stroke.

The NINDS t-PA stroke trial is the landmark trial which lead to the licensing of Alteplase in 3-h window period of stroke [35]. Subsequently ECASS [36] and ATLANTIS-B trials [37] evaluated the outcome within 6 h of symptom onset and the post-hoc analysis favored the earlier use is associated with improved outcome thus extending the window to 4.5 h. The benefit of Alteplase in the 3–4.5-h window has been reemphasized by the results of ECASS II trial [38]. Though the largest trial of thrombolysis showed the improved functional outcome of thrombolysis within 6 h, the benefit was more when treated within 3 h. The pooled analysis of multiple trials including NINDS, ATLANTIS reported no outcome benefit of using Alteplase more than 4.5-h window [39]. The benefit of a low dose of Alteplase was analyzed specifically in patients on prior antiplatelets, but ENCHANTED trial reported a neutral outcome. Further trials are necessary to identify the benefit of low dose Alteplase [40]. The other drugs Desmoteplase and Tenecteplase has also been studied. Studies reported variable outcome with Desmoteplase. Though NORTEST [41] trial did not favor Tenecteplase over Alteplase, the EXTEND-IA TNK trial showed that Tenecteplase has a higher incidence of reperfusion and better functional outcome compared to Alteplase within a 4.5-h window [42]. Tenecteplase might be considered as an alternative to Alteplase in patients with minor neurological impairment and no major intracranial occlusion.

Thrombolysis within 3 h window and 3–4.5 h window is initiated as per eligibility criteria (Table 12.7) [43]. If there are no absolute contraindications, one can proceed with thrombolysis after having considered the relative conditions. Additional conditions if any, has to be considered on a case-to-case basis (Table 12.8). Successful management of hypertension is essential to administer EVT. Uncontrolled

**Table 12.7** Eligibility for intravenous thrombolysis (IVT)

| Criterion | No | Yes |
|---|---|---|
| Time of Symptom onset / Last Known well **UNCLEAR** | No | Yes |
| Wake Up stroke | No | Yes |
| ICH in CT / History of ICH | No | Yes |
| Clinical features strongly suggestive of SAH irrespective of CT negative for SAH | No | Yes |
| Ischaemic Stroke / Severe Head Injury / Intracranial Surgery/Intraspinal Surgery in the last 3 months | No | Yes |
| Structural GI Malignancy or GI bleeding in the Past 21 days | No | Yes |
| Intracranial Intraaxial Neoplasm | No | Yes |
| Aortic Arch Dissection | No | Yes |
| Infective Endocarditis | No | Yes |
| Direct Thrombin Inhibitors/ factor Xa Inhibitors/ GP IIa/IIIb receptor Inhibitors / Therapeutic LMWH in 24 hrs | No | Yes |
| Coagulopathy *(Need not wait for results, when results are available and unfavourable STOP Alteplase)* (Platelet Count < 1 Lakh/cu mm, PT > 15 s, INR > 1.7, aPTT > 40s) | No | Yes |

**No to all** → Time Window

**Yes to any** → NOT ELIGIBLE FOR IVT

| Time Window | |
|---|---|
| **<3 hrs** | **3-4.5 hrs** |
| • Age >/= 18 Y<br>• BP < 185/110 mmHg<br>• CBG >50 mgs %<br>• No Frank Hypodensities in CT | • All eligibility of < 3 hrs AND<br>• Age </= 80 Y<br>• No H/O DM and Prior Stroke<br>• No H/O OAC<br>• NIHSS </= 25 |

Yes / No → **Check additional conditions on a case to case basis *(Table :8)***

**NOT ELIGIBLE FOR IVT**

**Table 12.8** Additional conditions for IVT (to be decided on a case-to-case basis)

| | |
|---|---|
| Extended 3- to 4.5-h Window (Age > 80 Year/On OAC/DM/ Prior stroke) | • For patients >80 years of age presenting in the 3- to 4.5-h window, IV Alteplase is safe and can be as effective as in younger patients<br>• For patients taking warfarin and with an INR ≤1.7 who present in the 3- to 4.5-h window, IV Alteplase appears safe and may be beneficial<br>• In AIS patients with prior stroke and diabetes mellitus presenting in the 3- to 4.5-h window, IV Alteplase may be as effective as treatment in the 0- to 3 h window and maybe a reasonable option |
| Severity 0- to 3 h Window: Mild non-disabling stroke | • Within 3 h from symptom onset, treatment of patients with mild ischemic stroke symptoms that are judged as non-disabling may be considered. Treatment risks should be weighed against possible benefits |
| Severity 3- to 4.5-h Window: Mild/ severe stroke | • For otherwise eligible patients with mild stroke presenting in the 3- to 4.5-h window, IV Alteplase may be as effective as treatment in the 0- to 3 h window and may be a reasonable option. Treatment risks should be weighed against possible benefits. The benefit of IV Alteplase between 3 and 4.5-h from symptom onset for patients with very severe stroke symptoms (NIHSS >25) is uncertain |
| Pre-existing disability | • Pre-existing disability does not seem to independently increase the risk of sICH after IV Alteplase, but it may be associated with less neurological improvement and higher mortality. Thrombolytic therapy with IV Alteplase for acute stroke patients with pre-existing disability (mRS score ≥ 2) may be reasonable, but decisions should take into account relevant factors, including quality of life, social support, place of residence, need for a caregiver, patients' and families' preferences, and goals of care. Patients with pre-existing dementia may benefit from IV Alteplase. Individual considerations such as life expectancy and premorbid level of function are important to determine whether Alteplase may offer a clinically meaningful benefit |
| Early improvement | • IV Alteplase treatment is reasonable for patients who present with moderate to severe ischemic stroke and demonstrate early improvement but remain moderately impaired and potentially disabled in the judgment of the examiner |
| Seizure at onset | • IV Alteplase is reasonable in patients with a seizure at the time of onset of acute stroke if evidence suggests that residual impairments are secondary to stroke and not a postictal phenomenon |
| Blood glucose | • Treatment with IV Alteplase in patients with AIS who present with initial glucose levels <50 or > 400 mg/dL that are subsequently normalized and who are otherwise eligible may be reasonable |
| Coagulopathy | • The safety and efficacy of IV Alteplase for acute stroke patients with a clinical history of potential bleeding diathesis or coagulopathy are unknown. IV Alteplase may be considered on a case-by-case basis<br>• IV Alteplase may be reasonable in patients who have a history of warfarin use and an INR ≤1.7 and/or a PT <15 s |
| Dural puncture | • IV Alteplase may be considered for patients who present with AIS, even in instances when they may have undergone a lumbar dural puncture in the preceding 7 days |
| Arterial puncture | • The safety and efficacy of administering IV Alteplase to acute stroke patients who have had an arterial puncture of a noncompressible blood vessel in the 7 days preceding stroke symptoms are uncertain |

(continued)

**Table 12.8** (continued)

| | |
|---|---|
| Recent major non head trauma | • In AIS patients with recent major trauma (within 14 days) not involving the head, IV Alteplase may be carefully considered, with the risks of bleeding from injuries related to the trauma weighed against the severity and potential disability from the ischemic stroke |
| Recent major surgery | • Use of IV Alteplase in carefully selected patients presenting with AIS who have undergone a major surgery in the preceding 14 days may be considered, but the potential increased risk of surgical-site hemorrhage should be weighed against the anticipated benefits of reduced stroke-related neurological deficits |
| GI and genitourinary bleeding | • Reported literature details a low bleeding risk with IV Alteplase administration in the setting of past (>21 days) GI/genitourinary bleeding. Administration of IV Alteplase in this patient population may be reasonable |
| Menstruation | • IV Alteplase is probably indicated in women who are menstruating who present with AIS and do not have a history of menorrhagia. However, women should be warned that Alteplase treatment could increase the degree of menstrual flow because the potential benefits of IV Alteplase probably outweigh the risks of serious bleeding in patients with recent or active history of menorrhagia without clinically significant anemia or hypotension, IV Alteplase administration may be considered. When there is a history of recent or active vaginal bleeding causing clinically significant anemia, then emergency consultation with a gynecologist is probably indicated before a decision about IV Alteplase is made |
| Extracranial cervical dissections | • IV Alteplase in AIS known or suspected to be associated with extracranial cervical arterial dissection is reasonably safe within 4.5-h and probably recommended |
| Intracranial arterial dissection | • IV Alteplase usefulness and hemorrhagic risk in AIS known or suspected to be associated with intracranial arterial dissection remain unknown, uncertain, and not well established |
| Unruptured intracranial aneurysm | • For patients presenting with AIS who are known to harbor a small or moderate-sized (<10 mm) unruptured and unsecured intracranial aneurysm, administration of IV Alteplase is reasonable and probably recommended. Usefulness and risk of IV Alteplase in patients with AIS who harbor a giant unruptured and unsecured intracranial aneurysm are not well established |
| Intracranial vascular malformations | • For patients presenting with AIS who are known to harbor an unruptured and untreated intracranial vascular malformation the usefulness and risks of administration of IV Alteplase are not well established. Because of the increased risk of ICH in this population of patients, IV Alteplase may be considered in patients with stroke with severe neurological deficits and a high likelihood of morbidity and mortality to outweigh the anticipated risk of ICH secondary to thrombolysis |
| CMBs | • In otherwise eligible patients who have previously had a small number (1–10) of CMBs demonstrated on MRI, administration of IV Alteplase is reasonable<br>• In otherwise eligible patients who have previously had a high burden of CMBs (>10) demonstrated on MRI, treatment with IV Alteplase may be associated with an increased risk of sICH, and the benefits of treatment is uncertain. Treatment may be reasonable if there is the potential for substantial benefit |

**Table 12.8** (continued)

| | |
|---|---|
| Extra-axial intracranial neoplasms | • IV Alteplase treatment is probably recommended for patients with AIS who harbor an extra-axial intracranial neoplasm |
| Acute MI | • For patients presenting with concurrent AIS and acute MI, treatment with IV Alteplase at the dose appropriate for cerebral ischemia<br>• Followed by percutaneous coronary angioplasty and stenting if indicated, is reasonable |
| Recent MI | • For patients presenting with AIS and a history of recent MI in the past 3 month, treating the ischemic stroke with IV Alteplase is reasonable if the recent MI was non-STEMI<br>• For patients presenting with AIS and a history of recent MI in the past 3 month, treating the ischemic stroke with IV Alteplase is reasonable if the recent MI was a STEMI involving the right or inferior myocardium<br>• For patients presenting with AIS and a history of recent MI in the past 3 month, treating the ischemic stroke with IV Alteplase may reasonable if the recent MI was a STEMI involving the left anterior myocardium<br>• Other cardiac diseases for patients with major AIS likely to produce severe disability and acute pericarditis, treatment with IV Alteplase may be reasonable. Urgent consultation with a cardiologist is recommended in this situation<br>• For patients presenting with moderate AIS likely to produce mild disability and acute pericarditis, treatment with IV Alteplase is of uncertain net benefit<br>• For patients with major AIS likely to produce severe disability and known left atrial or ventricular thrombus, treatment with IV Alteplase may be reasonable<br>• For patients presenting with moderate AIS likely to produce mild disability and known left atrial or ventricular thrombus, treatment with IV Alteplase is of uncertain net benefit<br>• For patients with major AIS likely to produce severe disability and cardiac myxoma, treatment with IV Alteplase may be reasonable<br>• For patients presenting with major AIS likely to produce severe disability and papillary fibroelastoma, treatment with IV Alteplase may be reasonable |
| Procedural stroke | • IV Alteplase is reasonable for the treatment of AIS complications of cardiac or cerebral angiographic procedures, depending on the usual eligibility criteria |
| Systemic malignancy | • The safety and efficacy of Alteplase in patients with current malignancy are not well established with systemic malignancy and reasonable (>6 month) life expectancy may benefit from IV Alteplase if other contraindications such as coagulation abnormalities, recent surgery, or systemic bleeding do not coexist |
| Pregnancy | • IV Alteplase administartion may be considered in pregnancy when the anticipated benefits of treating moderate or severe stroke outweigh the anticipated increased risks of uterine bleeding. (class IIb; LOE CLD)<br>• The safety and efficacy of IV Alteplase in the early postpartum period (<14 d after delivery) have not been well established |

(continued)

**Table 12.8** (continued)

| | |
|---|---|
| Ophthalmological conditions | • Use of IV Alteplase in patients presenting with AIS who have a history of diabetic hemorrhagic retinopathy or other hemorrhagic ophthalmic conditions are reasonable to recommend, but the potential increased risk of visual loss should be weighed against the anticipated benefits of reduced stroke-related neurological deficits |
| Sickle cell disease | • IV Alteplase for adults presenting with an AIS with known sickle cell disease can be beneficial |
| Illicit drug use | • Treating clinicians should be aware that illicit drug use may be a contributing factor to incident stroke. IV Alteplase is reasonable in instances of illicit drug use–associated AIS in patients with no other exclusions |
| Stroke mimics | • The risk of symptomatic intracranial hemorrhage in the stroke mimic population is quite low; thus, starting IV Alteplase is probably recommended in preference over delaying treatment to pursue additional diagnostic studies |

**Table 12.9** Risk of ICH after IVT

| NIHSS | Risk |
|---|---|
| 0–10 | 2–3% |
| 11–20 | 4–5% |
| >20 | 17% |

**Table 12.10** Administration of IV Alteplase

- Estimate Body weight (Actual Body weight if Known )
- Calculate total Dose : 0.9 mg /Kg ( NOT to exceed 90 mg )
- Mix In saline to make 1ml = 1 mg in a 50 ml syringe (For wt > 55 Kg use 2 x 50 ml Syringes). Take the calculated dose and discard the remaining
- 10% of the dose to be withdrawn in a 10 ml syringe and given as a bolus over 1 min
- Infuse remaining dose over 60 min. Flush the line with 10 ml saline at the same rate of infusion
- If the patient develops severe headache, acute hypertension, nausea, or vomiting or has a worsening neurological examination, discontinue the infusion (if IV Alteplase is being administered) and obtain emergency head CT scan
- Measure BP and perform neurological assessments every 15 min during and after IV Alteplase infusion for 2 h, then every 30 min for 6 h, then hourly until 24 h after IV Alteplase treatment
- Increase the frequency of BP measurements if SBP is >180 mmHg or if DBP is >105 mmHg; administer antihypertensive medications to maintain BP at or below these levels *(Page : 10)*
- Delay placement of nasogastric tubes, indwelling bladder catheters, or intra-arterial pressure catheters if the patient can be safely managed without them

**IV Alteplase : DOSE**
**1 mL = 1 mg of Alteplase**

| | Weight (Kg) | Total dose (mg or mL ) | Bolus (mg/or mL) over 1 min | Infusion (mL/hr or mg/hr) |
|---|---|---|---|---|
| **One 50 mg Vial** | 45 | 40 | 4.0 | 36.0 |
| | 50 | 45 | 4.5 | 40.5 |
| | 55 | 49 | 4.9 | 44.1 |
| **Two Vials (one 50 mg & one 20 mg)** | 60 | 54 | 5.4 | 48.6 |
| | 65 | 58 | 5.8 | 52.2 |
| | 70 | 63 | 6.3 | 56.7 |
| | 75 | 67 | 6.7 | 60.3 |
| **Two Vials (Two 50 mg)** | 80 | 72 | 7.2 | 64.8 |
| | 85 | 76 | 7.6 | 68.4 |
| | 90 | 81 | 8.1 | 72.9 |
| | 95 | 85 | 8.5 | 76.5 |
| | >/=100 | 90 | 9.0 | 81.0 |

hypertension increases the risks of symptomatic ICH (sICH) (Table 12.9). Administration of IV Alteplase should be based on patient weight (Table 12.10). Any BP > 185/110 mmHg should be treated aggressively to target <180/105 mmHg during and after IVT (Table 12.11). Major complications associated with IVT include

**Table 12.11** Management of hypertension

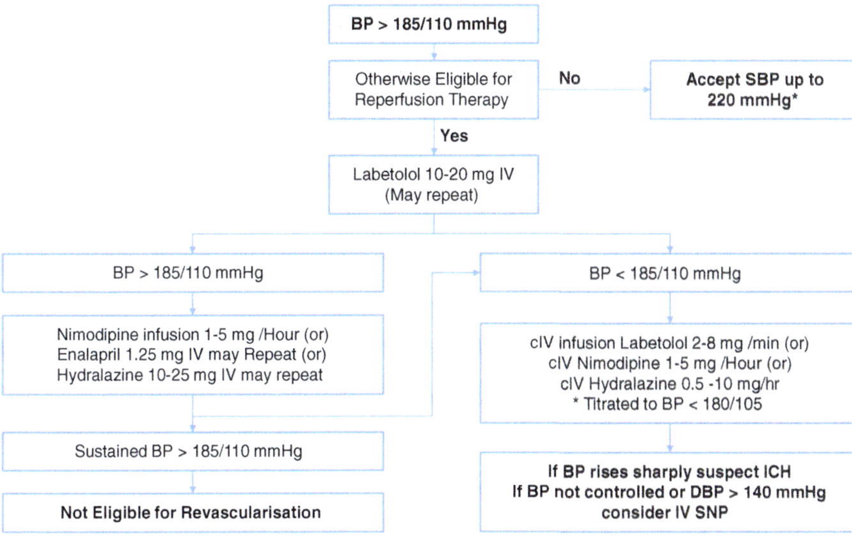


* Different treatment options may be appropriate in patients who have comorbid conditions that may benefit from acute reductions in BP such as acute coronary event, acute heart failure, aortic dissection, or preeclampsia/eclampsia.

**Table 12.12** Management of symptomatic ICH complicating IVT

- Stop Alteplase infusion
- CBC, PT (INR), aPTT, fibrinogen level, and type and cross-match
- Emergent head CT: Confirm ICH
- Cryoprecipitate (includes factor VIII): 10 U infused over 10–30 min (onset in 1 h, peaks in 12 h); administer additional dose for fibrinogen level of <200 mg/dL
- Consider 1 pooled platelet or SDP
- Tranexamic acid 1000 mg IV infused over 10 min OR ε-aminocaproic acid 4–5 g over 1 h, followed by 1 g IV until bleeding is controlled (peak onset in 3 h)
- Neurosurgery consultation
- Critical care management: including BP management, ICP, CPP, MAP, temperature, and glucose control

Intracerebral Hemorrhage, Systemic Hemorrhage, and Angioedema, which has to be quickly recognized and treated (Tables 12.12 and 12.13).

IV Alteplase is generally not recommended in ischemic stroke patients, where the time of onset of symptoms is not clear. In a recent WAKE-UP clinical trial, patients with MRI DWI findings of an ischemic lesion without clearly visible FLAIR signal (indicates the onset of stroke to be less than 4.5 h) are randomized to

**Table 12.13** Management of angioedema

| |
|---|
| • Maintain airway |
| – Endotracheal intubation may not be necessary if edema is limited to anterior tongue and lips |
| – Edema involving the larynx, palate, floor of mouth, or oropharynx with rapid progression (within 30 min) poses a higher risk of requiring intubation |
| – Awake fiberoptic intubation is optimal |
| – Nasal-tracheal intubation may be required but poses risk of epistaxis post-IV Alteplase |
| – Cricothyroidotomy is rarely needed and also problematic after IV Alteplase |
| • Discontinue IV Alteplase infusion and hold ACEIs |
| • Administer IV methylprednisolone 125 mg |
| • Administer IV diphenhydramine 50 mg |
| • Administer ranitidine 50 mg IV |
| • If there is further increase in angioedema, administer epinephrine (0.1%) 0.3 mL subcutaneously or by nebulizer 0.5 mL |
| • Icatibant, a selective bradykinin B2 receptor antagonist, 3 mL (30 mg) subcutaneously in abdominal area; additional injection of 30 mg may be administered at intervals of 6 h not to exceed a total of 3 injections in 24 h |

receive IVT versus placebo and the authors found favorable functional outcome at 90 days with IVT [44].

## 12.8 Endovascular Treatment (EVT)

Endovascular treatment (EVT) with newer stent retrievers and aspiration devices has revolutionized the management of major stroke with large vessel occlusion (Fig. 12.7). Clinical trials like MR CLEAN [45], EXTEND-IA [46], ESCAPE [47], REVASCAT [48], SWIFT PRIME [49], THRACE [50], THERAPY [51], PISTE [52], AND EASI [53] reported positive outcomes in LVO strokes. Till recently EVT was offered only for eligible patients presenting within 6 h of symptom onset who satisfies the eligibility criteria. With advanced additional neuroimaging like CT perfusion and MR perfusion carefully selected patients outside the 6 h window period up to 24 h can be eligible for EVT (Table 12.14). DAWN and DEFUSE-3 [54] trails have reported positive outcomes in this subset of patients who present after 6 h of symptom onset. Despite these late window studies, fast delivery of treatment remains crucial. The SWIFTPRIME trial reported that reperfusion within 150 min from symptom onset in the intervention arm led to a 91% estimated probability of functional independence, which decreased by 10% over the next hour and by 20% with every subsequent hour of delay [55].

Thrombolysis in Cerebral Infarction (TICI) scale grading is used to access the success of EVT. TICI range from 0 (no reperfusion) to 3 (normal). Procedural success is usually defined as achieving TICI 2b (antegrade partial perfusion of half or greater of the downstream ischemic territory) or TICI 3(Table 12.15) [56].

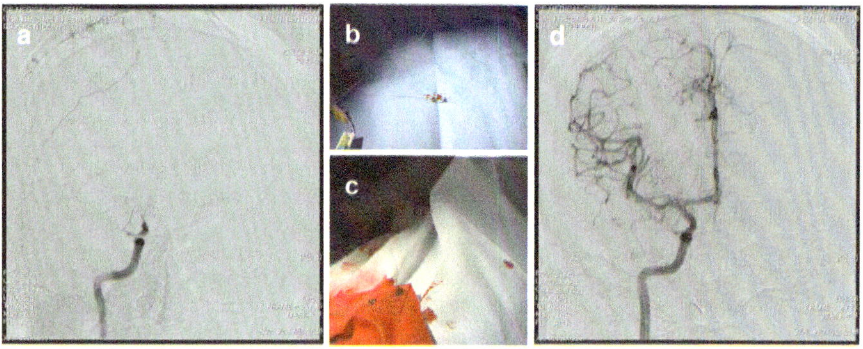

**Fig. 12.7** A 34-year-old male had a severe Stroke with NIHSS 24 and LSN of 4 h. DSA show LVO of the right ICA (**a**). Stent retriever (**b**) was used for Endovascular treatment (EVT). Thrombectomy was successful in the second pass (**c**). Post EVT DSA show filling of Right MCA and ACA, TICI Grade 3 (**d**)

**Table 12.14** Eligibility for Endovascular Treatment (EVT)

| Eligibility for EVT (< 6 hrs) | |
|---|---|
| **Standard Eligibility** | • Pre Stroke mRS 0-1<br>• Occlusion of ICA/ M1<br>• Age >/= 18Y<br>• NIHSS >/= 6<br>• ASPECTS >/= 6<br>• Groin Puncture can be initiated within 6 hrs |
| **Other Eligibility based on Case to case basis** | Occlusion of one of the below:<br>M2 , M3 MCA / ACA / PCA / VA / BA |
| | M1 or ICA occlusion and<br>• mRS >1<br>• ASPECTS < 6<br>• NIHSS<6 |
| | Contraindications to IV-tPA |

| Eligibility for EVT ( >6 hrs) | |
|---|---|
| **6-16 hrs**<br>• Age 18-90 Y<br>• NIHSS >/= 6<br>• Femoral Puncture 6-16 hrs<br>• mRS </= 2<br>• **CTA /MRA:** ICA/ MCA- M1 occlusion<br>(OR )<br>Tmax > 6 s Perfusion deficit consistent with an ICA or MCA-M1 occlusion<br>• **CTP/MRP :** Ischemic Core Volume <70 ml ,<br>Mismatch Ratio >/=1.8,<br>Mismatch Volume >/=15 ml<br>(OR)<br>MRI DWI Lesion volume <25 ml | **6-24 hrs**<br>• Age >/= 18 Y<br>• Failed / Contraindicated for Alteplase<br>• NIHSS >/= 10<br>• Pre Stroke mRS 0-1<br>• Groin Puncture can happen in 6-24 hrs<br>• Anticipated Life Expectance atleast 6 months<br>• < 1/3 rd MCA territory<br>• Intracranial ICA/ MCA-M1 Occlusion<br>• **Clinical Imaging Mismatch**<br>* Age >/= 80 Y, NIHSS >/= 10 AND Core < 21 ml /<br>* Age <80Y, NIHSS >/=10 AND Core 0-31 ml /<br>* Age < 80 Y, NIHSS >/= 20 AND Core 31-51 ml |
| **EVT Eligible** | |
| **Yes** | **No** |
| | |

## 12.8.1 Direct EVT Versus Bridging Therapy in Stroke Patients Eligible for IVT

The advantage of bridging therapy with IV thrombolysis before Mechanical Thrombectomy (MT) among patients with LVO has been studied. Fischer et al. stated that immediate and direct MT is equally effective and not inferior to bridging thrombolysis [57]. A subsequent meta-analysis of 13 studies favored bridging thrombolysis over direct MT (dMT) patients [58]. But this study has selection bias as they included both IVT eligible and ineligible patients. Further in a pooled

**Table 12.15** Modified Treatment in Cerebral Infarction (mTICI) score

- Grade 0: No perfusion
- Grade 1: Antegrade reperfusion past the initial occlusion, but limited distal branch filling with little or slow distal reperfusion
- Grade 2
  - Grade 2a: Antegrade reperfusion of less than half of the occluded target artery previously ischemic territory (e.g., in one major division of the middle cerebral artery and its territory)
  - Grade 2b: Antegrade reperfusion of more than half of the previously occluded target artery ischemic territory (e.g., in two major divisions of the MCA and their territories)
- Grade 3: Complete antegrade reperfusion of the previously occluded target artery ischemic territory, with absence of visualized occlusion in all distal branches

analysis of two stroke registries that included only patients who were eligible for IV thrombolysis, there was no difference in outcome between the two groups. But with internal carotid artery occlusion direct MT has lower mortality [59]. To exclude all selection bias, Kaesmacher et al. presented meta-analysis distinguishing between studies including dMT patients eligible for IVT and studies including dMT patients ineligible for IVT. Though dMT may offer comparable safety and efficacy as compared with IVT + MT, the results varied with less comparable groups [60]. SWIFT DIRECT and MR CLEAN NO IV are the two RCTs in process and these studies will throw up some light on the debate on bridging therapy. Always we should analyze for favorable factors and the decision should be individualized.

### 12.8.2 Bail Out Stents Following Failed Anterior Circulation Thrombectomy

Successful recanalization of emerging LVO is associated with favorable outcome. However, there is recanalization failure and 14–41% technical failure rate using a stent retriever, balloon guide catheter, or a combination of techniques [61]. Studies showed good safety and recanalization rates with stent placement. Stent deployment maintains vessel patency and improves outcome but necessitates antiplatelet therapy and risk of sICH. Wareham et al. in his analysis reported the rate of successful recanalization as 71% and favorable outcomes in 43% of the patients [62]. But the studies included were mostly retrospective and heterogeneous. However, use of self-expandable stents as a bailout procedure appears to be a reasonable approach.

## 12.9 Anesthesia for EVT

The technique of anesthesia for EVT depends upon based on multiple patient factors. Previously, a meta-analysis of 9 retrospective studies suggested that general anesthesia was associated with worse functional outcomes and higher mortality rates [63]. Recently, four prospective randomized controlled trials (GOLIATH [64], AnStoke [65], SIESTA [66], and EAST [67]) compared the use of general anesthesia versus conscious sedation for endovascular stroke treatment. They did not demonstrate any difference in neurological outcomes between the anesthesia types and found no delay in time to reperfusion in the general anesthesia group. Conscious sedation was associated with worse angiographic quality and more frequent patient movement, whereas general anesthesia was associated with a higher rate of successful reperfusion. Hypotension during EVT was an independent predictor for poor neurological outcome. Hence, regardless of anesthesia technique, a strict protocol for aggressive management of intraprocedural systemic blood pressure should be adopted during endovascular stroke treatment [68].

## 12.10 TIA and Minor Stroke

The historical epidemiological definition differentiating transient ischemic attacks and ischemic stroke based on the duration of their symptoms (less or more than 24 h) is now outdated because duration does not accurately predict the pathology. MRI studies have shown that symptom duration greater than 1 h is strongly associated with irreversible ischemia on diffusion-weighted MRI (DWI) and thus clinically defined transient ischemic attacks might not be transient on a tissue level. A transient ischemic attack is not a pathological entity itself but rather the mildest form on the spectrum of ischemic stroke syndrome presentations.

Fischer et al. defined minor stroke as patients with NIHSS less than 3 as they had the best short-term and medium-term outcomes [69]. All disabling strokes even though minor should be considered for reperfusion treatments. PRISM trial states that treatment with Alteplase vs aspirin did not increase the likelihood of favorable functional outcome at 90 days. But the trial was prematurely terminated hence we cannot draw any conclusions. In the SITS-ISTR and GWTG registry, good functional outcomes, mortality, and risk of sICH were the same in mild stroke treated in 0–3 and 3–4.5 h [70]. Hence treatment with IV Alteplase may be reasonable in mild stroke presenting in the 3- to 4.5-h window [14].

Generally a NIHSS of more than 5 points typically warrants thrombolysis in almost all cases; with NIHSS less than 5, patients premorbid quality of life and activities of daily living has to be taken into consideration to initiate thrombolysis. However, practice varies among clinicians, as some clinicians consider thrombolysis for minor stroke as standard of care while others consider it an unresolved research question. Patients with minor stroke are at risk of subsequent deterioration and disability [71]. Establishing the balance between risk and benefit is the impetus for ongoing randomized clinical trials of thrombolysis in minor stroke [72].

## 12.11 Malignant Infarction and Decompressive Craniectomy

Osmotic therapy can be used for patients with clinical deterioration from cerebral swelling associated with cerebral infarction is reasonable. In patients who develop symptoms of obstructive hydrocephalus from a cerebellar stroke, emergency ventriculostomy is a reasonable first step in the surgical management paradigm [73].

**Table 12.16** Indications for decompressive craniectomy

| Standard Indications |
|---|
| ☐ CT : Infarct of at least 50% of MCA territory (Or) ☐ MRI DWI : Infarct Volume > 145 cm³ |
| ☐ NIHSS > 15 |
| ☐ LOC (1a) : >/= 1 |
| ☐ Age : 18-60 years |
| ☐ With in 45 hours of symptom onset |
| ☐ Consent |

| Standard Exclusions |
|---|
| ❑ Pre Stroke mRS >/= 2 |
| ❑ B/L Fixed Dilated Pupils |
| ❑ Contralateral Ischemia |
| ❑ Other Brain Leisions that could affect outcome |
| ❑ Life Expectancy < 3 years |
| ❑ Other serious co-Existing Illness |
| ❑ Coagulopathy |

Remarks for DC outside standard indications:
- ❑ Age > 60 Years : to reduce mortality
- ❑ ------------------------------------------------
- ❑ ------------------------------------------------
- ❑ ------------------------------------------------

- ❑ Decompressive Craniectomy as a Life saving surgery in patients presenting with Mass effect and herniation
- ❑ EVD for obstructive HCP
- ❑ Decompressive sub occipital craniectomy for Cerebellar infarction , swelling and brainstem compression

Decompressive sub-occipital craniectomy with dural expansion should be performed in patients with cerebellar infarction causing neurological deterioration from brainstem compression despite maximal medical therapy. The outcome after cerebellar infarct can be good after sub-occipital craniectomy [74].

Malignant MCA infarction is a devastating event with substantial morbidity and mortality because of cerebral edema and raised intracranial pressure and risk of hemorrhagic transformation. Malignant MCA stroke is indicated by MCA territory stroke of >50% on CT, perfusion deficit of >66% on CT, infarct volume > 82 mL within 6 h of onset (on MRI) [75, 76, 77] DECIMAL [78], DESTINY [79], and HAMLET [80] trials and pooled analysis favored decompressive craniectomy over medical treatment in terms of mortality reduction, but functional outcome was not good [81]. DESTINY II trial investigated in patients of age > 60 years and reported mortality reduction but none of the survivors had good outcomes [82]. Hence decompressive hemicraniectomy (Table 12.16) can be considered in patients <60 years of age, within 48 h of stroke onset, although outcomes are still likely to be poor. Decompressive craniectomy is not preferable in malignant MCA stroke patients aged >60 years as survivors will be severely disabled.

## 12.12 Summary

Patients are preferably admitted in neurocritical care units or stroke units. Admission into specialized units with rehabilitation is associated with better outcomes. A standardized order sets as per the institution will ensure uniformity and better adherence to the set protocols. Antiplatelet is instituted typically after 24 h of intervention. Dual antiplatelet for minor stroke has been associated with improved outcomes. Patients are to be monitored for improvement, worsening of symptoms, development of cerebral infarction/swelling in ineligible or non-recanalized stroke, secondary complications (Aspiration Pneumonia/Fever/DVT). Dysphagia Screening, BP control, Glycaemic control, and General critical care measures are to be ensured. Follow-up of IVT/EVT with TCD/NIRS can be done in facilities where they are available. Malignant cerebral swelling despite osmotic therapy will require decompressive craniectomy as a lifesaving surgery and also to improve functional outcomes in young patients. Posterior circulation strokes with swelling and with obstructive hydrocephalus would need an EVD and posterior fossa decompression. Risk factor stratification and control of risk factors for the prevention of stroke are carried out before discharge.

## References

1. World Health Organization. The top 10 causes of death: factsheet. Geneva: World Health Organization; 2017. http://www.who.int/mediacentre/factsheets/fs310/en.
2. Feigin VL, Nguyen G, Cercy K. Global, regional, and country-specific lifetime risks of stroke, 1990 and 2016. New Engl J Med. 2018;379:2429–37.
3. World Stroke Organization Global Stroke Fact Sheet: Available at http://www.world-stroke.org.
4. Global Burden of Disease Stroke Statistics Worldwide for the year 2016. Available at http://ghdx.healthdata.org/gbd-results-tool.
5. Benjamin EJ, Blaha MJ, Chiuve SE, et al. Heart disease and stroke statistics—2017 update a report from the American Heart Association. Circulation. 2017;135:e146–603.
6. Saver JL, et al. Time is brain – quantified. Stroke. 2006;37:263–6.
7. Berglund A, Svensson L, Wahlgren N, von Euler M, HASTA Collaborators, et al. Face arm speech time test use in the prehospitalsetting, better in the ambulance than in the emergency medical communication center. Cerebrovasc Dis. 2014;37:212–6.
8. De Luca A, Giorgi Rossi P, Villa GF, Stroke Group Italian Society PreHospital Emergency Services, et al. The use of Cincinnati prehospital stroke scale during telephone dispatch interview increases the accuracy in identifying stroke and transient ischemic attack symptoms. BMC Health Serv Res. 2013;13:513.
9. Katz BS, McMullan JT, Sucharew H, Adeoye O, Broderick JP, et al. Design and validation of a prehospital scale to predict stroke severity: Cincinnati Prehospital stroke severity scale. Stroke. 2015;46:1508–12.
10. Noorian AR, Sanossian N, Shkirkova K, David S, et al. Los Angeles Motor Scales to identify large vessel occlusion prehospital validation and comparison with other screens. Stroke. 2018;49:565–72.
11. Jauch EC, Saver JL, Adams HP Jr, et al. Guidelines for the early management of patients with acute ischemic stroke: a guideline for healthcare professionals from the American Heart Association/American Stroke Association. Stroke. 2013;44:870–947.
12. Higashida R, Alberts MJ, Alexander DN, et al. Interactions within stroke systems of care: a policy statement from the American Heart Association/American Stroke Association. Stroke. 2013;44:2961–84.
13. Summers D, Leonard A, Wentworth D, et al. Comprehensive overview of nursing and interdisciplinary care of the acute ischemic stroke patient: a scientific statement from the American Heart Association. Stroke. 2009;40(8):2911–44.
14. Powers WJ, Rabinsten A, Ackerson T, et al. Guidelines for the early management of patients with acute ischemic stroke: a guideline for healthcare professionals from the American Heart Association/American Stroke Association. Stroke. 2018;49(3):e46–e110.
15. Roffe C, Nevatte T, Sim J, Stroke Oxygen Study Investigators and the Stroke Oxygen Study Collaborative Group, et al. Effect of routine low-dose oxygen supplementation on death and disability in adults with acute stroke: the stroke oxygen study randomized clinical trial. JAMA. 2017;318:1125–35.

16. Perini F, De Boni A, Marcon M, et al. Systolic blood pressure contributes to intracerebral haemorrhage after thrombolysis for ischemic stroke. J Neurol Sci. 2010;297:52–4.
17. Wohlfahrt P, Krajcoviechova A, Jozifovam M, et al. Low blood pressure during the acute period of ischemic stroke is associated with decreased survival. J Hypertens. 2015;33:339–45.
18. Lin CB, Peterson ED, Smith EE. Emergency medical service hospital prenotification is associated with improved evaluation and treatment of acute ischemic stroke. Circ Cardiovasc Qual Outcomes. 2012;5:514–22.
19. Lyden P, Raman R, Liu L, et al. National Institutes of Health scale certification is reliable across multiple venues. Stroke. 2009;40:2507–11.
20. Wardlaw JM, Seymour J, Cairns J, et al. Immediate computed tomography scanning of acute stroke is costeffective and improves quality of life. Stroke. 2004;35:2477–83.
21. Barber PA, Demchuk AM, Zhang J, Buchan AM. Validity and reliability of a quantitative computed tomography score in predicting outcome of hyperacute stroke before thrombolytic therapy. Lancet. 2000;355:1670–4.
22. Gupta AC, Schaefer PW, Chaudhry ZA, et al. Interobserver reliability of baseline noncontrast CT Alberta Stroke Program Early CT Score for intra-arterial stroke treatment selection. Am J Neuroradiol. 2012;33:1046–9.
23. Dzialowski I, Hill MD, Coutts SB, et al. Extent of early ischemic changes on computed tomography (CT) before thrombolysis: prognostic value of the Alberta stroke program early CT score in ECASS II. Stroke. 2006;37:973–8.
24. Hill MD, Demchuk AM, Goyal M, et al. Alberta stroke program early computed tomography score to select patients for endovascular treatment: interventional management of stroke (IMS) III trial. Stroke. 2014;45:444–9.
25. Aulicky P, Mikulík R, Goldemund D, et al. Safety of performing CT angiography in stroke patients treated with intravenous thrombolysis. J Neurol Neurosurg Psychiatry. 2010;81:783–7.
26. Chalela JA, Kidwell CS, Nentwich LM, et al. Magnetic resonance imaging and computed tomography in emergency assessment of patients with suspected acute stroke: a prospective comparison. Lancet. 2007;369:293–8.
27. Yu AY, Zerna C, Assis Z, et al. Multiphase CT angiography increases detection of anterior circulation intracranial occlusion. Neurology. 2016;87:609–16.
28. Barber PA, Hill MD, Eliasziw M, et al. Imaging of the brain in acute ischaemic stroke: comparison of computed tomography and magnetic resonance diffusion-weighted imaging. J Neurol Neurosurg Psychiatry. 2005;76:1528–33.
29. Greenberg SM, Vernooij MW, Cordonnier C, et al. Cerebral microbleeds: a guide to detection and interpretation. Lancet Neurol. 2009;8:165–74.
30. d'Esterre CD, Boesen ME, Ahn SH, et al. Time dependent computed tomographic perfusion thresholds for patients with acute ischemic stroke. Stroke. 2015;46:3390–7.
31. Bivard A, Kleinig T, Miteff F, et al. Ischemic core thresholds change with time to reperfusion: a case control study. Ann Neurol. 2017;82:995–1003.
32. Campbell BC, Christensen S, Levi CR, et al. Cerebral blood flow is the optimal CT perfusion parameter for assessing infarct core. Stroke. 2011;42:3435–40.
33. Campbell BC, Yassi N, Ma H, et al. Imaging selection in ischemic stroke: feasibility of automated CTperfusion analysis. Int J Stroke. 2015;10:51–4.
34. Nogueira RG, Jadhav AP, Haussen DC, et al. Trial investigators. Thrombectomy 6 to 24 hours after stroke with a mismatch between deficit and infarct. N Engl J Med. 2018;378(1):11–21.
35. Berkhemer OA, Fransen PS, Beumer D, et al. A randomized trial of intraarterial treatment for acute ischemic stroke. N Engl J Med. 2015;372(1):11–20.
36. Daemaerschalk BM, Kleindorfer DO, Adeoye OM, et al. Scientific rationale for the inclusion and exclusion criteria for intravenous alteplase in acute ischemic stroke. Stroke. 2016;47:581–641.
37. Hacke W, Kaste M, Bluhmki E, et al. Thrombolysis with alteplase 3–4.5 h after acute ischemic stroke. N Engl J Med. 2008;359:1317–29.
38. The National Institute of Neurological Disorders and Stroke rt-PA Stroke Study Group. Tissue plasminogen activator for acute ischemic stroke. N Engl J Med. 1995;333:1581–7.

39. Hacke W, Kaste M, Fieschi C, et al. Intravenous thrombolysis with recombinant tissue plasminogen activator for acute hemispheric stroke. The European Cooperative Acute Stroke Study (ECASS). JAMA. 1995;274(13):1017–25.
40. Robinson TG, Wang X, Arima H, et al. Low-versus standard-dose alteplase in patients on prior antiplatelet therapy: the enchanted trial (enhanced control of hypertension and thrombolysis stroke study). Stroke. 2017;48:1877–83.
41. Logallo N, Novotny V, Assmus J, et al. Tenecteplase versus alteplase for management of acute ischaemic stroke (NOR-TEST): a phase 3, randomised, open-label, blinded endpoint trial. Lancet Neurol. 2017;16:781–8.
42. Campbell BCV, Mitchell PJ, Churilov L, et al. Tenecteplase versus alteplase before thrombectomy for ischemic stroke. N Engl J Med. 2018;378:1573–82.
43. Daemaerschalk BM, Kleindorfer DO, Adeoye OM, et al. Scientific rationale for the inclusion and exclusion criteria for intravenous alteplase in acute ischemic stroke. Stroke. 2016;47:581–641.
44. Thomalla G, Simonsen CZ, Boutitie F, et al. MRI-guided thrombolysis for stroke with unknown time of onset. N Engl J Med. 2018;379:611–22.
45. Berkhemer OA, Puck SS, for the MR CLEAN investigators, et al. A randomized trial of intraarterial treatment for acute ischemic stroke. N Engl J Med. 2015;372:11–20.
46. Campbell BC, Mitchell PJ, Yan B, et al. A multicenter, randomized, controlled study to investigate EXtending the time for thrombolysis in emergency neurological deficits with intra-arterial therapy (EXTEND-IA). Int J Stroke. 2014;9:126–32.
47. Demchuk AM, Goyal M, Menon BK, et al. Endovascular treatment for small Core and anterior circulation proximal occlusion with emphasis on minimizing CT to recanalization times (ESCAPE) trial: methodology. Int J Stroke. 2015;10(3):429–38.
48. Jovin TG, Chamorro A, Cobo E, et al. Thrombectomy within 8 h after symptom onset in ischemic stroke [REVASCAT]. N Engl J Med. 2015;372:2296–306.
49. Saver JL, Jahan R, Levy EI, et al. Solitaire flow restoration device versus the Merci retriever in patients with acute ischaemic stroke (SWIFT): a randomised, parallel-group, non inferiority trial. Lancet. 2012;380:1241–9.
50. Bracard S, Ducrocq X, Mas JL, et al. Mechanical thrombectomy after intravenous alteplase versus alteplase alone after stroke (THRACE): a randomised controlled trial. Lancet Neurol. 2016;15(11):1138–47.
51. Mocco J, Zaidat OO, et al. Aspiration thrombectomy after intravenous alteplase versus intravenous Alteplase alone (THERAPY). Stroke. 2016;47(9):2331–8.
52. Muir KW, Ford GA, Messow C, on behalf of the PISTE Investigators, et al. Endovascular therapy for acute ischaemic stroke: the pragmatic ischemic stroke thrombectomy evaluation (PISTE) randomised, controlled trial. J Neurol Neurosurg Psychiatry. 2017;88:38–44.
53. Khoury NN, Darsaut TE, Ghostine J, et al. Endovascular thrombectomy and medical therapy versus medical therapy alone in acute stroke: a randomized care trial. J Neuroradiol. 2017;44(3):198–20.
54. Albers GW, Lansberg MG, Kemp S, et al. A multicenter randomized controlled trial of endovascular therapy following imaging evaluation for ischemic stroke. Int J Stroke. 2017;12(8):896–905.
55. Goyal M, Jadhav AP, Bonafe A, et al. Analysis of workflow and time to treatment and the effects on outcome in endovascular treatment of acute ischemic stroke: results from the swift prime randomized controlled trial. Radiology. 2016;279:888–97.
56. Yoo AJ, Simonsen CZ, Prabhakaran S, et al. Refining angiographic biomarkers of revascularization: improving outcome prediction after intra-arterial therapy. Stroke. 2013;44(9):2509–12.
57. Ebinger M, Winter B, Wendt M, et al. Effect of the use of ambulance-based thrombolysis on time to thrombolysis in acute ischemic stroke: a randomized clinical trial. JAMA. 2014;311:1622–31.
58. Walter S, Kostopoulos P, Haass A, et al. Diagnosis and treatment of patients with stroke in a mobile stroke unit versus in hospital: a randomised controlled trial. Lancet Neurol. 2012;11:397–404.

59. Hastrup S, Damgaard D, Johnsen SP, Andersen G, et al. Prehospital acute stroke severity scale to predict large artery occlusion: design and comparison with other scales. Stroke. 2016;47:1772–6.
60. Kamal N, Holodinsky JK, Stephenson C, et al. Improving door-to-needle times for acute ischemic stroke: effect of rapid patient registration, moving directly to computed tomography, and giving alteplase at the computed tomography scanner. Circ Cardiovasc Qual Outcomes. 2017;10(1):e003242.
61. Stroke Unit Trialists' Collaboration. Organised inpatient (stroke unit) care for stroke. Cochrane Database Syst Rev. 2007;17(4):CD000197.
62. Candelise L, Gattinoni M, Bersano A, Micieli G, Sterzi R, Morabito A, et al. Stroke-unit care for acute stroke patients: an observational follow-up study. Lancet. 2007;369:299–305.
63. Brinjikji W, Murad MH, Rabinstein AA, et al. Conscious sedation versus general anesthesia during endovascular acute ischemic stroke treatment: a systematic review and meta-analysis. AJNR Am J Neuroradiol. 2015;36:529.
64. Simonsen CZ, Yoo AJ, Sørensen LH, et al. Effect of general anesthesia and conscious sedation during endovascular therapy on infarct growth and clinical outcomes in acute ischemic stroke: a randomized clinical trial. JAMA Neurol. 2018;75:470–7.
65. Lowhagen H, Rentzos A, Karlsson JE, et al. General anesthesia versus conscious sedation for endovascular treatment of acute ischemic stroke (The AnStroke Trial). Stroke. 2017;48:1601–7.
66. Schonenberger S, Uhlmann L, Hacke W, et al. Effect of conscious sedation vs general anesthesia on early neurological improvement among patients with ischemic stroke undergoing endovascular thrombectomy: a randomized controlled trial. JAMA. 2016;316:1986–96.
67. Peng Y, Wu Y, Huo X, Endovascular Therapy for Acute Ischemic Stroke trial (EAST) group, et al. Outcomes of anesthesia selection in endovascular treatment of acute ischemic stroke. J Neurosurg Anesthesiol. 2019;31(1):43–9.
68. Talke OP, Sharma D, Heyer EJ, et al. Society for neuroscience in anesthesiology and critical care expert consensus statement: anesthetic management of endovascular treatment for acute ischemic stroke. J Neurosurg Anesthesiol. 2014;26:95–108.
69. Fischer U, Baumgartner A, Arnold M, et al. What is a minor stroke? Stroke. 2010;41(4):661–6.
70. Ahmed N, Wahlgren N, Grond M, et al. SITS Investigators. Implementation and outcome of thrombolysis with alteplase 3-4.5 h after an acute stroke: an updated analysis from SITS-ISTR. Lancet Neurol. 2010;9:866–74.
71. Coutts SB, Modi J, Patel SK, et al. What causes disability after transient ischemic attack and minor stroke? Results from the CT and MRI in the triage of TIA and minor cerebrovascular events to identify high risk patients (catch) study. Stroke. 2012;43:3018–22.
72. Bivard A, Huang X, Levi CR, et al. Tenecteplase in ischemic stroke offers improved recanalization: analysis of 2 trials. Neurology. 2017;89:62–7.
73. Raco A, Caroli E, Isidori A, et al. Management of acute cerebellar infarction: one institution's experience. Neurosurgery. 2003;53(5):1061–5.
74. Agarwalla PK, Stapleton CJ, Ogilvy CS, et al. Craniectomy in acute ischemic stroke. Neurosurgery. 2014;74(suppl 1):S151–62.
75. Dittrich R, Kloska SP, Fischer T, et al. Accuracy of perfusion-CT in predicting malignant middle cerebral artery brain infarction. J Neurol. 2008;255(6):896–902.
76. Oppenheim C, Samson Y, Manaï R, et al. Prediction of malignant middle cerebral artery infarction by diffusion-weighted imaging. Stroke. 2000;31(9):2175–81.
77. Kasner SE, Demchuk AM, Berrouschot J, et al. Predictors of fatal brain edema in massive hemispheric ischemic stroke. Stroke. 2001;32(9):2117–23.
78. Vahedi K, Vicaut E, Mateo J, on behalf of the DECIMAL Investigators, et al. Sequential-design, multicenter, randomized, controlled trial of early decompressive craniectomy in malignant middle cerebral artery infarction (DECIMAL trial). Stroke. 2007;38:2506–17.
79. Jüttler E, Schwab S, Schmiedek P, DESTINY Study Group, et al. Decompressive surgery for the treatment of malignant infarction of the middle cerebral artery (DESTINY): a randomized, controlled trial. Stroke. 2007;38(9):2518–25.

80. Hofmeijer J, Kappelle LJ, Algra A, Amelink GJ, Van Gijn J, Van der Worp HB, HAMLET investigators. Surgical decompression for space-occupying cerebral infarction (the Hemicraniectomy after middle cerebral artery infarction with life-threatening Edema trial [HAMLET]): a multicentre, open, randomised trial. Lancet Neurol. 2009;8(4):326–33.
81. Vahedi K, Hofmeijer J, Juettler E, et al. Early decompressive surgery in malignant infarction of the middle cerebral artery: a pooled analysis of three randomised controlled trials. Lancet Neurol. 2007;6:215–22.
82. Jüttler E, Unterberg A, Woitzik J, et al. DESTINY II investigators. Hemicraniectomy in older patients with extensive middle-cerebral-artery stroke. N Engl J Med. 2014;370(12):1091–100.

# Management of Status Epilepticus

# 13

K. N. Gopalakrishna and M. Radhakrishnan

## Key Points

- Status epilepticus (SE) is defined as continuous clinical/electroencephalographic seizure activity lasting for 5 min or more, or recurrent episodes of seizure activity in a 5-min interval without recovery to baseline neurological status between seizures.
- Status epilepticus may be convulsive, non-convulsive, refractory or super refractory.
- Etiology may be acute or chronic: Acute causes include CNS infections, anti-epileptic drug (AED) non-compliance, trauma, stroke, metabolic, etc. Chronic causes include neurodegenerative disorders, congenital malformations of the brain.
- Appropriate investigations to delineate the cause of seizures should be ordered and appropriate monitoring should be instituted.
- Management is aimed at aborting the seizure activity, preventing recurrences, and providing hemodynamic support to the patient.
- A wide range of anti-epileptic drugs including benzodiazepines and barbiturates are available for the management of SE.

## Case Scenario

A 34-year-old male patient presented to casualty with tonic-clonic seizures. He was treated with two doses of 0.1 mg/kg of intravenous (IV) lorazepam with in 5 min apart with oxygen supplementation and airway support, in addition, Phenytoin 20 mg/kg IV was administered over 30 min. On examination, the patient

K. N. Gopalakrishna · M. Radhakrishnan (✉)
National Institute of Mental Health and Neurosciences, Bengaluru, India


P. U. Bidkar, P. Vanamoorthy (eds.), *Acute Neuro Care*,
https://doi.org/10.1007/978-981-15-4071-4_13

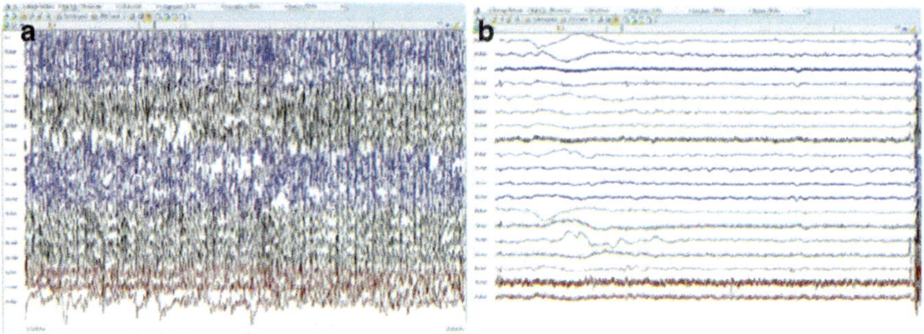

**Fig. 13.1** (**a**) EEG showing generalized seizure discharges; (**b**) EEG showing Burst suppression of electrical activity during ketamine bolus followed by infusion

was found unresponsive and continued to have seizures. The patient was intubated for airway protection, and IV Levetiracetam 30 mg/kg bolus was administered. The patient was put on mechanical ventilation, and he continued to have seizures. Intravenous anesthetic midazolam 0.2 mg/kg bolus was given followed by 0.2 mg/kg/h, titrated up to 0.6 mg/kg. Electroencephalogram (EEG) monitoring instituted to monitor for seizure activity. Laboratory workup was with in normal limit, and computed tomography (CT) brain did not reveal any intracranial bleed/mass or features of raised intracranial pressure. The patient continued to have clinical seizures once in every 40 min, for which a thiopental sodium bolus of 4 mg/Kg followed by infusion at 5 mg/kg/h was initiated. The patient continued to have focal motor seizures and EEG showed a generalization of the seizure (Fig. 13.1a). Ketamine 1 mg/kg bolus followed by 2 mg/kg/h of infusion was instituted for control of seizures clinically and electroencephalographically (Fig. 13.1b).

## 13.1 Introduction

Status epilepticus (SE) is a life-threatening neurological emergency associated with significant morbidity and mortality and requires immediate evaluation and treatment. Early termination of seizure activity decreases the chances of neuronal injury and improves the clinical outcome. It is recommended to have an in-house protocol involving a multi-disciplinary team (neurologist, intensivist, anesthetist) for the comprehensive management of SE.

## 13.2 Definition

SE is defined as continuous clinical/electroencephalographic seizure activity lasting for 5 min or more, or recurrent episodes of seizure activity in a 5-min interval without recovery to baseline neurological status between seizures [1].

## 13.3 Classification

The two main criteria for SE classification are based on the presence or absence of prominent motor symptoms and degree of impaired consciousness [2]. SE classification is described in Flow chart 13.1 [2].

- Convulsive SE (CSE): generalized tonic-clonic movements of the extremities and impairment of mental status (lethargy, confusion, coma).
- Non-convulsive SE (NCSE): seizure activity seen on an electroencephalogram (EEG), without accompanying clinical tonic-clonic movements [3].
- Refractory SE (RSE): continuing convulsive or non-convulsive seizure activity despite administration of adequate doses of first-line and second-line anti-epileptic drugs (AED) [4].
- Super refractory SE (SRSE): continued seizure activity for 24 h or more after the induction of anesthetic coma, including cases where SE recurs within 24 h of weaning/withdrawal of the anesthetic drugs [5].

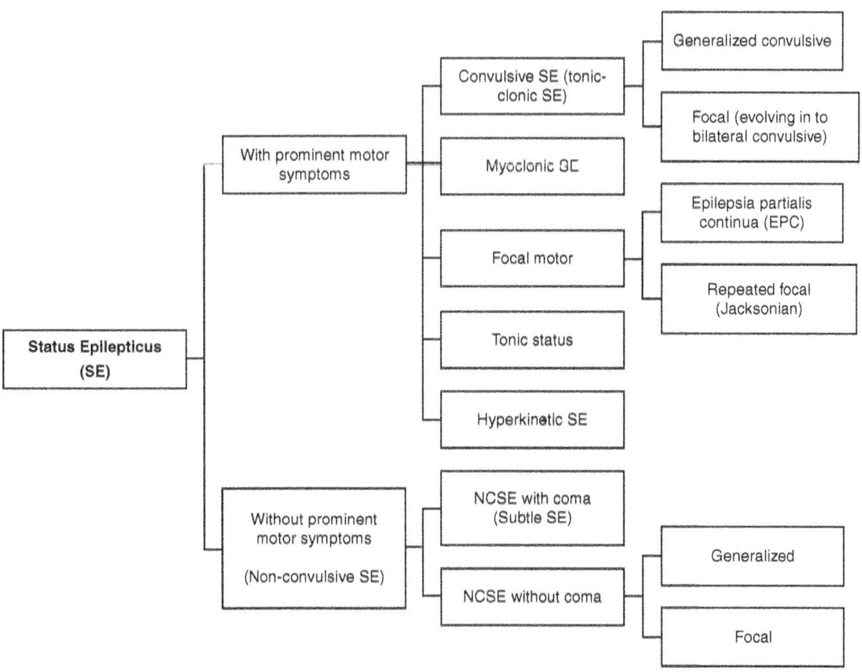


**Flow chart 13.1** SE classification [2]

## 13.4 Epidemiology

The incidence of SE has a bimodal age distribution with increased occurrence during infancy and in the age group above 60 years. The frequent causes of SE in Indian scenario include central nervous system (CNS) infections, an anti-epileptic drug (AED) non-compliance, and stroke [6, 7].

## 13.5 Pathophysiology

A seizure is a paroxysmal manifestation of the electrical discharge of the neurons in the cerebral cortex. An imbalance in the excitatory and inhibitory neurotransmitters within the network of cortical neurons leads to the sudden onset of net excitation [8]. SE occurs when intrinsic brain network is unable to terminate a seizure or when the neuronal environment becomes conducive to prolonged seizure activity.

At the cellular level, receptors on the surface of axons are in a highly dynamic state, moving onto (externalization), and away from (internalization) the axonal membrane. This "receptor trafficking" intensifies during SE and the overall effect is a reduction in the number of functional Gamma-aminobutyric acid (GABA) receptors in the cells involved in the seizure discharge. As GABA is the principal inhibitory transmitter, this reduction in GABA-ergic activity causes the seizures to become persistent [9]. Furthermore, the number of glutaminergic receptors at the cell surface increases, and the reduction in the density of the GABA receptors is itself triggered by activation of the glutaminergic receptor systems. Alteration in GABA receptor sensitivity induces drug resistance resulting in RSE. Mitochondrial failure or insufficiency is another reason for the failure of seizure termination [10].

## 13.6 Etiology [2, 11]

### 13.6.1 Acute

- Central nervous system infection (ex: meningitis, encephalitis, abscess)
- Metabolic (ex: Hypoglycemia, Hyponatremia, Hypocalcemia, Hepatic encephalopathy, Uremia)
- Cerebrovascular accidents (ex: stroke, cerebral venous sinus thrombosis)
- Traumatic brain injury
- Brain tumor
- Anoxic-ischemic injury (ex: post-cardiac arrest)
- Septic encephalopathy
- Drug effect (ex: Acute drug toxicity, low AED levels, withdrawal effect from alcohol/ benzodiazepines/barbiturates)
- Hypertensive encephalopathy
- Autoimmune encephalitis
- CNS inflammation
- Post neurosurgery (ex: pneumocephalus)

### 13.6.2 Chronic

- Pre-existing epilepsy with AED non-compliance or breakthrough seizures
- Neurodegenerative disorders (ex: Alzheimer's, amyloid angiopathy)
- Congenital malformation of the brain
- Encephalomalacia (due to stroke, head injury, prior neurosurgery)

## 13.7 Clinical Presentation

Seizure presentation can involve the sensory, motor, autonomic, and cognitive systems. Patients can present with either positive or negative symptoms. The positive symptoms include rhythmic tonic-clonic movements of the limbs, nystagmoid movements of eyes, and continuous flickering of a group of muscles. The negative symptoms include confusion, aphasia, comatose, and non-responsive, catatonia, and focal weakness (Todd's palsy) [1]. Sometimes SE can present as a global neurologic dysfunction not explained by imaging findings. As the duration of SE progresses, positive signs become minimal, and sometimes patients have only EEG evidence of SE [3].

### 13.7.1 Differential Diagnosis

- Movement disorders
- Posturing due to herniation
- Psychiatric disorders
- Transient global amnesia
- Acute encephalopathies (toxic, metabolic or infection)

## 13.8 Investigations

SE can result in systemic disturbances, and vice versa is also true. Investigations are done to identify readily treatable causes of SE (ex: hypoglycemia), to detect complications following SE and to diagnose the cause of SE (ex: imaging studies for encephalitis)

- Blood sugar, serum electrolytes (ex: sodium disturbances), serum calcium, magnesium
- Complete blood count (ex: infections), cerebrospinal fluid (CSF) analysis, CSF biomarkers for infections
- Brain imaging studies (CT, MRI)
- EEG, serum AED levels
- Others: liver function tests, metabolite screen for inborn errors of metabolism, drug toxicology screen (ex: cocaine, sympathomimetics, tricyclic antidepressants, alcohol), autoimmune disorder workup.

## 13.9 Monitoring

- Pulse oximetry, electrocardiogram, blood pressure (invasive during third-line therapy), respiratory rate, temperature, urine output, and arterial blood gas analysis.
- Continuous bedside EEG preferable when proceeding to third-line therapy.

## 13.10 SE Complications [12, 13]

The complications occuring due to continued seizures is listed in Table 13.1.

## 13.11 Management Goals [14–17]

- Abort seizure activity (First-line therapy, Table 13.2)
- Prevent seizure recurrence (Second-line AED therapy, Table 13.3)
- If seizure persists, escalate therapy (Third-line/other therapy, Table 13.4).
- General care: Support hemodynamics and respiration
- Investigate for systemic causes, focal cerebral pathology
- Monitor for seizure activity
- Treatment of complications

## 13.12 Treatment Principles [1, 14, 15]

- Most patients receive initial treatment in the hospital and referred to a specialty hospital in case the patient does not respond.
- It is better to give first-line and second-line AED therapy together so that the second-line drugs start having its effect by the time the first-line drug wears off (SE treatment algorithm described in Flow chart 13.2).

**Table 13.1** SE complications [12, 13]

| Systems | Possible complications |
|---|---|
| Respiratory | Neurogenic pulmonary edema, aspiration pneumonia |
| Cardiovascular | Arrhythmia, stress-induced cardiomyopathy |
| Musculoskeletal | Rhabdomyolysis, tongue injury, joint dislocations |
| Renal | Acute kidney injury |
| Autonomic | Hyperpyrexia, arrhythmias, sudden death |
| Metabolic | Metabolic acidosis, hyperglycemia, hyperkalemia |
| Cerebral | Brain edema, blood barrier disruption, hippocampus damage, brain atrophy, sclerosis |
| Treatment associated | Propofol infusion syndrome, hypotension, respiratory depression, nosocomial infections, paralytic ileus |

**Table 13.2** First-line anti-epileptic drugs

| | Lorazepam | Midazolam | Diazepam |
|---|---|---|---|
| Initial dose | IV 0.1 mg/kg (up to maximum of 4 mg per dose, can repeat in 5–10 min) | IV/IM0.15–0.2 mg/kg (up to max 10 mg),<br>Intranasal 0.2 mg/kg<br>Buccal 0.5 mg/kg | IV/IM 0.15 mg/kg (up to max 10 mg), can repeat in 5 min<br>Rectal 0.2–0.5 mg/kg |
| Route | IV | IV/IM/Intranasal/Buccal route | IV/IM/rectal |
| Adverse reactions | – Respiratory depression<br>– Hypotension | – Respiratory depression<br>– Hypotension | – Respiratory depression<br>– Hypotension |
| Important considerations | IV preparation contains propylene glycol, may cause metabolic acidosis | Short duration, caution in renal failure | IV preparation contains propylene glycol, may cause metabolic acidosis |

*IV* Intravenous, *IM* Intramuscular

**Table 13.3** Second-line anti-epileptic drugs

| | Phenytoin | Fosphenytoin | Sodium valproate | Levetiracetam |
|---|---|---|---|---|
| Initial dose | 20 mg/kg, IV administration up to 50 mg/min, additional dose of 5–10 mg/kg after 10 min | 20 mg/kg, IV administration up to 150 mg/min, additional dose 5–10 mg/kg after 10 min | 20–40 mg/kg, additional dose 20 mg/kg after 10 min | 20–60 mg/kg, max 4500 mg per dose |
| Maintenance | 5 mg/kg/day | 4–6 mg/kg/day | 10 mg/kg twice daily | 1–4 g/day |
| Route | IV | IV | IV | IV |
| Therapeutic range | 15–20 μg/mL | 15–20 μg/mL | 50–100 μg/mL | 5–45 μg/mL |
| Adverse reactions | Hypotension<br>Cardiac arrhythmias<br>purple glove syndrome<br>Gingival hypertrophy | Arrhythmias<br>Hypotension | Hepatotoxicity<br>Hyperammonemia<br>Thrombocytopenia<br>Ataxia<br>Pancreatitis | Irritability<br>Behavior problems<br>Anemia<br>Leukopenia |
| Drug interactions | Serum levels decreased by enzyme-inducing drugs.<br>Serum level increased by isoniazid, sulfonamides, fluoxetine | | Serum levels decreased by enzyme-inducing drugs | Not known significant interactions |

(continued)

**Table 13.3** (continued)

| | Phenytoin | Fosphenytoin | Sodium valproate | Levetiracetam |
|---|---|---|---|---|
| Important considerations | Compatible with saline only | Compatible with saline, ringer, and dextrose solutions | Avoid in liver disorders, porphyria, and coagulopathy | Safe in liver disease or coagulopathy |
| | *Phenobarbital* | *Lacosamide* | *Topiramate* | *Clobazam* |
| Initial dose | 20 mg/kg, additional 10 mg/kg after 10 min | 200–400 mg | 200–400 mg | 5–10 mg |
| Maintenance | 1–5 mg/kg/h | 100–200 mg BD | 100–200 mg BD | 20–30 mg/day |
| Route | IV | IV | Enteral route | Enteral route |
| Therapeutic range | 10–40 μg/mL | Not established | 2–20 μg/mL | |
| Adverse reaction | Sedation<br>Respiratory depression | PR interval prolongation in ECG | Metabolic acidosis<br>Glaucoma<br>Renal stones | Sedation<br>Ataxia<br>Skin rash |
| Drug interaction | Enzyme induction | Serum levels decreased by enzyme induced drugs | Serum levels decreased by enzyme-inducing drugs | Serum level increased by CYP2C19 inhibitors |
| Important considerations | Decrease the effect of warfarin, steroids, theophylline, and digoxin | Limited experience in SE treatment | Avoid use with other carbonic anhydrase inhibitors | |

*IV* Intravenous, *IM* Intramuscular

**Table 13.4** Third-line anti-epileptic drugs

| | Midazolam | Propofol | Thiopental | Ketamine |
|---|---|---|---|---|
| Initial dose | 0.2 mg/kg | 1–2 mg/kg | 2–7 mg/kg | 1–2 mg/kg |
| Maintenance | 0.05–2 mg/kg/h | 2–10 mg/kg/h | 0.5 to 5 mg/kg/h | 2–7 mg/kg/h |
| Route | IV | IV | IV | IV |
| Adverse reaction | Hypotension<br>Respiratory depression | Hypotension<br>Propofol infusion syndrome<br>Infections | Hypotension<br>Paralytic ileus<br>Nosocomial infections | Hypertension<br>Raised ICP/IOP<br>arrhythmias |
| Important considerations | Tachyphylaxis with prolonged infusion, cautious in renal disorders | Requires ventilator support, Adjust daily calorie intake (propofol contains 1.1 kcal/mL) | Requires ventilator and vasopressor support | Contraindicated in patients with severe hypertension |

*IV* intravenous, *IM* intramuscular, *ICP* intracranial pressure, *IOP* intraocular pressure

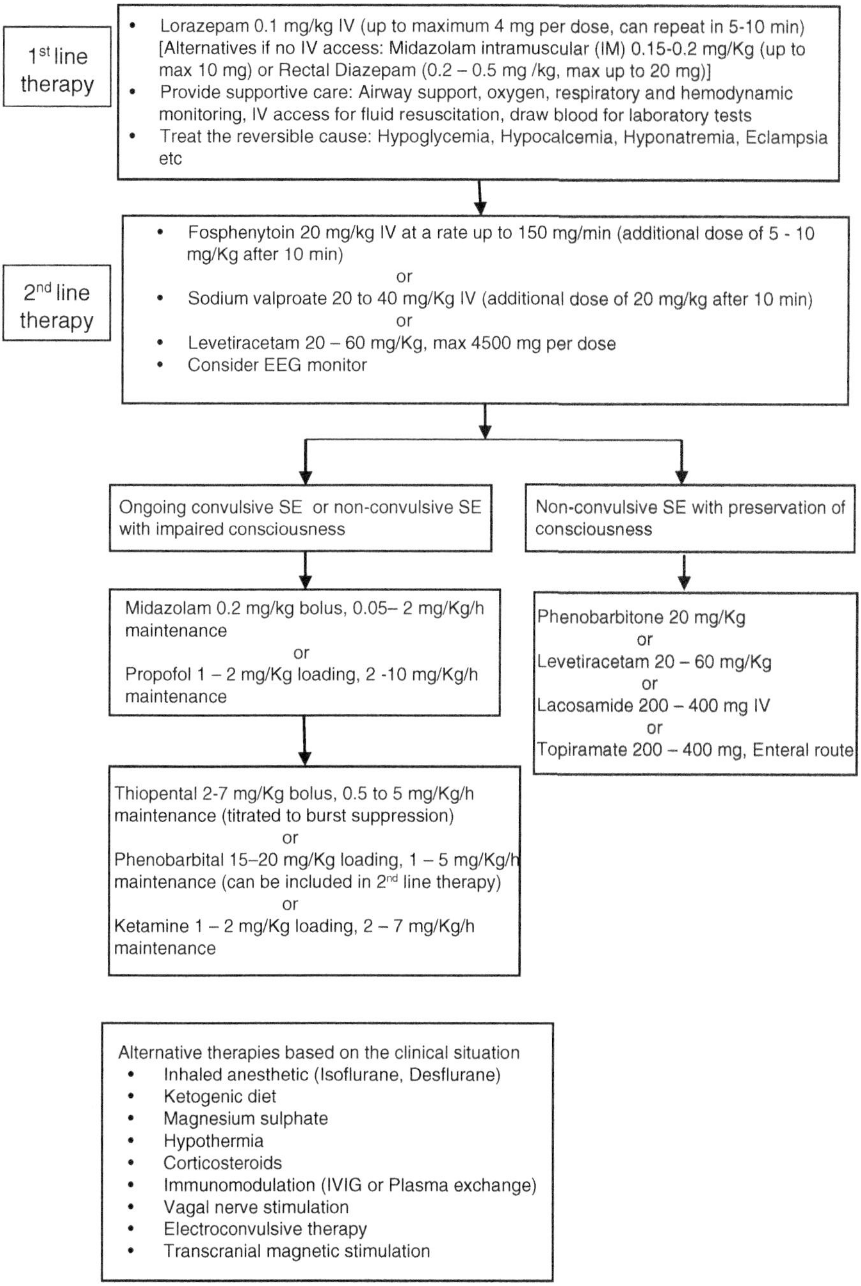


**Flow chart 13.2** Status epilepticus treatment algorithm [14, 26, 27]

- When giving phenytoin, stick to the 50 mg/min infusion to avoid adverse hemodynamic effects. The infusion should be even slower if the patient is hypothermic.
- When given multiple drugs, drug interaction should be kept in mind to avoid over/under dosage. Phenytoin and carbamazepine reduce the availability of other drugs, while valproate increases the availability of other AEDs.
- Physical compatibility is also an issue when infusions are given in the same IV lines. (ex: Thiopentone precipitates ketamine, Phenytoin is not compatible with dextrose containing solutions). It is better to have a pamphlet listing out the possible drug interaction so that everyone in the treating team is aware of it.
- It is better to start ketamine early as an adjuvant to third-line therapy to reduce the dose of IV anesthetics and also to maintain hemodynamic stability.
- If managed by anesthetists, RSE can also be controlled with volatile anesthetic agents like isoflurane [18]. It can achieve faster and good control of seizure activity. Anesthesia machine used in the operation theater can be used for this purpose (note: nursing staff in the ICU might not be familiar). The dose can be titrated by monitoring minimum alveolar concentration (MAC) and EEG. The other advantage of using isoflurane is that even after prolonged administration, unlike thiopentone, it gets washed off from the body much faster.
- A patient receiving IV anesthetics are prone to infections as all these medications suppress the immune system. Patients might succumb to infections even if the seizures are controlled due to these medications. It is better to start high dose of empiric antibiotics.
- Patients receiving third-line medications are prone to hemodynamic instability. They frequently require vasopressors and it is better to place an arterial line for monitoring.
- The management of the underlying etiology of SE (ex: CNS infection, low antileptic levels, stroke, electrolyte imbalance) is essential for seizure termination.
- Patients with autoimmune encephalitis might improve with methylprednisolone and immunoglobulins.
- When imaging studies suggest cerebral edema, administer osmotic diuresis, but to be careful with electrolyte disturbance.
- Along with described medications, intravenous magnesium sulfate might be tried for seizure control (4gm IV bolus followed by 2-4gm/h infusion). Note: keep serum level < 6 mEq/L and monitor blood pressure and renal function.
- Pyridoxine is an important co-factor in the GABA synthesis. Supplementation of pyridoxine 100 mg/day might be beneficial.
- When using high dose thiopental administration, it is better to avoid enteral feeding as it is known to cause paralytic ileus.
- Atleast 24–48 h of seizure-free EEG or Burst suppression must be achieved before tapering third-line medications. Duration and amount of dose reduction depend on the half-life of medications administered and the possible drug interactions. A useful dictum is to aim for a 20% dose reduction every 4–6 h.

## 13.13 Prognosis

Despite comprehensive medical management, in-hospital mortality due to SE is between 9% and 21% [19–21]. Patients with prolonged SE (more than 1 h) and myoclonic SE have higher mortality [22]. RSE patients have a poor outcome with the mortality rate ranges between 22% and 60% [21, 23–25]. In the case of NCSE, the mortality ranges from 18% to 50% [14].

## Multiple Choice Question

1. The clinical/electroencephalographic seizure activity lasting longer than what period of time is defined as status epilepticus?
   (a) 5 min
   (b) 30 min
   (c) 45 min
   (d) 60 min
2. The following neurotransmitter alteration most likely observed with status epilepticus
   (a) Increased GABA, Increased Glutamate
   (b) Decreased GABA, Decreased Glutamate
   (c) Decreased GABA, Increased Glutamate
   (d) Increased GABA, Decreased Glutamate
3. All of the following drugs are used in the management of status epilepticus except?
   (a) Lorazepam
   (b) Phenytoin
   (c) Levetiracetam
   (d) Carbamazepine
4. Following anticonvulsant medications not suitable for administration via rectal route in children.
   (a) Diazepam
   (b) Phenobarbitone
   (c) Sodium valproate
   (d) Propofol
5. Alternative therapies for Refractory Status epilepticus include all except:
   (a) Vagal Nerve Stimulation
   (b) Transcranial magnetic stimulation
   (c) ketamine
   (d) Theophylline
6. The most common Status Epilepticus etiology in Indian adult population?
   (a) Stroke
   (b) Central nervous system infections

   (c) Anti-epileptic drug non-compliance
   (d) Neurodegenerative disorders
7. A 28-year-old male patient presented to casualty with generalized seizure activity that has lasted for more than 5 min. Which of the following is the first-line drug of choice to terminate seizure
   (a) Phenytoin
   (b) Sodium valproate
   (c) Lorazepam
   (d) Levetiracetam
8. Which of the following third-line anticonvulsant agent is appropriate for refractory status epilepticus
   (a) Fosphenytoin
   (b) Topiramate
   (c) Midazolam
   (d) Lacosamide
9. The following anti-epileptic drug which has no known significant interaction with enzyme-inducing drugs
   (a) Sodium valproate
   (b) Phenytoin
   (c) Levetiracetam
   (d) Topiramate
10. The therapeutic range of serum phenytoin level is
   (a) 15–20 μg/mL
   (b) 40–60 μg/mL
   (c) 100–120 μg/mL
   (d) 1–2 μg/mL

Answers: 1. (a), 2. (c), 3. (d), 4. (d), 5. (d), 6. (b), 7. (c), 8. (c), 9. (c), 10. (a).

## References

1. Brophy GM, Bell R, Claassen J, Alldredge B, Bleck TP, Glauser T, et al. Guidelines for the evaluation and management of status epilepticus. Neurocrit Care. 2012;17(1):3–23.
2. Trinka E, Cock H, Hesdorffer D, Rossetti AO, Scheffer IE, Shinnar S, et al. A definition and classification of status epilepticus--Report of the ILAE Task Force on Classification of Status Epilepticus. Epilepsia. 2015;56(10):1515–23.
3. Caricato A, Melchionda I, Antonelli M. Continuous electroencephalography monitoring in adults in the intensive care unit. Crit Care. 2018;22(1):75.
4. Mayer SA, Claassen J, Lokin J, Mendelsohn F, Dennis LJ, Fitzsimmons BF. Refractory status epilepticus: frequency, risk factors, and impact on outcome. Arch Neurol. 2002;59(2):205–10.
5. Shorvon S, Ferlisi M. The treatment of super-refractory status epilepticus: a critical review of available therapies and a clinical treatment protocol. Brain. 2011;134(Pt 10):2802–18.
6. Kalita J, Nair PP, Misra UK. A clinical, radiological and outcome study of status epilepticus from India. J Neurol. 2010;257(2):224–9.
7. Santhosh NS, Sinha S, Satishchandra P. Epilepsy: Indian perspective. Ann Indian Acad Neurol. 2014;17(Suppl 1):S3–s11.

8. Bromfield EB, Cavazos JE, Sirven JI. Basic mechanisms underlying seizures and epilepsy. Landover: American Epilepsy Society; 2006.
9. Arancibia-Carcamo IL, Kittler JT. Regulation of GABA(A) receptor membrane trafficking and synaptic localization. Pharmacol Ther. 2009;123(1):17–31.
10. Cock HR, Tong X, Hargreaves IP, Heales SJ, Clark JB, Patsalos PN, et al. Mitochondrial dysfunction associated with neuronal death following status epilepticus in rat. Epilepsy Res. 2002;48(3):157–68.
11. Berg AT, Berkovic SF, Brodie MJ, Buchhalter J, Cross JH, van Emde BW, et al. Revised terminology and concepts for organization of seizures and epilepsies: report of the ILAE Commission on Classification and Terminology, 2005-2009. Epilepsia. 2010;51(4):676–85.
12. Varelas PN, Mirski MA. Seizures in the adult intensive care unit. J Neurosurg Anesthesiol. 2001;13(2):163–75.
13. Gullapalli B. Status epilepticus. In: Suarez JI, editor. Critical care neurology and neurosurgery. Totowa: Humana Press; 2004. p. 449–68.
14. Al-Mufti F, Claassen J. Neurocritical care: status epilepticus review. Crit Care Clin. 2014;30(4):751–64.
15. Claassen J, Goldstein JN. Emergency neurological life support: status epilepticus. Neurocrit Care. 2017;27(Suppl 1):152–8.
16. Unterberger I. Status epilepticus: do treatment guidelines make sense? J Clin Neurophysiol. 2016;33(1):10–3.
17. Shorvon S. The treatment of status epilepticus. Curr Opin Neurol. 2011;24(2):165–70.
18. Zeiler FA, Zeiler KJ, Teitelbaum J, Gillman LM, West M. Modern inhalational anesthetics for refractory status epilepticus. Can J Neurol Sci. 2015;42(2):106–15.
19. Alldredge BK, Gelb AM, Isaacs SM, Corry MD, Allen F, Ulrich S, et al. A comparison of lorazepam, diazepam, and placebo for the treatment of out-of-hospital status epilepticus. N Engl J Med. 2001;345(9):631–7.
20. Claassen J, Lokin JK, Fitzsimmons BF, Mendelsohn FA, Mayer SA. Predictors of functional disability and mortality after status epilepticus. Neurology. 2002;58(1):139–42.
21. Novy J, Logroscino G, Rossetti AO. Refractory status epilepticus: a prospective observational study. Epilepsia. 2010;51(2):251–6.
22. Logroscino G, Hesdorffer DC, Cascino GD, Annegers JF, Bagiella E, Hauser WA. Long-term mortality after a first episode of status epilepticus. Neurology. 2002;58(4):537–41.
23. Claassen J, Hirsch LJ, Emerson RG, Mayer SA. Treatment of refractory status epilepticus with pentobarbital, propofol, or midazolam: a systematic review. Epilepsia. 2002;43(2):146–53.
24. Claassen J, Hirsch LJ, Emerson RG, Bates JE, Thompson TB, Mayer SA. Continuous EEG monitoring and midazolam infusion for refractory nonconvulsive status epilepticus. Neurology. 2001;57(6):1036–42.
25. Rossetti AO, Reichhart MD, Schaller MD, Despland PA, Bogousslavsky J. Propofol treatment of refractory status epilepticus: a study of 31 episodes. Epilepsia. 2004;45(7):757–63.
26. Hocker SE. Status Epilepticus. Continuum (Minneap Minn). 2015;21(5 Neurocritical Care):1362–83.
27. Pichler M, Hocker S. Management of status epilepticus. In: Wijdicks EFM, Kramer AH, editors. Hand book of clinical neurology: critical care neurology part 1, vol. 140. Amsterdam: Elsevier; 2017. p. 131–51.

# 14 Acute Non-traumatic Weakness

Venkataramaiah Sudhir and Kamath Sriganesh

**Key Points**

- The cause of non-traumatic weakness can lie anywhere between the brain and the muscle
- A thorough history and clinical examination is of paramount importance
- Maintenance of airway, breathing and circulation takes precedence over establishing a diagnosis, although undue delay should be avoided
- Localisation of the neurological deficit should be attempted at the earliest
- Investigations should be based upon clinical suspicion and should be targeted towards appropriate management
- Attempt should be made to as certain treatable causes of the weakness such as infections or toxins

**Case Scenario**

A 40-year-old male presented to the emergency department with history of severe cramps, abdominal pain, diarrhoea and vomiting. He also complained of blurring of vision, dizziness, generalised weakness and mild difficulty in breathing. He had difficulty in speaking coherently. On examination his pulse rate was 90 beats per minute, BP was 160/90 mmHg and respiratory rate was 18. Neurological examination showed generalised weakness with slowing of reflexes. The attending physician ordered a CT scan, blood investigations and placed the patient under observation. The patient deteriorated over a period of 6 h with complete flaccid paralysis requiring intubation and mechanical ventilation to support respiration.

V. Sudhir · K. Sriganesh (✉)
National Institute of Mental Health and Neurosciences, Bengaluru, India



P. U. Bidkar, P. Vanamoorthy (eds.), *Acute Neuro Care*,
https://doi.org/10.1007/978-981-15-4071-4_14

The preliminary blood investigations were normal and CT brain did not show any abnormalities. Hence, the physician ordered for a toxicology screening. On interviewing the family, the patient was found to have consumed a portion of canned pickles the day before. Botulin toxins were detected in the blood and mouse bioassay also confirmed presence of toxins in the injected serum.

## 14.1 Introduction

The disorders which fall into this group of emergencies can range from a seemingly minor medical condition to a rapidly progressing fatal disease [1]. To make matters difficult the cause of the disease can lie anywhere between the brain to the muscle including the brainstem, anterior horn cells, peripheral nerve, and the neuromuscular junction [2]. However, in a Swiss observational study of patients presenting with acute weakness to the emergency department, non-neurological causes were observed to be the most common reasons for acute non-traumatic weakness [3]. The importance of a comprehensive history and a thorough clinical examination, therefore, cannot be overstressed. Figure 14.1 demonstrates an approach to a patient with diffuse weakness.

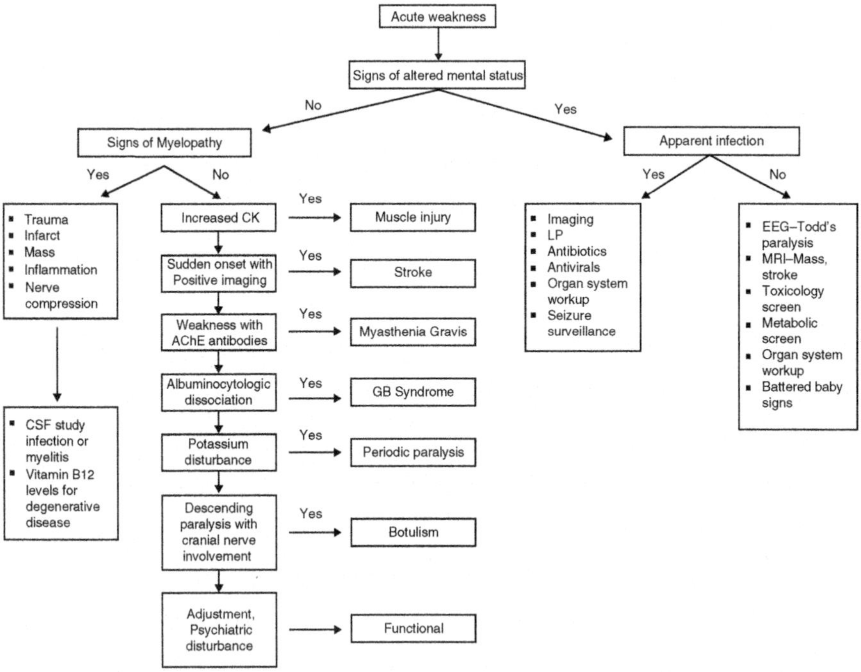


**Fig. 14.1** Approach to a patient with diffuse weakness

In a given patient who is not maintaining circulation and oxygenation, resuscitation and restoration of homeostasis takes immediate precedence. Airway, breathing and circulatory issues are addressed with simultaneous laboratory investigations with a plan for imaging at the earliest following stabilization of the patient's condition [4].

## 14.2 Initial Management

This should include rapid assessment along the following lines [2].

- Document the duration of onset of signs of neurological illness which includes when the patient was last known to be well.
- Assess airway and breathing, intervene, and secure airway if needed.
- Assess circulation and initiate circulatory support if needed.
- Obtain a GCS or FOUR score and document the same.
- Check blood sugar.
- If exposure to poison/toxins are suspected, document the type and duration of exposure.
- Arterial blood gases will give information about oxygenation, ventilation, electrolytes status, acid-base status, and hemoglobin.
- If stroke is suspected, a stroke scoring is done, and the stroke team is intimated.

In patients with acute neuromuscular disorders, weakness of the diaphragm, intercostal muscles, upper airway obstruction and inability to protect the lower airway due to weakness of the oropharyngeal muscles leads to respiratory crisis. Assessment of ventilation and intervention to support breathing with or without airway access is an immediate requirement [2]. Airway protection will be paramount when there is absent gag and cough reflexes with poor swallowing effort indicating cranial nerve dysfunction. If the cranial nerves are found to be intact on examination with the patient able to protect the airway, weakness is mainly restricted to the diaphragm and the intercostal muscles, then non-invasive ventilation (NIV) can be attempted initially [5]. If gas exchange is not being effectively maintained by NIV and the patient is not comfortable, not co-operating for NIV, then invasive airway access may be obtained for mechanical ventilation [2].

After the patient is rendered stable, detailed neurological examination, laboratory investigations and imaging should be directed at localizing the lesion for subsequent management.

## 14.3 Basic Overview for Possible Localisation of a Lesion

Lesions arising in the CNS (brain and the spinal cord) and the neuromuscular junction are the most critical and important since specific treatment modalities are available. Abnormal or absent sensation can give valuable information and can help in ruling out lesions originating from a peripheral nerve. Examining the reflexes will add to the information.

After the basic neurological examination, refer to the following tables for probable anatomical localization. Possible causes of acute onset monoplegia are enumerated in Tables 14.1 and 14.2 informs localization and pattern of weakness with possible aetiologies. Table 14.3 informs localization of pathology based on sensory deficits.

**Table 14.1** Acute monoplegia—Upper limb vs Lower limb

| Acute onset monoplegia lower limb | Acute onset monoplegia upper limb |
|---|---|
| 1. Stroke- involving Anterior Cerebral artery distribution | 1. Stroke, affecting the superior division of contralateral middle cerebral artery territory, affecting parietal lobe, or unpaired anterior cerebral artery |
| 2. Superior sagittal Sinus thrombosis | 2. Parietal lobe injury following trauma |
| 3. Frontal lobe traumatic brain injury | 3. Brachial plexus injury. |
| 4. Infections of the frontal lobe | 4. Injury to multiple cervical nerve roots |
| 5. Trauma to the lumbosacral plexus, diabetic lumbosacral plexopathy | 5. Functional or psychogenic |
| 6. Functional or psychogenic | |

**Table 14.2** Possible localisation of weakness [2]

| Localisation | Sensory symptoms/ signs | Reflexes | Pattern of weakness | Aetiologies |
|---|---|---|---|---|
| Brain/spinal cord | ± | ↑ | Distal > proximal | Acute stroke, SAH, seizure, hypertensive encephalopathy, epidural abscess, tumour, spinal cord infarct |
| Motor neuron/ Anterior horn cell | No sensory loss | ↑ in ALS; ↓ in polio | Muscular atrophy | Polio, ALS |
| Spinal nerve/ peripheral nerve | +++ | ↓ ↓ | Distribution of the nerve | GBS, vasculitis |
| Neuromuscular junction | No sensory loss | Intact | Predominantly proximal | OP poisoning, myasthenia gravis, tick borne diseases, botulism |
| Muscle | No sensory loss | Intact | Proximal | Rhabdomyolysis |

*SAH* sub arachnoid hemorrhage, *ALS* amyotrophic lateral sclerosis, *GBS* Guillain-Barré syndrome, *OP* organo phosphorus

**Table 14.3** Localisation based on sensory deficits

| Sensory deficit | | | | | |
|---|---|---|---|---|---|
| Brain | | | | | Nerve |
| Cortex | Sub cortex | Thalamus | Brainstem | Spinal cord | Radiculopathies |
| Parietal Lobe | Corona Radiata | | Midbrain | Any level of the spinal column | Neuropathies (mono/poly) |
| | Internal Capsule | | Pons | | DRG involvement |
| | | | Medulla | | Plexus injury |

*DRG* dorsal root ganglion

## 14.4 Approaches to Specific Disorders

1. **Monoplegia and Hemiplegia:**

   Monoplegia and hemiplegia are fairly common disorders presenting to the emergency or the outpatient departments. Weakness of one extremity (upper or lower) is termed as monoplegia, while the weakness of one entire side of the body (left or right side) is termed as hemiplegia. A detailed history taking concerning onset, duration, progression of weakness is crucial to narrow down on the possible etiology [6].

### 14.4.1 Causes of Monoplegia and Hemiplegia

1) Though stroke is the major cause of acute hemiplegia differential diagnosis of other aetiologies should be kept in mind. The possible causes of acute onset hemiplegia are enumerated below [6].
   1. Stroke
   2. Thrombosis of the intracerebral venous sinuses.
   3. CNS infections.
   4. Head injury causing damage to the motor cortex, deeper structures like basal ganglia, thalamus, and brainstem.
   5. Acute bleed into a brain tumour.
   6. Demyelinating illness, such as ADEM (acute disseminated encephalomyelitis) or MS (multiple sclerosis).
   7. Todd's paresis.
   8. Metabolic derangements in blood sugar and electrolytes.
   9. Functional or psychogenic

A non-contrast CT scan will give information related to bleed/ trauma and a diffusion weighted MRI scan will be the investigation of choice if an acute ischemic insult is suspected.

Blood sugar levels and electrolytes should be corrected and serially monitored. Since acute hemiplegia and monoplegia are commonly due to stroke, approach towards management will be discussed in detail in the section dealing with stroke.

**2) Quadriparesis with or without sensory involvement** [2]:

Etiology:

1) Compression of the spinal cord
   (a) Disc herniation—Imaging, surgery
   (b) Epidural abscess—Imaging, culture and sensitivity, antibiotic therapy, surgery
   (c) Hematoma—Imaging, surgery
   (d) Tumour—Imaging, steroids, chemotherapy, surgery
2) Spinal cord infarction.
3) Transverse myelitis.
4) Glucose and electrolyte abnormalities.

**3) Anterior horn cell disorders:**

Two main diseases involve the anterior horn cell, poliomyelitis and West Nile Virus infection. India has completed 5 years as a Polio-free nation as on January 2016. There exists no cure for polio and management is reserved to control of acute symptoms until the infection runs its natural course [7].

Acute symptoms of overt clinical disease include fever, muscular pain, and asymmetric proximal muscular paralysis with no change in sensation. Patients with respiratory muscle involvement may need intubation and support of ventilation. Muscular pains can be controlled by analgesics.

West Nile Virus infection is not prevalent in India, and is mainly restricted to North America.

**4) Proximal muscle weakness:**

These disorders predominantly affect the proximal muscle groups of the upper and lower limbs with or without the involvement of the axial muscles [2, 8].

The causes for proximal muscle weakness include the following:

1. Toxicities—Statins, alcohol, corticosteroids
2. Metabolic—Electrolyte disorders (periodic paralyzes), endocrine disorders
3. Malignancy
4. Infections—Retrovirus, influenza, hepatitis B/C, enteroviruses
5. Idiopathic.
6. Sarcoidosis.

Management:

- Conduct a detailed clinical history and physical examination and testing the proximal group of muscles.
- Exclude distal muscle weakness
- Look for dermatological signs—rashes on chest/shoulders/eyelids
- Investigations—CK is elevated >50 times, statin levels, cortisol levels, electrolytes, hormone assay, muscle imaging, nerve muscle conduction studies, muscle biopsy.

Treatment:

- Patients in acute respiratory distress; assess the need for intubation and ventilation and obtain airway access.
- Seek the offending agent; cessation of the agent will reduce the symptoms along with symptomatic management.
- Correct electrolyte disturbances and stop agents like diuretics which might be the cause of the electrolyte disorder.

**5) Distal Muscle weakness:**

Predominantly involve small muscles of the hand and feet [9–12]
Causes:

1. Nerve entrapment/compression
2. Vasculitis
3. Toxicity

Presentation:

- Altered sensation with or without pain, weakness with or without atrophy of muscles, weight loss, and fever in vasculitis.
- Lower limbs predominantly involved in vasculitis
- Progressive weakness from distal to proximal may be seen in toxicities.

Management:

- Investigation: comprehensive vasculitis screening, nerve conduction studies, toxicology screening, biopsy (nerve/muscle)
- Acute pain management with analgesics and agents specific to neuropathic pain.
- Nerve exploration and release in case of entrapment.
- Symptomatic management and supportive care.

### 6) Guillain–Barre syndrome (GBS):

GBS is the most common form of acute paralytic disorder in India and worldwide which can rapidly progress to a life-threatening disease [13]. In almost all of the cases an infective etiology is present with Campylobacter jejuni infection being the commonest [14]. Pathologically, axonal and demyelinating subtypes of GBS are described. Demyelinating neuropathy is the commonest presentation.

*Presentation*:

- Acute onset and rapid progression of limb weakness, symmetrical in distribution with or without sensory involvement.
- Bulbar involvement can present with ophthalmoplegia, ataxia, areflexia, cranial nerve dysfunction, respiratory distress along with limb weakness.
- CSF study will show classic albumin cytological dissociation, a high CSF protein content, and normal leucocyte count.
- Nerve conduction studies can be used for confirmation and classification.

*Treatment:*

- Airway, breathing, and circulation to be addressed in patients presenting with ascending weakness and bulbar symptoms. The patient needs to be closely observed with monitoring of vital parameters and measurement of vital capacity (Single breath count can be used as a valuable bedside tool).
- Intravenous immunoglobulins and/or plasma exchange are the mainstay of specific therapy. Supportive treatment, early physiotherapy, DVT prophylaxis are to be initiated once the patient is stabilized.

### 7) Neuromuscular Junction disorders:
#### a. Myasthenia Gravis:

Autoimmune disorder presenting with fluctuating muscle weakness predominantly involving ocular and bulbar muscles. Antibodies target the post-synaptic acetyl choline receptors [15].

Presentation:

- Patients present with weakness, double vision, swallowing difficulty, inability to support the neck and dysarthria. Patients in myasthenic/cholinergic crisis present with respiratory failure and require airway access and mechanical ventilation.
- A positive edrophonium test, demonstration of auto antibodies against the Ach receptor, and diminishing response strength on repeated nerve stimulation will clinch the diagnosis.

Management:

- Supportive therapy, immunosuppression, neostigmine and pyridostigmine form the mainstay of treatment. Patients with a thymoma may benefit by thymectomy.

**b. Botulism:**

A foodborne disease caused by a toxin released 24–48 h following consumption of Clostridium Botulinum contaminated food material. Presynaptic acetyl choline release will be affected by the toxin [16, 17].

Presentation:

- Bulbar muscle involvement with weakness descending to the periphery, and ocular muscle involvement with autonomic dysfunction. Sensation will be intact, reflexes might be absent and overt respiratory failure occurs in severe toxin release.
- Diagnosis is based on a history of contaminated food intake and demonstration of the toxin in serum and other body fluids.

Management:

- Supportive therapy with or without mechanical ventilation and specific anti-toxin.

The other causes affecting NMJ include snakebite envenomation and drug induced, a detailed discussion can be found elsewhere.

**8) Aortic dissection:**

Painless aortic dissection leading to muscle weakness/paralysis is rare but a possible occurrence. Acute sharp chest pain with elevated blood pressure is the usual presentation of aortic dissection. Aortic dissection causes separation of intercostal arteries from the lumen of the aorta thereby decreasing or shutting off blood supply to the spinal cord. The great radicular artery of Adamkiewicz arising from the posterior intercostal artery supplies the lower two-thirds of the spinal cord through the anterior spinal artery. In case of damage or obstruction of blood flow, this can result in the anterior spinal artery syndrome characterized by weakness of the lower limbs and loss of bowel and bladder control [18–20].

To summarise, if a patient presents with sharp chest pain, pallor and pulseless lower limbs, weakness/paralysis of the lower limbs, loss of bowel and bladder control, co-existing hypertension—dissection of the aorta has to be suspected [21, 22].

Investigations:

- Basic biochemistry, hematology with blood grouping and cross-matching. Chest X-ray may show a widened mediastinum. Echocardiogram—Transthoracic/transoesophageal and a CT aortogram will be diagnostic. A CT brain can detect ischemic changes in the brain.

Management:

- Opioid analgesic for pain
- Reduce elevated blood pressure with vasodilators ± beta-blockers with invasive pressure monitoring.

- Type A (Ascending aortic aneurysms) need immediate surgical intervention.

9) **Disorders affecting the muscles:**
   a. **Periodic paralysis (PP):**

Periodic paralysis is a genetic disorder occurring from mutation in the ion channels in the muscles [23]. The prevalence of these disorders is very low. Of all the periodic paralysis, hypokalemic periodic paralysis is rather more common. We shall restrict to Hypokalemic PP in this chapter, readers can find the data regarding other PPs elsewhere.

Presentation:

- Intermittent flaccid muscular weakness with normal periods in between irregular episodes.
- Sensation is intact.
- Triggering factors include a high carbohydrate diet, strenuous physical activity, stress, and fasting.

Investigations:

- ECG, serum potassium levels <3.5 mEq/l (may not be always present), creatinine kinase may be elevated.

Management:

- Oral high dose potassium (40–60 mEq)/IV potassium
- Acetazolamide

Other causes of periodic paralysis:

- Hyperkalemic PP
- Andersen–Tawil syndrome
- Thyrotoxicosis

b. **Dermatomyositis:**

Inflammatory muscle disorder characterized by skin lesions. Muscular weakness will be restricted to proximal muscles and rarely extends to distal muscles. The rash of dermatomyositis is classic and is called as the 'heliotrope rash' presenting as red to purple on the eyelids [24].
Investigations:

- Elevated muscle enzymes—CK-MB, muscle biopsy and electrophysiological studies of the muscle.

**Table 14.4** Toxicities with muscle weakness

| | |
|---|---|
| Organophosphate compounds | Mainly used as pesticides<br>Poisoning will cause initial cholinergic crisis (excessive lacrimation, salivation) followed by muscular paralysis. Occasionally muscular paralysis may present after a gap of 3–4 weeks of poisoning called as 'intermediate syndrome'<br>Management is restricted to removal of the agent from the stomach by aspiration and symptomatic management to contain the cholinergic crisis with anticholinergics. Ventilatory support may be needed if the paralysis ascends and involves the respiratory muscles [25] |
| Arsenic | Axonal patter of neuropathies following accidental or homicidal ingestion<br>Acute poisoning presents as acute gastrointestinal symptoms—abdominal pain, diarrhea, vomiting<br>Serum and urine arsenic levels will be increased<br>Chelating agents can be used for treatment along with supportive care [4] |
| Other heavy metals | Present mainly with gastroinestinal symptoms. Central nervous system symptoms may be present in acute heavy metal toxicity—encephalopathy, cerebral edema. Arrhythmias and metabolic acidosis with kidney injury may also be present<br>Complete serum biochemistry and heavy metal levels in the serum have to be obtained<br>Gastric lavage, chelating agents and supportive therapy are the mainstay of management with referral to toxicology specialist [4] |

Management:

- Corticosteroids
- Immunosuppression
- Immunoglobulin therapy if other treatments fail.

10) Toxicities causing muscular weakness: Muscle weakness from toxicities and their clinical presentations are presented in Table 14.4.
11) Weakness due to electrolyte disorders:

Severe electrolyte disorders can manifest as weakness and should be excluded with laboratory assessment in the emergency room before further costly, time-consuming and invasive investigations for identifying the cause for generalized weakness are carried out. The two most commonly reported acute electrolyte related weakness in the emergency room include hypokalemia and hypoglycemia.

### 14.4.2 Hypokalemic Weakness and Paralysis [26, 27]

Hypokalemic paralysis was defined as an acute onset flaccid paralysis associated with low plasma potassium (<3.5 mEq/L) [26]. Acute weakness from hypokalemia can present as mild generalized weakness to severe paralysis. Severe hypokalemia may be associated with cardiac arrhythmias and respiratory muscle weakness which is a medical emergency. The cause could be idiopathic or systemic diseases such as thyrotoxicosis, renal tubular acidosis, Sjogren syndrome, gastrointestinal losses, Gitelman's syndrome, and Barium poisoning. In the Indian scenario, dengue has been an important cause for acute weakness from hypokalemia. Hypokalemia is easy to detect by measurement of serum potassium level and if present, should be managed with enteral or intravenous potassium chloride administration depending on severity and acuity of manifestation, which results in rapid improvement of the weakness. The causes and key findings in differentiating hypokalemia related weakness are listed below.

Familial idiopathic hypokalemic periodic paralysis [28]

- Recurrent episodes of weakness with hypokalemia
- Normal acid-base balance
- Absence of secondary factors

Thyrotoxic Hypokalemic paralysis

- Recurrent episodes of acute flaccid paralysis
- Low serum potassium levels with normal pH
- Hyperthyroidism

Renal tubular acidosis

- Hypokalemia
- Hyperchloremia, metabolic acidosis, normal anion gap
- Urine pH > 5.5 during systemic acidosis

Dengue associated weakness

- Acute onset fever
- Motor weakness
- Hypokalemia and rapid improvement of symptoms with potassium correction
- Positive dengue serology

Gitelman's syndrome

- Metabolic alkalosis blood pH >7.45, serum bicarbonate >29 mEq/l
- Hypokalemia (serum potassium <3 mEq/L)
- Hypomagnesemia (serum magnesium <1.8 mg/dL)
- Hypocalciuria (urine calcium <100 mg/24 h)

Sjogren syndrome

- Decreased saliva and tear secretion
- Renal tubular acidosis
- Hypokalemic flaccid paralysis

Management of Hypokalemic Weakness and Paralysis

### 14.4.3 Hypoglycemic Hemiplegia

Severe hypoglycemia (serum glucose <50 mg%) can contribute to acute weakness mimicking stroke. The most common focal neurological sign is usually unilateral motor weakness accompanied by alteration in consciousness. Immediate blood glucose measurement excludes or confirms the etiology for such a presentation. The clinical presentation resolves immediately after the administration of high concentration glucose containing solutions [29, 30].

Other electrolyte disorders causing acute weakness are rare and reported in Table 14.5.

**Table 14.5** Electrolyte disorders causing acute muscle weakness [31, 32]

| Electrolyte abnormality | Diagnosis | Neurological manifestation related to weakness |
|---|---|---|
| Hyponatremia | Serum sodium <135 mEq/L | Muscle cramps, hyporeflexia |
| Hypernatremia | Serum sodium >145 mEq/L | Weakness, hyperreflexia |
| Hypokalemia | Serum potassium <3.5 mmol/L | Weakness, paraesthesia, normal reflexes |
| Hyperkalemia | Serum potassium >5.5 mmol/L | Weakness, hyporeflexia, paraesthesia |
| Hypocalcemia | Serum calcium <8 mg/dL | Tetany, Chvostek's sign, Trousseau sign, opisthotonus |
| Hypercalcemia | Serum calcium >10.5 mg/dL | Weakness (proximal), hyperreflexia, rigidity |
| Hypomagnesemia | Serum magnesium <0.6 mmol/L | Tetany, hyperreflexia |
| Hypermagnesemia | Serum magnesium >0.6 mmol/L | Acute flaccid paralysis, areflexia |
| Hypophosphatemia | Serum phosphorus <0.8 mmol/L | Perioral paraesthesia, acute paralysis including axial muscles, areflexia |

## Multiple Choice Question

1. All of these are a cause of periodic paralysis except,
   (a) Hyperkalemic periodic paralysis
   (b) Andersen–Tawil syndrome
   (c) Thyrotoxicosis
   (d) Botulism
2. Characteristics of infantile botulism include all except
   (a) Fever
   (b) Vomiting
   (c) Symmetrical weakness and profound hypotonia
   (d) Fixed dilated pupils
3. Proximal symmetric weakness of muscles with a heliotrope rash and swelled up hand, sensation being normal is seen in
   (a) Diabetic neuropathy
   (b) Radiculopathy
   (c) Dermatomyositis
   (d) Periodic Paralysis
4. Mees lines (horizontal hypopigmented lines across all nails) is a feature of
   (a) Arsenic poisoning
   (b) Lead toxicity
   (c) Dermatomyositis
   (d) Botulism
5. All of the following are appropriate in the management of weakness due to Anterior spinal artery syndrome except.
   (a) T2 weighted MRI to delineate the arterial territory.
   (b) Corticosteroids
   (c) Supportive therapy
   (d) Antiplatelet agents in patients with vascular disorders
6. The ideal antidote for organo-phosphorous compound is
   (a) Atropine
   (b) Pralidoxime
   (c) Flumazenil
   (d) Naloxone
7. Sudden onset hemiplegia with contralateral loss of pain and temperature sensations are a feature of,
   (a) Hemiplegic migraine
   (b) Brown-Sequard syndrome
   (c) Heavy metal poisoning
   (d) Acute porphyria
8. A 35-year-old female patient with a history of recent viral disease presented to the emergency with weakness and sensory disturbances below T2 level. Her weakness progressed slowly over days. She also complained of pain the back

and bladder and bowel control were also lost. MRI revealed a segmental spinal lesion. The most probable diagnosis is?
   (a) Spinal Cord infarction
   (b) Transverse Myelitis
   (c) Guillain–Barre syndrome
   (d) Heavy metal toxicity.
9. Which of these naturally occurring toxins is responsible for muscular paralysis and even death in some cases after consumption of Puffer Fish?
   (a) Histamine
   (b) Ciguatoxin
   (c) Shellfish toxin
   (d) Tetrodotoxin
10. A 50-year-old gentleman who was a hypertensive on medication suddenly complained of severe chest pain both on the anterior and posterior aspect of the chest wall. By the time he reached the emergency he was profusely sweating and had developed monoplegia of the left hand. He described his pain as 'searing' chest pain. What could be the diagnosis?
   (a) Myocardial Infarction
   (b) Aortic dissection
   (c) Musculoskeletal pain
   (d) Severe pleuritis

Answers: 1. (d), 2. (a), 3. (c), 4. (b), 5. (b), 6. (b), 7. (b), 8. (b), 9. (d), 10. (b)

## References


1. Yeager S, Miller C. Acute nontraumatic weakness: overview of central nervous system differential diagnosis. AACN Adv Crit Care. 2014;25(3):251–65.
2. Caulfield AF, Flower O, Pineda JA, Uddin S. Emergency neurological life support: acute non-traumatic weakness. Neurocrit Care. 2017;27(Suppl 1):29–50. https://doi.org/10.1007/s12028-017-0450-3.
3. Ganti L, Rastogi V. Acute generalized weakness. Emerg Med Clin North Am. 2016;34(4):795–809.
4. Nayak R. Practical approach to the patient with acute neuromuscular weakness. World J Clin Cases. 2017;5(7):270–9. https://doi.org/10.12998/wjcc.v5.i7.270.
5. Rabinstein AA. Noninvasive ventilation for neuromuscular respiratory failure: when to use and when to avoid. Curr Opin Crit Care. 2016;22(2):94–9.
6. Kumar S, Kaul S. Approach to a patient with hemiplegia and monoplegia. Available at http://www.apiindia.org/pdf/progress_in_medicine_2017/mu_27.pdf.
7. Jacob John T, Vashishtha VM. Eradicating poliomyelitis: India's journey from hyperendemic to polio-free status. Indian J Med Res. 2013;137(5):881–94.
8. Suresh E, Wimalaratna S. Proximal myopathy: diagnostic approach and initial management. Postgrad Med J. 2013;89(1054):470–7.
9. Dimachkie MM, Barohn RJ. Distal myopathies. Neurol Clin. 2014;32(3):817–42. https://doi.org/10.1016/j.ncl.2014.04.004.
10. Neal S, Fields KB. Peripheral nerve entrapment and injury in the upper extremity. Am Fam Physician. 2010;81:147–55.

11. Mathew L, Talbot K, Love S, Puvanarajah S, Donaghy M. Treatment of vasculitic peripheral neuropathy: a retrospective analysis of outcome. QJM. 2007;100:41–51.
12. London Z, Albers JW. Toxic neuropathies associated with pharmaceutic and industrial agents. Neurol Clin. 2007;25:257–76.
13. Meena AK, Khadilkar SV, Murthy JM. Treatment guidelines for Guillain–Barre syndrome. Ann Indian Acad Neurol. 2011;14:S73–81.
14. Alter M. The epidemiology of Guillain-Barré syndrome. Ann Neurol. 1990;27(Suppl):S7–S12.
15. Juel VC. Myasthenia gravis: management of myasthenic crisis and perioperative care. Semin Neurol. 2004;24:75–81.
16. Varma JK, Katsitadze G, Moiscrafishvili M, et al. Signs and symptoms predictive of death in patients with foodborne botulism—Republic of Georgia, 1980–2002. Clin Infect Dis. 2004;39:357–62.
17. Chalk C, Benstead TJ, Keezer M. Medical treatment for botulism. Cochrane Database Syst Rev. 2011;16(3):CD008123.
18. Hagan PG, Nienaber CA, Isselbacher EM, et al. The International Registry of Acute Aortic Dissection (IRAD): new insights into an old disease. JAMA. 2000;283:897–903.
19. Gaul C, Dietrich W, Friedrich I, Sirch J, Erbguth FJ. Neurological symptoms in type A aortic dissections. Stroke. 2007;38:292–7.
20. Tsai TT, Nienaber CA, Eagle KA. Acute aortic syndromes. Circulation. 2005;112:3802–13.
21. Colak N, Nazli Y, Alpay MF, Akkaya IO, Cakir O. Painless aortic dissection presenting as paraplegia. Tex Heart Inst J. 2012;39(2):273–6. PMID: 22740752.
22. Park C-B, Jo D-J, Kim M-K, Kim S-H. Paraplegia due to acute aortic coarctation and occlusion. J Korean Neurosurg Soc. 2014;55(3):156–9.
23. Venance SL, Cannon SC, Fialho D, et al. The primary periodic paralyses: diagnosis, pathogenesis and treatment. Brain. 2006;129:8–17.
24. Lorizzo LJ 3rd, Jorizzo JL. The treatment and prognosis of dermatomyositis: an updated review. J Am Acad Dermatol. 2008;59:99–112.
25. Eddleston M, Buckley NA, Eyer P, Dawson AH. Management of acute organophosphorus pesticide poisoning. Lancet. 2008;371:597–607.
26. Garg RK, Malhotra HS, Verma R, Sharma P, Singh MK. Etiological spectrum of hypokalemic paralysis: A retrospective analysis of 29 patients. Ann Indian Acad Neurol. 2013;16(3):365–70.
27. Kumar Singh A, Kumar Maurya P, Kulshreshtha D, Deepak Thakkar M, Kumar TA. Analysis of clinical and metabolic profile of acute neuromuscular weakness related to Hypokalemia. Acta Neurol Taiwanica. 2017;26(3):97–105.
28. Statland JM, Fontaine B, Hanna MG, Johnson NE, Kissel JT, Sansone VA, Shieh PB, Tawil RN, Trivedi J, Cannon SC, Griggs RC. Review of the diagnosis and treatment of periodic paralysis. Muscle Nerve. 2018;57(4):522–30. https://doi.org/10.1002/mus.26009. Published online 2017 Nov 29.
29. Ohshita T, Imamura E, Nomura E, Wakabayashi S, Kajikawa H, Matsumoto M. Hypoglycemia with focal neurological signs as stroke mimic: clinical and neuroradiological characteristics. J Neurol Sci. 2015;353(1–2):98–101.
30. Wallis WE, Donaldson I, Scott RS, Wilson J. Hypoglycemia masquerading as cerebrovascular disease (hypoglycemic hemiplegia). Ann Neurol. 1985;18(4):510–2.
31. Riggs JE. Neurologic manifestations of electrolyte disturbances. Neurol Clin. 2002;20:227–39.
32. Sebastian S, Clarence D, Newson C. Severe hypophosphataemia mimicking Guillain–Barre syndrome. Anaesthesia. 2008;63:873–5.

# Meningitis and Encephalitis

15

Vasudha Singhal and Prasanna Udupi Bidkar

**Key Points**

- Acute inflammation of meninges is termed meningitis, and it may be bacterial, viral, or fungal in origin
- *Neisseria Meningitidis* and *Streptococcal pneumoniae* are the commonest bacteria causing meningitis in adults. The elderly and the immunosuppressed are at risk of infection from *Streptococcus pneumoniae* and *Listeria monocytogenes*
- In patients with a high clinical suspicion of meningitis or encephalitis, parenteral antibiotics should be started immediately, without waiting for a brain imaging or lumbar puncture
- Current guidelines recommend the use of IV dexamethasone in a dose of 10 mg (0.15 mg/kg in children) every 6 h for a duration of 2–4 days, started just before or at the same time as antibiotic therapy
- A lumbar puncture is indicated in all patients with suspected meningitis for assessing the CSF opening pressure and analysis
- CSF pleocytosis (counts usually >1000/mm$^3$) with neutrophilic predominance, low glucose (<40 mg/dL, or <2/3rd of serum glucose levels), and a positive gram's stain are diagnostic of bacterial meningitis.

V. Singhal (✉)
Medanta-the Medicity, Gurugram, India

P. U. Bidkar
Jawaharlal Institute of Postgraduate Medical Education and Research, Pondicherry, India


P. U. Bidkar, P. Vanamoorthy (eds.), *Acute Neuro Care*,
https://doi.org/10.1007/978-981-15-4071-4_15

**Case Scenario**

A 26-year-old male presented to the emergency department (ED) with a history of headache and fever since the past 1 day, and altered sensorium for the past 6 h. His past medical history revealed a history of sinusitis. On physical examination, the patient was confused, with a stiff neck, but no focal neurological deficits. His vitals revealed a heart rate of 102 beats/min, blood pressure 106/64 mmHg, respiratory rate 26/min, $SpO_2$ 99%, and temperature 38.8 °C. On arrival in the ED, the patient was resuscitated with IV fluids, antipyretics were administered for temperature control, and blood samples were sent for routine laboratory investigations, along with blood cultures. A shot of dexamethasone 10 mg IV was administered, and parenteral antibiotics—Inj Ceftriaxone 2 g IV and Inj Vancomycin 1 g IV were begun prophylactically. The patient was shifted to the ICU for close neuromonitoring. A diagnostic lumbar puncture was performed, which revealed a cell count of 5600 cells/cu mm with 98% neutrophils, glucose 20 mg/dL, and proteins 1244. The gram's stain showed gram positive cocci, and the CSF PCR revealed *Streptococcus pneumoniae*. Ceftriaxone 2 g IV 'q12 h Vancomycin 1 g IV BD were continued, along with dexamethasone 10 mg IV q6 h. The patient improved neurologically over the next 2 days, and was shifted to the ward. The CSF culture & sensitivity also revealed *Streptococcus pneumoniae*, which was sensitive to both ceftriaxone and vancomycin. Steroids were administered for 3 days and then stopped. Antibiotics were continued for 14 days, and the patient was discharged with no residual deficits.

## 15.1 Introduction

Meningitis and encephalitis are the two infectious neurological emergencies that need prompt recognition and treatment, to prevent significant morbidity and mortality in the affected population. While meningitis refers to the neurologic syndrome arising due to the inflammation of meninges, encephalitis is caused by the inflammation of the brain parenchyma. Preventing long-term neurological sequelae in this central nervous system (CNS) infections are critically dependent upon early diagnosis and timely initiation of appropriate therapy. The approach to these patients involves a good medical history and detailed examination, including the patient's demographics and immune status.

Acute inflammation of meninges may be bacterial, viral, or fungal in origin. Bacterial meningitis occurs when the organisms invade the subarachnoid space through bacteremia via the nasopharyngeal epithelium or a contiguous spread from dental or sinus infections [1]. Recent neurosurgery, head trauma, indwelling implants like ventriculoperitoneal shunts, and immunosuppression may predispose to this clinical condition. The advent of successful *Hemophilus Influenzae type B (Hib)* and conjugate pneumococcal vaccination has resulted in a significant decrease in the incidence of bacterial meningitis in the pediatric population. However, prior vaccination status does not preclude infection from other strains [2]. The elderly and the immunosuppressed are at risk of infection from *Streptococcus pneumoniae* and

*Listeria monocytogenes*. Nosocomial pathogens, like *Staphylococcus* and gram-negative organisms are increasingly becoming more common as causative pathogens in hospital-acquired meningitis [3, 4].

Meningitis caused by viral infections is usually self-limiting and less severe. The most common causative organisms include enteroviruses (Coxsackie A and B), followed by herpes simplex virus-1&2 (HSV-1&2), varicella-zoster, and arboviruses [5]. HSV encephalitis, though represents only 10–15% of viral encephalitis cases, carries high morbidity and mortality if not treated early. Fungal meningitis is usually secondary to systemic mycosis and is most commonly caused by the *Cryptococcus* species in an immunocompromised patient.

Tuberculous meningitis, caused by *Mycobacterium tuberculosis*, is one diagnosis that must be considered in the Indian scenario. It, however, has a subacute or chronic course, and the patients usually present to the emergency department with a neurological complication, such as elevated intracranial pressure, hydrocephalus, vasculitic infarcts, acute seizures or hyponatremia, resulting in an altered sensorium or a neurological deficit. Tuberculous meningitis to date remains a diagnostic challenge, and the diagnosis is empirical in a significant number of patients.

The present article attempts to focus on the rapid identification of patients with meningitis in the first "golden" hour of arrival to the emergency, adequate resuscitation in the initial hours, interpretation of cerebrospinal fluid (CSF) results, and guidelines for the initiation of appropriate antibiotics and steroids.

## 15.2 Clinical Presentation

The clinical triad of fever, meningismus, and altered sensorium, typically thought to be diagnostic of meningitis, is seen in <50% of patients. Most patients, however, would have two of the four symptoms of headache, fever, neck stiffness, and altered mentation [6]. The cortical brain function may be affected in encephalitis, resulting in focal neurological deficits and seizures. The presence of seizure activity is considered an independent predictor of mortality. Multiple cerebral infarcts secondary to vasculitis or venous thrombosis may cause cerebral edema and a decreased level of consciousness on clinical presentation. A petechial or purpural rash at the time of presentation may point towards meningococcal meningitis. Systemic complications like septic shock, pneumonia, and disseminated intravascular coagulation may occasionally be seen in the sicker subgroup. Herpes simplex encephalitis has a predilection for the temporal and orbitofrontal lobes, resulting in a clinical picture of altered consciousness, personality change, memory loss, confusion, or olfactory hallucinations. Neonates with meningitis may present with irritability, decreased feeding, vomiting, and listlessness [7].

The classically described signs of meningeal irritation, such as the *Kernig's* (extending the knee on a flexed hip at 90° to elicit pain in the back and legs) and *Brudzinski's* (forced flexion of the neck to elicit reflex flexion of the hip), have a low sensitivity, but the specificity may be high, suggesting a high likelihood of meningitis if these signs are present. Another test, the *jolt accentuation test*, elicited by the exacerbation of a baseline headache with the horizontal rotation of the neck maybe sensitive for meningitis, but not too specific [8, 9].

## 15.3 Golden Hour Management

### 15.3.1 Initial Assessment and Resuscitation

Any patient presenting to the emergency department with symptoms and signs suggestive of meningitis or encephalitis should have a basic vital check along with blood glucose, and the ABC of resuscitation followed. The vitals should include temperature, heart rate, blood pressure, respiratory rate, oxygen saturation, and the Glasgow Coma Score (GCS). Intravenous access should be immediately secured in all patients for resuscitation. Patients with depressed mentation may be at risk of aspiration and may need intubation for airway protection. Blood samples that need to be sent for laboratory analysis include complete blood count (CBC), coagulation profile, liver, and renal function tests, and serum lactate, besides blood cultures.

In all patients presenting with shock, initial fluid resuscitation with 20–30 mL/kg of fluid bolus should be given, and the vitals and GCS reassessed at frequent intervals. Inotropes may be used to support blood pressure if the patient is not fluid responsive.

### 15.3.2 Parenteral Antibiotics

In patients with a high clinical suspicion of meningitis or encephalitis, parenteral antibiotics should be started immediately, without waiting for a brain imaging or lumbar puncture, as the CSF sterilization takes 4–6 h after the initiation of antibiotics even with the most sensitive organisms. Early initiation of antibiotic therapy within 1 h of triage has been proven to improve mortality in patients with sepsis [10]. The antibiotic therapy should be broad-spectrum, covering both gram-negative and gram-positive organisms, should have a reasonable penetration in the CSF, and should be bactericidal (Table 15.1). A third-generation cephalosporin like ceftriaxone (2 g IV q12 h) and vancomycin (1 g IV q12 h) are reasonable choices, to begin with. In patients with

**Table 15.1** Etiological and recommended therapy in bacterial meningitis

| Age group | Causative pathogens | Empirical therapy |
|---|---|---|
| Infants and children | *S pneumoniae, N meningitidis* | Ceftriaxone 50 mg/kg IV, plus<br>Vancomycin 15 mg/kg IV |
| Adults | *S pneumoniae, N meningitidis* | Ceftriaxone 2 g IV q 12 h, plus<br>Vancomycin 15 mg/kg q 12 h |
| Elderly | *S pneumoniae, N meningitidis, L monocytogenes* | Ampicillin 2 g IV q 6 h, plus<br>Ceftriaxone 2 g IV q 12 h, plus<br>Vancomycin 15 mg/kg q 12 h |
| Immunocompromised | *S pneumoniae, N meningitidis,Hinfluenzae*, aerobic gram-negative bacilli | Ampicillin 2 g IV q 6 h, plus<br>Ceftazidime 2 g IV q8 h or<br>Cefepime 2 g IV q8 h, plus<br>Vancomycin 15 mg/kg q 12 h |
| Nosocomial | *S aureus, S epidermidis*, aerobic gram-negative bacilli | Ceftazidime 2 g IV q8 h or<br>Cefepime 2 g IV q8 h, plus<br>Vancomycin 15 mg/kg q 12 h |

suspected ventriculoperitoneal shunt infections, a cephalosporin with antipseudomonal activity (such as cefepime or ceftazidime), or meropenem should be considered to cover resistant gram-negative organisms like *Pseudomonas* and *Acinetobacter* species, along with vancomycin. Ampicillin (2 g IV q4 h) may be added in elderly and immunosuppressed patients to cover *Listeria monocytogenes* [11]. In patients with suspected herpes encephalitis, acyclovir (10 mg/kg q8 h) should be initiated empirically, and the dose adjusted based on renal functions. Acyclovir may be withdrawn after the exclusion of herpes encephalitis, as it is not effective against other viral encephalitic syndromes. In immunocompromised patients with suspected fungal meningitis, liposomal amphotericin B in a dose of 3–5 mg/kg IV daily may be considered.

### 15.3.3 Steroids

The empiric use of steroids (dexamethasone), concurrently with antibiotics, in all adults suspected with bacterial meningitis, may be reasonable to prevent the release of inflammatory cytokines triggered by bacterial lysis [12]. Recent studies have shown corticosteroid benefit in reducing the incidence of deafness and reduced mortality in adults older than 55 years of age in developed countries, particularly in *Streptococcus pneumoniae* meningitis. Current guidelines recommend the use of IV dexamethasone in a dose of 10 mg (0.15 mg/kg in children) every 6 h for a duration of 2–4 days, started just before or at the same time as antibiotic therapy [13]. It should, however, be continued only in patients with cultures positive for pneumococci, and should not be given to patients who have previously received antibiotics. Patients with suspected herpes simplex encephalitis and tuberculous meningitis also benefit from steroid therapy by controlling cerebral edema [14, 15].

## 15.4 Diagnostic Workup

In the absence of clear contraindications, patients suspected to have meningitis or encephalitis should undergo a lumbar puncture (LP) for cerebrospinal fluid (CSF) analysis (Fig. 15.1).

**Role of CNS Imaging:** The Infectious Diseases Society of America (IDSA) guidelines recommend obtaining a head computed tomography (CT) before LP in patients at risk of brain herniation following lumbar puncture, such as those with an intracranial mass lesion, hydrocephalus, cerebral edema, or midline shift. The high risk patient population includes patients who are elderly (age >60 years), immunocompromised, have a prior history of CNS disease (such as a mass lesion, stroke or focal lesion), presented with a history of a new-onset seizure within the past 1 week, or have abnormal neurological findings (such as papilledema, depressed level of consciousness or focal neurological deficits) [11, 16].

**CSF Analysis:** A lumbar puncture is performed with a measurement of the CSF opening pressure (in the left lateral decubitus position), and CSF sent for cytology

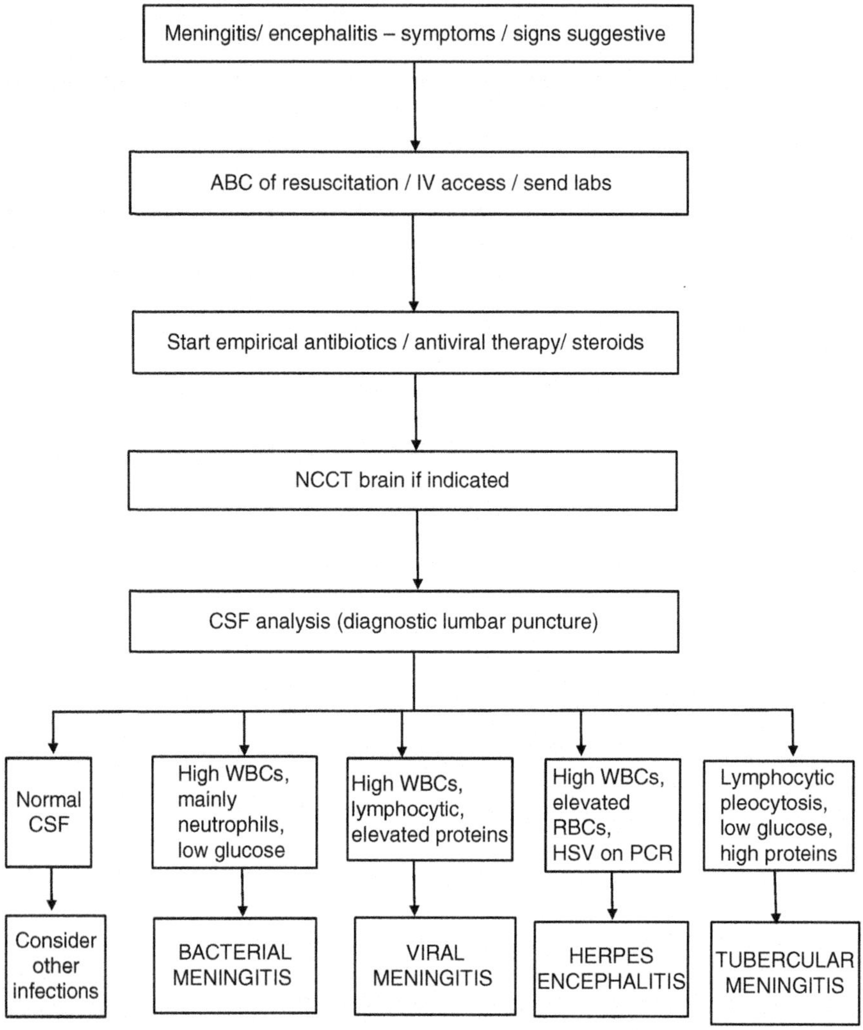


**Fig. 15.1** Meningitis and encephalitis algorithm

(number and type of cells), biochemistry (glucose, protein, chloride), lactate, gram's stain, and culture & sensitivity. Polymerase chain reaction (PCR) assay for bacterial DNA (*Neisseria, H influenzae, S pneumoniae, Streptococcus agalactiae,* and *Listeria*), viral meningitis panel (*herpes simplex, cytomegalovirus, enterovirus, varicella zoster*), and *Cryptococcus* are a useful aid for the rapid detection of causative pathogens. CSF adenosine deaminase (ADA), *Mycobacterium tuberculosis* PCR, and nucleic acid amplification tests help in the diagnosis of tuberculous meningitis.

CSF pleocytosis (counts usually >1000/mm$^3$) with neutrophilic predominance, low glucose (<40 mg/dL, or < 2/third of serum glucose levels), and a positive

**Table 15.2** CSF findings in bacterial, viral, tubercular, and fungal meningitis

| CSF parameter | Normal | Bacterial meningitis | Viral meningitis | Tubercular meningitis | Fungal meningitis |
|---|---|---|---|---|---|
| Opening pressure | 80–160 mmHg | Elevated | Normal | Normal | Normal or elevated |
| Cell count | <5 cells/cu mm | >1000/mm$^3$ | <1000/mm$^3$ | 100–500/mm$^3$ | 100–500/mm$^3$ |
| Cell predominance | Nil | Neutrophils | Lymphocytes | Lymphocytes | Lymphocytes |
| CSF glucose | >2/3rd of serum glucose | Low | Normal | Low | Low |
| CSF proteins | < 45 mg/dL | Elevated | Normal/elevated | Elevated | Elevated |

gram's stain are diagnostic of bacterial meningitis (Table 15.2). The opening pressures are usually high (>200 mmHg). CSF lactate concentration (>4 mmol/L) has an additional diagnostic value in hospital-acquired bacterial meningitis, though it may lack specificity in community-acquired cases [17]. Viral meningitis presents with a lymphocytic pleocytosis and elevated protein content in the CSF. The red blood cell count in CSF may be markedly elevated in HSV-1 encephalitis, as the CSF is hemorrhagic. PCR for HSV detection is highly sensitive and specific in diagnosing this condition. Tuberculous meningitis typically presents with lympho cytic pleocytosis, with decreased glucose and elevated proteins. In immunocompromised patients with cryptococcal meningitis, the CSF opening pressure may be high, and serological detection of the antigen is sensitive and relatively specific for Cryptococcus.

## 15.5 Further Management

In patients with CSF diagnostic of bacterial meningitis, antibiotics should be continued, depending on the organism and culture, and acyclovir stopped if initiated. Steroids may be given for 4 days, particularly in pneumococcal meningitis. Patients should be looked in for a concomitant bloodstream infection, and treatment for sepsis continued. Intracranial pressure should be closely monitored and treated with osmotic agents, if need be.

Cases who have tested positive for herpes encephalitis should receive acyclovir. The treatment for nonherpetic encephalitis is, however, largely supportive, with close neuromonitoring [18].

Many patients may present to the emergency with complications of meningitis, such as hydrocephalus (in fungal, Listeria, and tuberculous meningitis), stroke (secondary to vasculitis), hyponatremia (cerebral salt wasting or syndrome of inappropriate antidiuretic hormone), seizures, etc. These should be carefully diagnosed and managed, taking into consideration the etiology of the complication.

## 15.6 Conclusion

The early diagnosis of meningitis and encephalitis is critical for its early management and reducing mortality resulting from the disease process. Changing microbial resistance patterns and the introduction of newer diagnostic modalities and antimicrobial agents have led to the evolution of the treatment of this disease. The importance of the first hour, however, remains unchanged, and the most crucial in determining outcomes.

## 15.7 Summary

- Acute inflammation of meninges is termed meningitis, and it may be bacterial, viral, or fungal in origin.
- *Neisseria Meningitidis* and *Streptococcal pneumoniae* are the commonest bacteria causing meningitis in adults. The elderly and the immunosuppressed are at risk of infection from *Streptococcus pneumoniae* and *Listeria monocytogenes*.
- Nosocomial pathogens, like *Staphylococcus* and gram-negative organisms, are increasingly becoming more common as causative pathogens in hospital-acquired meningitis.
- HSV encephalitis, though represents only 10–15% of viral encephalitis cases, carries high morbidity and mortality if not treated early.
- Tuberculous meningitis to date remains a diagnostic challenge, and the diagnosis is empirical in a significant number of patients.
- Most patients with bacterial meningitis have two of the four symptoms of headache, fever, neck stiffness, and altered mentation.
- In patients with a high clinical suspicion of meningitis or encephalitis, parenteral antibiotics should be started immediately, without waiting for a brain imaging or lumbar puncture.
- Current guidelines recommend the use of IV dexamethasone in a dose of 10 mg (0.15 mg/kg in children) every 6 h for a duration of 2–4 days, started just before or at the same time as antibiotic therapy.
- IDSA guidelines recommend obtaining a head CT before lumbar puncture in patients at risk of brain herniation.
- A lumbar puncture is indicated in all patients with suspected meningitis for assessing the CSF opening pressure and analysis.
- CSF pleocytosis (counts usually $>1000/mm^3$) with neutrophilic predominance, low glucose ($<40$ mg/dL, or $< 2/3$rd of serum glucose levels), and a positive gram's stain are diagnostic of bacterial meningitis.
- PCR for HSV detection is highly sensitive and specific in diagnosing this condition.
- Tuberculous meningitis typically presents with lymphocytic pleocytosis, with decreased glucose and elevated proteins. CSF adenosine deaminase (ADA), *Mycobacterium tuberculosis* PCR and nucleic acid amplification tests further aid in the diagnosis.
- Early initiation of antibiotic therapy is the cornerstone for reducing mortality in patients with meningitis.

**Checklist for Patients with Meningitis**

- Detailed history and examination—symptoms/signs suggestive of meningitis
- Check vitals
- Begin ABC of resuscitation
- Secure intravenous access—treat shock
- Send labs—CBC/coagulation/LFT/RFT/serum lactate/blood cultures
- Administer steroids followed by parenteral empirical antibiotics
- Consider antivirals (acyclovir) if herpes encephalitis suspected
- NCCT head if abnormal neurological examination
- Lumbar puncture—assess opening pressure and CSF analysis

## Multiple Choice Questions (MCQs)

1. Which of the following is the least common identifiable cause of bacterial meningitis in *neonates*?
   (a) *Streptococcus agalactiae*
   (b) *E.Coli*
   (c) *Listeria monocytogenes*
   (d) *Pseudomonas aeruginosa*
2. What is the recommended prophylactic antibiotic regime for an 84-year-old immunocompromised adult presenting with fever and altered sensorium?
   (a) Ceftriaxone only
   (b) Ceftriaxone/Vancomycin
   (c) Ceftriaxone/Vancomycin/Ampicillin
   (d) Vancomycin only
3. A patient with suspected bacterial meningitis is shifted to the ICU after receiving a 3-day course of antibiotics elsewhere. Which of the following statements about the administration of steroids is true?
   (a) Administer dexamethasone 10 mg IV irrespective of the antibiotic status
   (b) Administer dexamethasone if the patient shows focal neurological deficits
   (c) Do not administer dexamethasone if the patient has already received antibiotics
   (d) Administer dexamethasone if the patient is elderly and immunocompromised
4. Which of the following CSF findings distinguishes tubercular meningitis from bacterial meningitis?
   (a) Low glucose
   (b) High proteins
   (c) Lymphocytic pleocytosis
   (d) High cell count
5. Which of the following CSF parameters may be diagnostic in nosocomial meningitis after a recent neurosurgery?
   (a) Raised lactates
   (b) High proteins

   (c) Elevated cells
   (d) Neutrophilic dominance
6. A 45-year-old female presented to the ED with seizures and altered sensorium. Based on clinical suspicion, she was started on Inj Ceftriaxone 2 g IV BD and Inj Acyclovir 750 mg TDS, and a diagnostic LP was performed. Which of these parameters need daily monitoring?
   (a) Liver function tests
   (b) Renal function tests
   (c) Platelet count
   (d) Coagulation profile
7. In which of the following case scenarios, a brain CT scan is *not* indicated prior to performing a diagnostic LP?
   (a) GCS 12
   (b) Age 50 years
   (c) Seizure at presentation
   (d) History of prior stroke
8. A patient presenting with seizures and altered sensorium was begun on Inj Acyclovir based on clinical suspicion of viral encephalitis. A diagnostic LP was performed, and the CSF PCR revealed enterovirus. What is the most appropriate line of management?
   (a) Continue Acyclovir for 7 days
   (b) Stop acyclovir and continue supportive therapy
   (c) Administer acyclovir and dexamethasone till the patient improves clinically
   (d) Continue acyclovir for at least 14–21 days
9. Which of the following regions of the brain may be most affected in HSV encephalitis as seen on an MRI?
   (a) Temporal and orbitofrontal lobes
   (b) Basal ganglia
   (c) Limbic system
   (d) Thalamus
10. What is the antifungal agent of choice in cryptococcal meningitis?
   (a) Echinocandins
   (b) Voriconazole
   (c) Liposomal amphotericin B
   (d) Flucytosine

Answers: 1. (d), 2. (c), 3. (c), 4. (c), 5. (a), 6. (b), 7. (b), 8. (b), 9. (a), 10. (c).

## References

1. Tintinalli JE, Stapczynski JS. Tintinalli's emergency medicine: a comprehensive study guide. 7th ed. New York: McGraw-Hill; 2011.
2. Pruitt AA. Neurologic infectious disease emergency. Neurol Clin. 2012;30:129–59.
3. Durand ML, Calderwood SB, Weber DJ, et al. Acute bacterial meningitis in adults. A review of 493 episodes. N Engl J Med. 1993;328:21–8.
4. Kourbeti IS, Jacobs AV, Koslow M, et al. Risk factors associated with postcraniotomy meningitis. Neurosurgery. 2007;60:317–25.

5. Fitch MT, Abrahamian FM, Moran GJ, Talan DA. Emergency department management of meningitis and encephalitis. Infect Dis Clin N Am. 2008;22(1):33–52.
6. Attia J, Hatala R, Cook DJ, et al. The rational clinical examination. Does this adult patient have acute meningitis? JAMA. 1999;282(2):175–81.
7. Saex-Llorens X, McCracken GH Jr. Bacterial meningitis in children. Lancet. 2013;361:2139–48.
8. Thomas KE, Hasbun R, Jekel J, et al. The diagnostic accuracy of Kernig's sign, Brudzinski's sign, and nuchal rigidity in adults with suspected meningitis. Clin Infect Dis. 2002;35(1):46–52.
9. Nakao JH, Jafri FN, Shah K, et al. Jolt accentuation of headache and other clinical signs: poor predictors of meningitis in adults. Am J Emerg Med. 2014;32(1):24–8.
10. Proulx N, Fréchette D, Toye B, et al. Delays in the administration of antibiotics are associated with mortality from adult acute bacterial meningitis. QJM. 2005;98(4):291–8.
11. Tunkel AR, Hartman BJ, Kaplan SL, et al. Practice guidelines for the management of bacterial meningitis. Clin Infect Dis. 2004;39:1267–84.
12. van de Beek D, de Gans J. Dexamethasone in adults with community-acquired bacterial meningitis. Drugs. 2006;66(4):415–27.
13. Brouwer MC, McIntyre P, Prasad K, van de Beek D. Corticosteroids for acute bacterial meningitis. Cochrane Database Syst Rev. 2015;9:CD004405.
14. Donald PR, Toorn RV. Use of corticosteroids in tuberculous meningitis. Lancet. 2016;387:2585–7.
15. Estebanez CR, Lizarraga KJ, Merenda A. A systematic review on the role of adjunctive corticosteroids in herpes simplex virus encephalitis: is timing critical for safety and efficacy? Antivir Ther. 2014;19:133–9.
16. Glimaker M, Johansson B, Grindborg O, et al. Adult bacterial meningitis: earlier treatment and improved outcome following guideline revision promoting prompt lumbar puncture. Clin Infect Dis. 2015;60(8):1162–9.
17. Sakushima K, Hayashino Y, Kawaguchi T, et al. Diagnostic accuracy of cerebrospinal fluid lactate for differentiating bacterial meningitis from aseptic meningitis: a meta-analysis. J Infect. 2011;62(4):255–62.
18. Kennedy PG. Viral encephalitis: causes, differential diagnosis, and management. J Neurol Neurosurg Psychiatry. 2004;75(Suppl 1):i10–5.

The manufacturer's authorised representative in the EU is Springer Nature Customer Service Centre GmbH, Europaplatz 3, 69115 Heidelberg, Germany. If you have any concerns regarding our products, please contact ProductSafety@springernature.com

Printed and bound by CPI Group (UK) Ltd, Croydon, CR0 4YY

30/07/2026

02181721-0001